Ocular Toxicology

Ocular Toxicology

Edited by

Ingo Weisse
Boehringer Ingelheim KG
Ingelheim, Germany

Otto Hockwin
University of Bonn
Bonn, Germany

Keith Green
Medical College of Georgia
Augusta, Georgia

and

Ramesh C. Tripathi
South Carolina Eye Institute
Columbia, South Carolina

Associate Editors

Martine Cottin

Pierre Duprat

Robert L. Peiffer, Jr.

Alfred Wegener

Springer Science+Business Media, LLC

Library of Congress Cataloging-in-Publication Data

Ocular toxicology / edited by Ingo Weisse ... [et al.] ; associate
  editors Martine Cottin ... [et al.]
      p. cm.
    "Proceedings of the Fourth Congress of the International Society
  of Ocular Toxicology (ISOT), held October 9-13, 1994, in Annecy,
  France"--T.p. verso.
    Includes bibliographical references and index.
    ISBN 978-0-306-45133-1   ISBN 978-1-4615-1887-7 (eBook)
    DOI 10.1007/978-1-4615-1887-7
    1. Ocular toxicology--Congresses.   I. Weisse, Ingo.
  II. International Society of Ocular Toxicology. Congress (4th :
  1994 : Annecy, France)
    [DNLM: 1. Eye Diseases-- chemically induced--congresses.
  2. Disease Models, Animal--congresses. 3. Eye--drug effects-
  -congresses. 4. Irritants--toxicity--congresses.   WW 140 O213
  1995]
  RE901.T670642 1995
  617.7'1--dc20
  DNLM/DLC
  for Library of Congress   95-37108
                                                                   CIP

Proceedings of the Fourth Congress of International Society of Ocular Toxicology (ISOT),
held October 9–13, 1994, in Annecy, France

ISBN 978-0-306-45133-1

© 1995 Springer Science+Business Media New York
Originally published by Plenum Press, New York in 1995

10 9 8 7 6 5 4 3 2 1

PREFACE

On behalf of the editorial board and the organizing committee of the 4th congress of the International Society of Ocular Toxicology (ISOT), held in Annecy/Veyrier du Lac, France, October 9 - 13, 1994, we are pleased to present to the ocular toxicology community this indexed volume of our congress proceedings. The 4th congress was designed primarily to facilitate and update the knowledge in ocular electrophysiology and ocular pharmacokinetics, in both the clinical and preclinical aspects. The outcome of this 4th congress, established in this volume, is a useful contribution to the methodology in both fields and will hopefully assist in the evaluation and interpretation of ocular findings recorded in animal studies on drugs and other chemicals, in order to protect human health. Undoubtedly, work on the mechanisms of ocular toxicology in the process of pharmaceutical development must continue and these proceedings, embodying the presented papers, will add to the data base.

The editors, the congress organizing committee and the members of the International Society of Ocular Toxicology thank the speakers who gave their time, knowledge, and expertise to assist us in this project. The following manuscripts contain the main substance of each of the platform presentations and, in some cases, much more. Moreover, our thanks go to all the participants coming from a range of backgrounds - regulatory, academic and industrial - for their attention and excellent contributions during the discussion.

Finally, we will use this preface to announce the next ISOT congress, which will be held in Asheville, North Carolina, USA, in October 1996. More information about Asheville will be distributed by our current President, Prof. Keith Green, later in this year.

I. Weisse   O. Hockwin   K. Green   R.C. Tripathi

BOARD OF DIRECTORS, ISOT, 1993/1994

President	Dr. Ingo Weisse, Ingelheim/Rh., Germany
President-elect	Prof. Keith Green, Augusta, GA
Past President	Prof. Sidney Lerman, New York, NY
Secretary-Treasurer	Prof. Ramesh C. Tripathi, Columbia, SC
Directors	Dr. Pierre Duprat, Riom, France
	Prof. Kazuyuki Sasaki, Kanazawa, Japan
	Dr. Hiroshi Suda, Osaka, Japan

ORGANIZING COMMITTEE, 1994

Chairman	Prof. Otto Hockwin, Bonn, Germany
Members	Dr. Martine Cottin, Aulnay Sous Bois, France
	Dr. Pierre Duprat, Riom, France
	Dr. Helmut Sterz, Fleury Les Aubrais Cedex, France
	PD Dr. Alfred Wegener, Bonn, Germany
	Dr. Ingo Weisse, Ingelheim/Rh., Germany

CONTENTS

B. Ocular Pharmacokinetics

C. Lens/Cataract

D. In Vitro Methods

E. Regulatory Affairs

F. Miscellaneous

WELCOME AND OPENING OF THE CONGRESS

Ingo Weisse

Department of Experimental Pathology and Toxicology
Boehringer Ingelheim KG
D-55218 Ingelheim/Rh., Germany

On behalf of the Board of Directors and the Organizing Committee I would like to extend a very warm welcome to all those attending the 4th Congress of the International Society of Ocular Toxicology (ISOT) and thank you all for coming to this beautiful, historic town of Annecy, and to the marvellous congress center of the Fondation Marcel Merieux, here in Veyrier du Lac.

I would like to greet all the colleagues from our host country, France, and the ISOT members and guests from 11 other countries:

Belgium	Great Britain	Russia	Switzerland
Finland	Italy	Sweden	USA
Germany	Japan	Spain	

We are especially pleased that guests from Russia have the opportunity to join us. We also welcome colleagues from the former German Democratic Republic and are delighted that, for the first time, they are also able to attend. The happy political developments of the last few years have washed away the previously almost insurmountable frontiers of Eastern Europe so that our Congress in Annecy is a convincing example of the fact that today science knows no boundaries, either for specialties or for countries.

We very much regret that our President-elect for the years 1995/1996, Prof. K. Green, Medical College of Georgia, Augusta, USA, and one of the Directors of our ISOT Board, Prof. K. Sasaki, Kanazawa Medical University, Ushinada, Japan, cannot be present at our Congress for health reasons. We wish both colleagues all the best and a speedy recovery. Similarly, it was unfortunately impossible for our Past President, Prof. S. Lerman, New York Medical College, Valhalla, USA, to attend this meeting either.

Ocular Toxicology - as we understand it today - is a relatively recent discipline in medical science (Green, 1992). With the increasing number of new drugs, ocular devices, agrochemicals, food additives, household chemicals and cosmetics in the past 3 or 4 decades, the problem of side-effects in the eye has become more evident and presents even more difficulties in understanding. I would like to remind you once again of three examples of drug-related ocular toxicity in man from the 50s and early 60s which are almost certainly familiar to you. These three events are not only characteristic of the origins of ocular toxicology and of the difficulties confronting drug manufacturers, toxicologists, clinical ophthalmologists, and regulatory authorities, but they also make it possible to demonstrate the progress ocular toxicology has made to date:

Example 1:
In 1954, NP 207, a phenothiazine derivative, was introduced on to the market for use as a tranquilizer in man. It was soon withdrawn when retinotoxic side-effects, such as night blindness, reduced visual acuity, and visual field constriction, became apparent in patients, usually 2 - 3 months after starting the oral clinical therapy (Verrey, 1956; Goar and Fletcher, 1956). Toxicological studies carried out previously and retrospectively in various species revealed that comparable retinopathy could be established within 6 - 7 weeks in cats only, but not in the more routinely used experimental animal species, such as albino or pigmented rats, dogs, rabbits or guinea pigs (Meier-Ruge and Cerletti, 1966).

Example 2:
Again in the 1950s, triparanol (MER-29) was introduced as a drug to reduce blood cholesterol in patients with hypercholesterolaemia. It was withdrawn from clinical use in April 1962. In addition to skin lesions, loss of hair and libido, the main ocular side-effect in man associated with the oral application of this drug was the formation of anterior and posterior subcapsular cataracts, in general, with a latency of 8 - 9 months (Laughlin and Carey, 1962). Retrospectively, cataracts were reproduced within 3 months in rats (v. Sallmann et al., 1963) and within 5 - 7 months in dogs, but not in monkeys (Bellows, 1963).

Example 3:
Another drug which caused a lot of controversy with regard to ocular toxicity in man in the 1960s was dimethyl sulfoxide (DMSO). On the basis of its supposed analgesic and anti-inflammatory properties and its fairly common use as a pharmaceutical vehicle, over 100,000 individuals were treated with DMSO on an investigational medical basis in the United States from 1964 - 1965. At the same time the first reports were published in England, dealing with nuclear lens changes and refractive errors in dogs chronically treated with DMSO (Rubin and Mattis, 1966). Because of the uncontrolled nature of many clinical trials and the large number of individuals exposed to DMSO, the US Food and Drug Administration (FDA) withdrew it from clinical investigation in November 1965. Although the lens toxicity findings originally noted in dogs were later confirmed in rabbits, pigs and monkeys (Wood et al., 1967; Rubin and Barnett, 1967; Barnett and Noel, 1967), no counterpart has yet been found in human lenses. After well-conducted ophthalmological studies (Gordon and Kleberger, 1968; Hanna et al., 1977) and following a re-evaluation of the DMSO findings by an ad-hoc committee, DMSO was subsequently released again, but limited to special therapeutic indications in man.

Further examples of serious drug reactions to the eye in humans in the 70s could be added. We only have to think of the likely involvement of clioquinol in SMON-syndrome reported in Japan (Tsubaki et al., 1971) or of the oculomucocutaneous syndrome due to practolol, established in England (Wright, 1975).
These - in the meantime - historical examples provided impetus and incitement, (1) not only to determine the efficacy of a drug, but also to consider its safety when a new drug application (NDA) is submitted to the regulatory authorities for approval for marketing. (2) They also taught us that , from an oculotoxicological point of view, the extrapolation of animal data from standard toxicological studies in a rodent and a non-rodent species to man has its hazards and pitfalls. (3) Furthermore, as a consequence, these historical examples made clear that research on ocular toxicity must be based on multidisciplinary efforts, not

only including reliable animal models or validated in-vitro test systems, but also routine postmarketing surveillance of drug safety including clinical follow-up examinations of patients in different clinical disciplines, and compilation of possible ocular side-effects over years in "early warning systems", such as registers (Venning, 1983).

The latter point of involvement and interest of various scientific disciplines in research in ocular toxicology is not only established by the richly diverse membership of our Society, but also exemplified by the broad audience at our present meeting here in Annecy, including clinical ophthalmologists, physicians, chemists, biochemists, veterinarians, biologists, and pharmacists, representing academia, the chemical industry in the broadest sense, and the regulatory authorities.

I am quoting our President-elect Keith Green (1992), when I repeat that in the past 20 years ocular toxicology has undergone encouraging progress in various fields:

First, today we have very diversified literature based on clinical observations and experience, as well as experimental laboratory data, which contains not only case reports, but also results of mechanistic investigations on ocular toxicology. Extensive and detailed lists of toxic eye responses caused by topically or systemically administered drugs, chemical agents, air pollutants, or occupational hazards have been published. I must mention here the excellent books by Grant (1962), Fraunfelder (1976,1989), Hockwin and Koch (1977), and Chiou (1992), and the Proceedings of the International Society for Eye Research, from the 2nd meeting held in Jerusalem edited by Dikstein (1977).

Secondly, in the last 20 years there has also been a vast expansion of methods and techniques used to study ocular toxicology: for instance, the Scheimpflug slit-image densitography and nuclear magnetic resonance spectroscopy for examining early, not yet visible lens changes or monitoring lens metabolism, the in-vivo and in-vitro specular microscopy for assessing toxic reactions of the corneal endothelium, ocular fluid analyses with HPLC, or the combined use of electrophysiological and microscopical techniques for the objective assessment of different structures of the retina or the optic nerve.

In addition to these advances in the investigational methods in our discipline, the significant development of a variety of noteworthy in-vitro methods must be mentioned. Some of these promising in-vitro test systems can already supplement the rabbit eye irritation test according to Draize et al. (1944). Other in vitro methods can be used as screening tests to study cytotoxicity or mechanisms of action, and to evaluate the toxic potential of xenobiotics. Enucleated eyes, isolated corneal, lens, or retinal preparations, cultures of corneal, lens, or retinal cells are used in the same way as non-eye tissues or non-eye cells such as the chick chorioallantoic membrane, mouse or human fibroblasts, peritoneal mast cells, HeLa cells, or the argarose diffusion in the EYTEX system. In general, these in-vitro tests offer the possibility of saving living animals, as well as time and money. Despite the inherent disadvantage that in-vitro tests cannot replace the eye as a complex organ with a wide variety of responses to toxic insults in a living organism, in-vitro ocular toxicological testing represents an active field of research which is well on the way to developing and consolidating ocular toxicity testing strategies which will hopefully replace the Draize test in the future. These more sophisticated approaches and the standard methods have been put together in the "Manual of Oculotoxicity Testing of Drugs" edited by Hockwin, Green and Rubin (1992) and they are also comprehensively summarized in the books by Hayes (1985) and Chiou (1992).

As the third essential point, I have to refer to one institution which has contributed substantially to the progress in, and to the establishment and dissemination of, knowledge in the field of ocular toxicology during the last two decades, namely the US-National Registry of Drug-Induced Ocular Side Effects. Founded in 1976 by a contract between the US FDA and the University of Arkansas Medical Center, this information system has been run since then by Prof. F. T. Fraunfelder. The Registry accumulates information on all possible drug-induced ocular side-effects in man. It also compiles data from related publications all over the world and makes this information available to clinicians and research workers in academia and industry. In other words, the Registry monitors, as a warning system, the so-called "probationary years" of new and older drugs during their clinical use. Now that I have mentioned the name of Prof. Fritz T. Fraunfelder twice, it is a great pleasure and an honour for me to welcome him as a participant in our Congress here in Annecy and we look forward with interest to hearing the latest from the Registry.

Last but not least, I must introduce our <u>Internationational Society of Ocular Toxicology (ISOT)</u> as a new driving force in the field of ocular toxicology. The major goals of our young Society are (1) to foster communication between the research workers in academia and industry, (2) to be a platform for the interchange of the most recent information on ocular toxicology, and (3) to accelerate the development of methods which can be applied in the research field in all aspects of ocular toxicology. Following a series of meetings on drug-induced ocular side-effects and ocular toxicology held in the United States from 1977 to 1984 in Little Rock, Portland, Milwaukee, and Augusta, it was during the 5th International Symposium in Bonn/Meckenheim (1986) where an Initiating Committee decided that it would be desirable to found an International Society of Ocular Toxicology.

Table 1. Meetings on "Drug-induced ocular side-effects on ocular toxicology" held before the foundation of International Society of Ocular Toxicology (ISOT)

1977	Little Rock/Arkansas	(host: Dr. F.T. Fraunfelder)
1980	Portland/Oregon	(host: Dr. F.T. Fraunfelder)
1982	Milwaukee/Wisconsin	(host: Dr. H.F. Edelhauser)
1984	Augusta/Georgia	(hosts: Dr. D.S. Hull/Dr. K. Green)
1986 (May 13-16)	Bonn/Meckenheim [ISOT initiating committee]	(host: Dr. O. Hockwin)

participants: ≈ *120 (12 countries)*
speeches/posters: *42 / 17*
published: *Concepts of Toxicology, Vol. 4, Karger, Basle 1987. O. Hockwin (ed.)*

The 15 founder members of the ISOT, coming from 6 countries, represent a mixture of scientists from universities and the chemical industry.

Table 2. Initiating Committee of International Society of Ocular Toxicology (ISOT)

P.K. Basu, Toronto, Canada	S. Lerman, Atlanta, USA
F.T. Fraunfelder, Portland, USA	L.F. Rubin, Philadelphia, USA
K. Green, Augusta, USA	K. Sasaki, Ushinada, Japan
R. Heywood, Huntingdon, G.B.	G. Schlüter, Wuppertal, Germany
O. Hockwin, Bonn, Germany	W. Schnitzlein, Ludwigshafen, Germany
P.D. Kaplan, Irvine, USA	I. Weisse, Ingelheim, Germany
H. Kilp, Köln, Germany	P. Wright, London, G.B.
P. Lapalus, Nice-Cedex, France	

It is thanks to Prof. O. Hockwin's unique status in academic medicine, his outstanding personality, and his untiring efforts and devotion, that our Society was formally inaugurated at the Toronto meeting in 1988. As the "father of the idea" it was only natural that Prof. Hockwin should serve as our first president.

The meeting in Toronto was the 1st International Congress of our Society. Successful meetings in Deidesheim and Sedona followed at two-year intervals. Participants from various countries, and speeches or posters concerning different research disciplines on the eyes, such as clinical ophthalmology, biochemistry, physiology, pharmacology, biophysics, and pathology or in-vitro methodology, reflected the diverse interests at our Society and contributed much to the understanding of ocular toxicology.

Table 3. Meetings organized by the International Society of Ocular Toxicology (ISOT)

1988 (June 6-8)	Toronto/Canada		(host: Dr. P. Basu)
	participants:	≈ 109 (12 countries)	
	speeches/posters:	47 / 25	
	published:	Lens and Eye Toxicity Res. 6 (1,2), 1989, S. Lerman, O. Hockwin, K. Sasaki (eds.)	
1990 (May 20-24)	Deidesheim/Germany		(host: Dr. O. Hockwin)
	participants:	≈ 105 (15 countries)	
	speeches/posters:	55 / 18	
	published:	Lens and Eye Toxicity Res. 7 (3,4), 1992, S. Lerman, O. Hockwin, K. Sasaki (eds.)	
1992 (Nov. 15-19)	Sedona/Arizona		(host: Dr. S. Lerman, Dr. K. Green)
	participants:	≈ 95 (8 countries)	
	speeches/posters:	47 / 30	
	published:	Lens and Eye Toxicity Res. 9 (3,4), 1992, S. Lerman, O. Hockwin, K. Sasaki (eds.)	

The main subjects to be covered at our 4th Congress here in Annecy are "Electrophysiology of the eye" and "Ocular Pharmacokinetics". I warmly welcome our invited speakers, very experienced and renowned colleagues, who will update our knowledge in both the clinical and preclinical aspects of these fields:

Prof. E. Zrenner, University of Tübingen, Germany
Prof. K. Kawasaki, Kanazawa University Medical School, Kanazawa, Japan
Prof. B. Clerc, Ecole National Veterinaire D'Alfort, France
Prof. R.L. Peiffer, University of North Carolina, Chapel Hill, USA
Prof. M.F. Saettone, University of Pisa, Italy
Dr. M. Kojima, Kanazawa Medical University, Ushinada, Japan

I also extend a grateful and special welcome to all speakers and poster authors who have given their expertise and their time, willingly and unselfishly, for the good of our meeting. Congresses are the testing place for scientific work and at the same time give us the opportunity to meet each other. I would like to encourage every one of the ISOT members and guests to take advantage of this opportunity and get to know one another.

Before closing I would particularly like to welcome the accompanying ladies, who will have a wonderful opportunity to experience the beauty of the town and its surroundings.

Finally, the arrangement of a meeting and its success depend not only on the speakers, but also on the local organization. I would like therefore to thank the Fondation Marcel

Merieux, Dr. L. Valette, and especially Mrs. J. Camy-Buffavand very much for making it possible to hold our Congress in this modern conference center in beautifully renovated old buildings, here in this magnificent place, Veyrier du Lac. I thank you for your hospitality and once again extend a very warm welcome to all participants.

REFERENCES

Barnett, K.C. and Noel, P.R.B., 1967, Dimethyl sulphoxide and lens changes in primates, *Nature* 214:1115 (June 10).

Bellows, J.G., 1963, Lens opacities produced by cataractogenic agents, *Amer. J. Ophthal.* 55:537.

Chiou, G.C.Y., 1992, Ophthalmic Toxicology, Raven Press Ltd., New York.

Dikstein, S., 1977, Drugs and Ocular Tissues, S. Karger, Basle, Paris, London, New York, Sydney.

Draize, J.H., Woodward, G. and Calvery, H., 1944, Methods for the study of irritiation and toxicity of substances applied topically to the skin and mucous membranes, *J. Pharmacol. Exp. Ther.* 82:377.

Fraunfelder, F.T. 1976, Drug-induced Ocular Side Effects and Drug Interactions, Lea and Febiger, Philadelphia.

Fraunfelder, F.T., 1989, Drug-induced Ocular Side Effects and Drug Interactions, 3rd ed., Lea and Febiger, Philadelphia.

Goar, E.L. and Fletcher M.C., 1956, Toxic chorioretinopathy following the use of NP 207, *Trans. Amer. Ophthal. Soc.* 54: 129.

Gordon, D.M. and Kleberger, K.E., 1968, The effect of dimethyl sulphoxide (DMSO) on animal and human eyes, *Arch. Ophthal.* 79:423.

Grant, W.M., 1962, Toxicology of the Eye, Charles C. Thomas Publisher, Springfield, Illinois.

Green, K., 1992, A brief history of ocular toxicology, *Lens and Eye Tox. Res.* 9:153.

Green, K., 1992, History of ophthalmic toxicology, in: Ophthalmic Toxicology, G.C.Y. Chiou, ed., Raven Press Ltd., New York.

Hanna, C. and Fraunfelder, F.T., Meyer, M.S., 1977, Effects of dimethyl sulphoxide on ocular inflammation, *Ann. Ophthalmol.* 9:61.

Hayes, A.W., 1985, Toxicology of the Eye, Ear, and other Special Senses, Raven Press Ltd., New York.

Hockwin, O., Green, K. and Rubin, L.F., 1992, Manual of Ocular Toxicity Testing of Drugs, Gustav Fischer Verlag, Stuttgart, Jena, New York.

Hockwin, O. and Koch, H-R., 1977, Arzneimittelnebenwirkungen am Auge, Gustav Fischer Verlag, Stuttgart, New York.

Laughlin, R. and Carey, T., 1962, Cataracts in patients treated with triparanol, *J. Amer. Med. Assoc.* 181:339.

Meier-Ruge, W. and Cerletti, A., 1966, Zur experimentellen Pathologie der Phenothiazin-Retinopathie, *Ophthamologica (Basel)* 151: 512.

Rubin, L.F. and Barnett, K.C., 1967, Ocular effects of oral and dermal applications of dimethyl sulfoxide in animals, *Ann. N.Y. Acad. Sci.* 141:333.

Rubin, L.F. and Mattis, P.A., 1966, Dimethyl sulphoxide: Lens changes in dogs during oral administration, *Science* 153:83.

Tsubaki, T., Honma, Y. and Hoshi, M., 1971, Neurological syndrome associated with clioquinol, *Lancet* 1:696.

v. Sallman, L., Grimes, P. and Collins, E., 1963, Triparanol induces cataract in rats, *Arch. Ophthal.* 70:522.

Venning, G.R., 1983, Identification of adverse reactions to new drugs. IV - Verification of suspected adverse reactions, *Brit. Med. J.* 286:544.

Verrey, F., 1956, Dégénérescence pigmentaire de la rétine d'origine médicamenteuse, *Ophthalmologica (Basle)* 131:296.

Wood, D.C., Sweet, D., Van Dolah, J., Smith, J.C. and Contaxis, I., 1967, A study of DMSO and steroids in rabbit eyes, *Trans. N.Y. Acad. Sci.* 141:346.

Wright, P., 1975, Untowarded effects associated with practolol administration: oculomucocutaneous syndrome, *Brit. Med. J.* 1:595.

THE ERG, EOG, AND VEP IN RATS

Andrew M. Geller[1], Catherine M. Osborne[2], and Robert L. Peiffer[2]

[1]Center for Environmental Medicine and Lung Biology
[2]Department of Ophthalmology
University of North Carolina at Chapel Hill

INTRODUCTION

The critical analysis of the physiological, functional, and anatomical responses of the eye to the introduction of exogenous compounds is an integral part of many toxicity studies. Clinical studies conducted with biomicroscopy, indirect ophthalmoscopy, and histopathology allow for the detection of anatomical changes. Electrophysiology and psychophysics provide functional measures of the visual system that complement anatomical analysis.

This paper discusses three sets of electrophysiological techniques, electroretinograms (ERG), electro-oculograms (EOG), and visual evoked potentials (VEP), and their use as measures of oculotoxicity in several common species of animals, with particular emphasis on rats. These techniques measure the massed responses of large populations of cells. The ERG represents light responses of the cells of the retina. The EOG measures slow changes in the standing potential across the retinal pigment epithelium (RPE). The VEP records potentials generated by the cells of the visual cortex and therefore tests the integrity of the visual system from the level of sensory transduction through to the visual cortex. For each procedure, we have summarized the techniques of recording, the origins of the waveforms, and the effects of anesthetics and neurotoxicants.

ELECTRORETINOGRAM

The ERG is an evoked-response recorded at the cornea that represents the mass response of cells discharging in the retina in response to both light flashes and changing patterned stimuli. Methods of recording vary as to the type of stimulation and form of corneal electrode used. For the flash ERG, xenon arc lamps, tungsten-halogen lamps, and light emitting diodes (LEDs) are the most commonly used light sources. These are sometimes used in conjunction with fiber optic cables to transmit the illumination to the cornea. Light can then either be focused in the plane of the pupil to achieve a Maxwellian view or can be diffused across the entire retina by transmitting the light onto a ganzfeld dome. For recording from the rat, the ganzfeld is commonly constructed by backlighting a half table tennis ball placed with its concave side facing the eye. A stimulus generator that can form temporally-modulated checkerboard or grating patterns on a CRT is generally

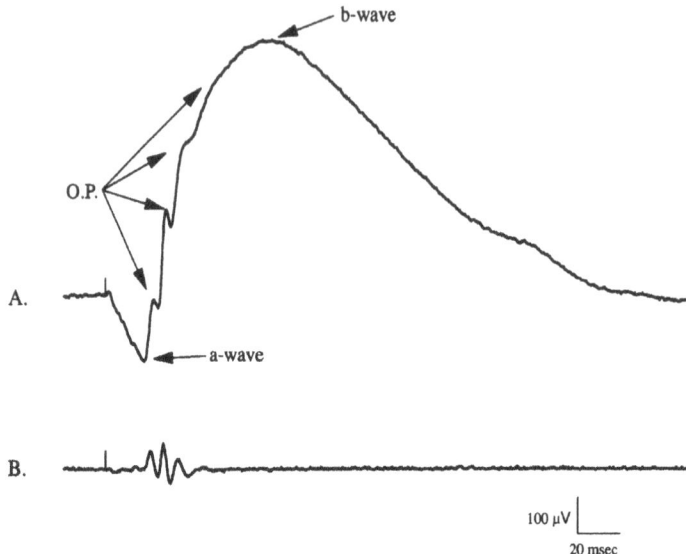

Figure 1A. Corneal electroretinogram recorded from adult male Long-Evans rat following single flash of light. The active electrode was a platinum-iridium wire loop (4 mm in diameter) placed in contact with the cornea, referenced to a subdermal needle electrode placed in the medial canthus. The light flash was generated by a Grass PS22 photostimulator (setting 16), channeled through a fiber optic bundle to a microscope objective, and focused in the plane of the dilated pupil (i.e. Maxwellian view), stimulating a circular region 37 degrees in diameter on the retina. Stimulus intensity was 14.29 lux-sec measured at the cornea. The ERG was amplified 1000X, analogue filtered (0.1 - 1000 Hz, 6 dB/octave rolloff), and sampled at 5000 Hz.

Vertical line at 20 ms denotes time of flash. Arrows indicate peaks of a- and b-waves and oscillatory potentials (O.P.). A-wave amplitude is measured from baseline to the a-wave peak. B-wave amplitude is measured from the a-wave peak to b-wave peak at intensities where the a-wave is present, from baseline otherwise. Implicit latency time is measured from stimulus onset to the peak of the ERG component of interest. The sampling duration was not long enough to record a c-wave in this example.
B. Same as above, but filter bandwidth adjusted to 100 - 1000 Hz to isolate the oscillatory potentials.

used for pattern stimulation to elicit the pattern ERG (PERG).

A variety of designs have been used for the corneal electrode. Cotton wick electrodes are sometimes favored for use in small animals such as the rat because of the difficulty in constructing a contact lens with such a minute diameter and steep curvature (Rosner et. al., 1993; Sandberg et. al., 1988). Gold and platinum-iridium wire loops are also used (Maertins et. al., 1993; Kiyosawa, et. al., 1993; Katz and Fox, 1991). Specially constructed contact lenses provide excellent electrical contact (Lachapelle and Blain, 1990) while yielding larger waveforms with relatively high signal-to-noise ratio (Mustonen and Sulg, 1980; Johnson and Massof, 1981). Some contact lenses serve as bipolar electrodes, referencing the corneal surface to the underside of the eye lid (Bush and Reme, 1992). Contact lenses have been used in rabbits (Chuang et. al., 1992; Nao-I et. al., 1986), rats (Imai and Tanakamaru, 1993; Hawlina and De Villiers, 1992; Stanford et. al., 1992; Penn et. al., 1989), cats (Narfstrom et. al., 1989), and monkeys (Jarkman et. al., 1985). The reference and the ground electrodes are commonly subcutaneous needle electrodes. The reference may be placed at the lateral or medial canthus, or in the ear, while the ground may be placed in the ear, the tongue, the leg, or the scruff of the neck (Cillino et. al., 1993; Maertins et. al, 1993b; Katz and Fox, 1991; Massof and Jones, 1972).

8

Flash Electroretinogram

The typical flash ERG waveform consists of a negative a-wave and positive b-wave of relatively short latency, and a positive c-wave at somewhat longer latency (figure 1a). In typical dark-adapted recording, the b-wave becomes evident at approximately 1 log unit higher intensity than absolute threshold. A-wave threshold is at light intensity levels approximately 2.5 log units greater than b-wave threshold (Bush and Reme, 1992; Fox and Farber, 1988).

The a-wave is an early corneal negative component. It is generally considered to reflect the voltage generated by the photoreceptors when they hyperpolarize in response to light. Recent models of the visual transduction process in rod photoreceptors, i.e. the conversion of the light stimulus into a neural impulse, have successfully linked a-wave parameters to the molecular and cellular physiology of the photoreceptors (Breton, et. al., 1993; Hood and Birch, 1993a, 1993b, 1990), and show promise for permitting a greater characterization of pathological or toxicological processes in these cells (Cideciyan and Jacobson, 1994). Unlike the rod a-wave, the cone-driven a-wave likely reflects inner as well as outer retinal contributions (Sieving and Bush, 1994).

The a-wave is distinct from two other corneal negative potentials, the short-latency early receptor potential (ERP) and the long-latency scotopic threshold response (STR). The ERP is generated with stimuli bright enough to bleach a significant percentage of the visual pigment, has a latency on the order of 0.7 μsec, and is thought to reflect charge displacement in the outer segment during the cascade of photochemical reactions following quantum absorption. This rapid, early deflection allows the approximation of the number of visual pigment molecules that are activated by light quanta (q) entering the eye (Steinberg et. al., 1991), but care must be taken in measuring the ERP because of the chance of photoelectric artifact (Sieving, et. al., 1978).

The STR is different from the rod a-wave in that it is the only ERG component present near rod absolute threshold, generated at light levels 4.0 log units less than those needed to generate a-waves in humans (Sieving and Wakabayashi, 1991) and albino (Bush and Reme, 1992) and pigmented rats (Hawks, et. al., 1994; Hubbard and Naarendorp, 1994). The STR has also been recorded in cat and monkey (Sieving, et. al., 1986; Wakabayashi, et. al., 1988), but not in rabbit. Its latency, on the order of 80 to 200 ms,

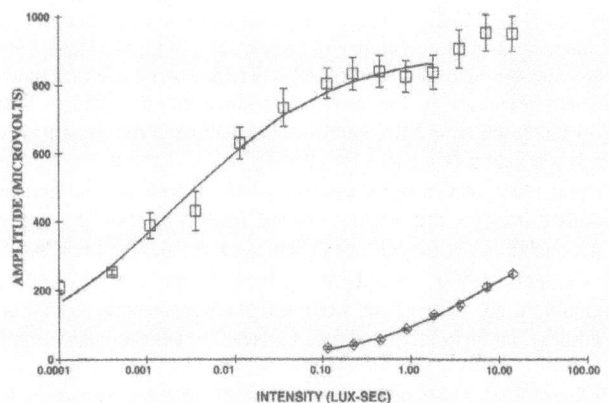

Figure 2. Amplitude-intensity functions for a- and b-waves recorded from adult male Long Evans rats (n = 5). Smooth curves are fits to data of Naka-Rushton equation (Birch, 1989); b-wave fit is to lower intensity (up to first asymptote) data. Squares: a-waves; diamonds: b-waves. Error bars indicate ± 1 standard error.

is long compared to the brief latency of the a-wave (Sieving and Nino, 1988; Wakabayashi, et. al., 1988). The sensitivity of the STR is likely a product of its post-receptoral origins. The weak receptor response is amplified through lateral interconnections in the proximal retina (Steinberg, et. al., 1991; Sieving, et. al., 1986). Current evidence points to an origin for the STR in the amacrine cell layer (Sieving, 1991). Although the STR is not currently used in neurotoxicology, it may prove to be a useful tool in detecting adverse changes in the inner retina.

The positive wave that appears immediately following the a-wave is the b-wave; it reflects the interaction between bipolar cells and Müller-type glial cells (Steinberg, et. al., 1991). In the rat, b-wave amplitude increases with flash intensity until approximately a-wave threshold, then plateaus as a-wave amplitude grows, and finally increases again (figure 2). Loss of the b-wave generally suggests a problem with the synaptic relay between the rod photoreceptors and the more proximal retinal components (Sandberg, 1994).

Smaller wave forms, known as oscillatory potentials (OP), are superimposed upon the ascending limb of the b-wave and can be isolated with appropriate filter settings (figure 1a, b). Current source density analysis in primates (Heynen, et. al., 1985) and the correlation between the earliest developmental appearance of OPs and the maturation of inner retinal synapses in rat suggest an origin for the OPs in inner retina (el Aziz and Wachtmeister, 1992, 1991a, 1991b, 1990). The first of these wavelets, OP1, was found to be a good indicator of anesthetic depth in the rabbit (Tashiro et. al., 1986); the second of these inflections (OP2) has been found to directly correlate with absolute intensity in rabbits (Lachapelle, et. al., 1990); the third may best reflect adaptational processes (Peachey, et. al. 1991).

The third major component of the ERG is a sustained potential termed the c-wave. This is a late (350 - 450 ms), slow ERG event that reflects the release of K^+ by the apical membrane of the retinal pigment epithelium after the photoreceptor light response. Though once believed to be unrecordable in non-pigmented retinas, this component of the ERG was observed in dark-reared albino rats (Graves et al., 1985). Parallels have been drawn between the c-wave and the standing potential of the eye (Textorius and Gottvall, 1992).

The flash ERG has proven to be a sensitive indicator of retinal neurotoxicity due to adult and developmental low-level lead exposure in rats. Lead exposure decreased the amplitude of the a- and b-wave components of the ERG and increased latency (Fox, et. al., 1991; Fox and Rubenstein, 1989; Fox and Farber, 1988). ERG studies have also demonstrated a change in increment thresholds and the rate of recovery of dark adaptation with lead (Fox and Katz, 1992). Changes in the a- and b-wave amplitudes have also been noted in rats dosed with methyl mercury (Gitter, et. al., 1988; Gramoni, 1980).

Solvent exposure also altered the ERG. Trichloroethylene and methylchloroform produced transient increases in the c-wave (Jarkman et. al., 1985). Prenatal ethanol exposure in rats increased cone ERG latencies and decreased rod sensitivity and the range and rate of dark adaptation (Katz and Fox, 1991).

Organophosphate pesticides have been reported to both increase and decrease a- and b-wave amplitudes, though this effect may be independent of the organophosphates' inhibition of acetylcholinesterase activity (Yoshikawa, et. al. 1990; reviewed in Boyes, et. al.,1994 and Dementi, 1994). Fenthion reduced a- and b-wave amplitudes in both pigmented and albino rats. The albino strain showed a more rapid reduction in amplitude as a function of time, but also produced much greater between animal variability (Imai, et. al., 1983).

The different ERG components are differentially affected by anesthetics. Halothane (HAL), alone or in combination with other anesthetics, depresses both a-and b-wave amplitudes. In rats, HAL alone depressed b-waves relative to a lower concentration of halothane combined with nitrous oxide (NO$_2$) (Wasserschaff and Schmidt, 1986). In dogs, a- and b-wave intensity thresholds were lower with ketamine hydrochloride / xylazine (K/X) than with thiopentone / HAL / NO$_2$. At suprathreshold intensities, only the latter treatment had an effect, reducing a-wave amplitudes (Kommonen, et. al., 1988). Urethane preserved the form of the ERG (Millar, et. al., 1989; Wioland and Bonaventure, 1985), but repeated subcutaneous dosing with urethane caused toxic retinopathy (Grant, 1986). OP amplitudes were depressed and peak latencies increased by the use of pentobarbital, methoxyflurane, halothane, and enflurane anesthesia (Maertins, et. al., 1993; Tashiro, et. al., 1986).

Pattern Electroretinogram

The PERG is generated by retinal stimulation with grating or checkerboard patterns. The pattern may be modulated in counterphase (contrast reversal) so that a pattern is always present, or in onset-offset, wherein the patterned field is alternated with a uniform field of identical space average luminance. Stray light outside of the retinal image of the pattern remains constant and therefore does not contribute to the response (Berninger and Arden, 1988).

The PERG is thought to be generated at the retinal ganglion cell level. The PERG shows spatial tuning, which suggests neural sources with antagonistic spatial organization (Vaegan, et. al., 1990; Hess and Baker, 1984). The origin of the PERG was investigated by sectioning the optic nerve (ON) in cat (Maffei and Fiorentini, 1981) and later in rat (Domenici, et. al., 1991). The waveform degenerated with the subsequent degeneration of the ganglion cell layer while flash and flicker electroretinograms were unaffected, though more recent reports show evidence of a residual pattern response with ON section, likely due to the retinal illuminance response (Berninger and Arden, 1988; Tobimatsu, et. al., 1989). Sieving and Steinberg (1987) provided evidence that the PERG is generated by local luminance responses in proximal retina by advancing electrodes through the vitreous and retina and performing current source density analysis.

The PERG can be segregated into a pattern specific response (PSR) and a retinal illumination response (Thompson and Drasdo, 1987; Drasdo, et. al. 1987a, 1987b). The PSR is uncovered by weighting the illuminance response by the spatial and temporal contrast attenuation factors of the eye, then subtracting it from the raw PERG. In humans, the PSR waveform remaining after the subtraction shows a change in spatial tuning with retinal eccentricity, as is expected with patterned stimuli.

To the authors' knowledge, the PERG has not been used in toxicology. According to one study (Vaegan and Burne, 1987), it is impossible to achieve a PERG in albino rats. It is clear, however, that conditions which effect the ganglion cells or regions specialized for pattern vision in foveate species have an effect on the PERG. For example, the PERG is attenuated by optic atrophy due to glaucoma or trauma in humans while the flash ERG is not (Bach, et. al., 1992). The PERG is also affected by maculopathies, suggesting the predominant contribution to the PERG of the densely-packed ganglion cells of the macular region (Maffei and Fiorentini, 1990).

Pharmacological agents also affect the PERG. Chlorpromazine, an antidopaminergic drug, increased the latency of the PERG in humans (Bartel, et. al., 1990). Ketamine/xylazine anaesthesia produced a high frequency shift in the peak of the PERG spatial frequency tuning curve measured in cats, relative to anaesthesia by urethane, alphaxalone/alphadone, pentobarbitone/xylazine, or halothane (Vaegan, et. al. 1990).

11

ELECTRO-OCULOGRAM

The EOG, first observed by Dubois-Reymond in 1849 (Peiffer, et. al., 1981), measures the voltage difference between the anterior and posterior poles of the eye (Sandberg, 1994). It examines the integrity of the RPE-photoreceptor complex. The RPE presents high electrical resistance; any current generated on the neural retina side of the RPE yields a large change in voltage with reference to an electrode on the outside of the eye. Changes in potassium levels driven by the photoreceptor light response yield a delayed depolarization of the basal membrane of the RPE, which produces a light-sensitive slow oscillation in potential called the light peak, at about 300 seconds (Steinberg et. al., 1985, 1983). A second, light-insensitive component of the EOG, is visualized as the dark trough (figure 3). This component mainly reflects the barrier function of the RPE; it is independent of the functional status of the photoreceptors (Fishman, 1990). Uncovering the dark trough requires at least fifteen minutes in the dark as the standing potential of the eye changes. These slow changes in potential allow the EOG to be used to quantify voltage changes across the eye resulting from a change from dark to light adaptation. The light rise:dark trough ratio increases with increasing luminance (Fishman, 1990).

Measurement of the EOG requires placement of electrodes at each canthus. A saccade will result in a sharp spike in the EOG recording as the anterior and posterior poles of the eye shift position in relation to the recording electrodes. As the light-adapted state of the eye changes, the size of the spike changes. The largest amplitude spike in the light is the light peak, the smallest in the dark, the dark trough (Fishman, 1990).

There are few examples in the literature of measuring dark-light adaptation EOGs in animals. One example, however, is the chicken. Measurement required the animal to be paralyzed with curare or gallamine and maintained under urethane anesthesia. Starting from a dark-adapted baseline, EOGs were recorded through thirty minutes each of light and dark adaptation by mechanically rotating the eye through horizontal oscillations of thirty degrees of arc at a rate of sixty per minute (Rudolph et. al.,1989; Wioland et. al., 1990).

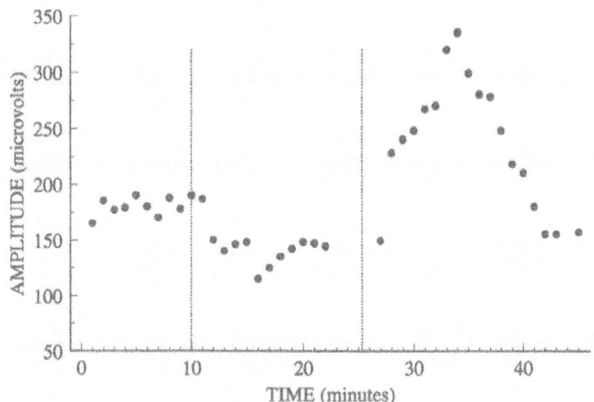

Figure 3. EOG recording. Region to the left of dotted lines shows baseline standing potential in ordinary room lighting. Region between dotted lines indicates period in the dark. Minimum amplitude in this region indicates dark trough. Region to right of dotted lines indicates period of light adaptation. Maximum amplitude in this region indicates light peak. After Finkelstein and Gouras, 1969.

Most human pharmacological studies have relied on patients with therapeutic complications to various treatments or who have volunteered for studies testing the effects of receptor antagonists in the catecholaminergic and indoleaminergic systems (Pall et. al., 1989; Hodgkins et. al., 1992; Maruiwa et. al., 1992). Such antagonists have also been tested in animals, such as the chicken and the cat, generating similar increases in the EOG basal values and amplitudes (Velasquez-Moctezuma et. al., 1991; Wioland et. al., 1990; Rudolph et. al., 1990, 1989). Exogenous compounds, such as haloperidol, iron dextran and metoclopramide, caused a decrease in the light rise:dark trough ratio in both humans and animals (Hodgkins et. al.,1992; Maruiwa et. al., 1992; Wioland et. al., 1990).

The EOG is also utilized to record eye movements. In studies analyzing rapid eye movement (REM) and sleep-wakefulness, unrestrained animals with wire electrodes chronically implanted at both canthi are allowed to experience free movement and natural sleep patterns, during which EOG data is collected. This preparation has been used in rats (Sato et. al., 1993; Kametani and Kawamura, 1990; Yang, et. al., 1990; Arito et. al., 1988), rabbits (Mondelski, 1991; Pivik, et. al. 1987; Kovalzon, et. al., 1986), cats (Marini, et. al. 1992; Mamelak, et. al. 1991), dogs (Xi, et. al., 1993), and monkeys (Erny et al., 1984). Acute preparations are possible, however, as demonstrated in the dog (Hendricks et. al., 1991) with a pair of 27 gauge needle electrodes implanted immediately prior to recording. These measures have demonstrated a loss of cerebellar activity as a result of exposure to compounds such as cholinergic antagonists, cocaine, ouabain, and toluene (Sato et al., 1993; Peters et. al., 1992; Velasquez-Moctezuma et. al., 1991; Burchfield et. al., 1990; Arito, et. al., 1988).

The EOG generated by optokinetic nystagmus (OKN) has also been recorded in many animals. In rats, OKN is induced by placing the rat on a rotating turntable inside of a drum or screen with a static pattern of vertical stripes (Larsby et. al., 1986). In other species, such as the cat or monkey, the awake, restrained animal is presented with a sinusoidal pseudorandom pattern projected onto a screen approximately 0.5 m in front of the test subject (Borel and Lacour, 1992) or can be placed with its head in a rotating drum, the surface of which presents either stripes or a pattern of dark dots randomly distributed on a white background (Flandrin et. al., 1990). Monkeys have also been trained to run around a circular track while recordings are obtained of compensatory oculo-motor activity from electrodes implanted subcutaneously at the canthal regions of each eye (Solomon and Cohen, 1992).

VISUAL EVOKED POTENTIAL

VEPs have been utilized in animal research for over 25 years as a method for analyzing the function of the visual neural pathway in its entirety. The cortical VEP waveform represents the thalamocortical input and spread of neural activity through the lamina of the primary visual cortex as well as activity generated in other visual areas. Recording the VEP in animals generally requires more invasive techniques for obtaining data than does the ERG. In most animal studies, electrodes are chronically implanted in the skull above the visual cortex. This insures that correct positioning is maintained throughout the duration of the testing procedure and allows recording from an unanesthetized animal. The epidural contact also increases the strength of the recorded signal over cutaneous or subcutaneous electrodes, though the latter have been used successfully in cats (Sims and Laratta, 1988).

The VEP, like the electroretinogram, has several different forms, determined by the type of visual stimulus presented to the subject. The two most widely used in neurotoxic

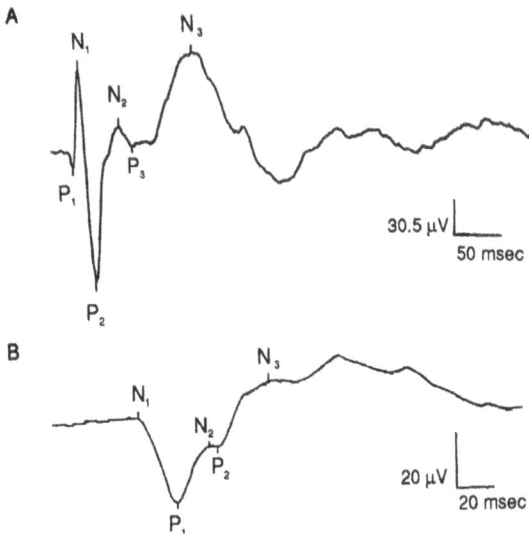

Figure 4 A. Group average flash evoked potential recorded from visual cortex of adult male Long Evans rats (n = 11) with stainless steel screw electrodes in contact with dura. The active electrode was located 1 mm anterior and 4 mm lateral (left) of lambda. The reference and ground electrodes were located 2 mm anterior and 2 mm lateral (right and left) of bregma. The stimulus was a 10 μsec flash of approximately 356 lux-sec produced by a Grass PS22 Photic Stimulator (strobe setting = 16) mounted exterior to the mirrored test chamber (Herr, et. al., 1991) delivered at 0.3 Hz. Ambient illumination was 100 lux. White noise was present to mask noise associated with the strobe discharge. The response of each animal was analogue filtered (0.8 -1000 Hz, 6 dB/octave rolloff), amplified 10,000x, and sampled at 2048 Hz. 50 trials/animal were averaged.

B. Group average pattern reversal potential from adult male Long Evans rats (n = 10). Electrodes placed as above. Awake rats were restrained in a harness and positioned in front of a screen subtending 69 x 74° of visual angle. The stimulus consisted of a square wave grating of fundamental spatial frequency of 0.5 cycle/deg modulated at 0.3 Hz. The response of each animal was analog filtered (0.8 -100 Hz, 6 dB/octave rolloff), amplified 10,000x, and sampled at 2000 Hz. 200 trials/animal were averaged.

Thanks to Dr. David W. Herr for generously donating this figure.

examinations are the flash evoked potential (FEP) and the pattern evoked potential (PEP). Much of the data available on the generators of the VEP comes from work on primates. To provide a general description of the waveforms, we have adopted a notation which subscripts the main positive and negative peaks in integer order, e.g. N_1, N_2. Subscripting with the actual latency of the peak, e.g. N_{160}, provides more detail for describing specific results.

Flash Evoked Potential

The FEP is similar to the flash ERG in that the stimulus is a brief flash of light which may be varied in intensity (Herreros de Tejada et. al., 1992; Dyer, 1986). The most important features of the FEP waveform are the latencies and amplitudes of the early components, from 0 to 200 ms (figure 4A) (Dyer, 1986). The major initial peak is a negative peak (N_1) with latency on the order of 30 ms (Boyes and Dyer, 1984, 1983b). The latency of this peak and the smaller positive peak (P_1) preceding it decreases with increasing intensity (Boyes, et. al., 1985). The amplitudes of these peaks increase monotonically with intensity (Boyes, et. al., 1985; Herreros de Tejada, et. al., 1992).

In primates and rats, the initial major negative deflection N_1 is generated mainly in the thalamocortical recipient layer (Dyer, 1986; Kraut, et. al., 1985). The middle components of the waveform, P_2 and N_2, likely reflect activity in stellate cells of layer 4 and the supragranular layer of the visual cortex (rev. in Herr and Boyes, in press). N_3 (i.e. N_{160}) may represent input from a reverberating thalamocortical circuit (rev. in Herr and Boyes, in press). N_3 is also noteworthy because it changes as a function of the number of times the animal was tested (Herr, et. al., 1991) and with the animal's level of arousal (Dyer, et. al., 1988).

In larger animals, such as the dog, cat, and rabbit, the FEP response is elicited from the entire retina by placing the animal in a restraining device with a flash unit held approximately 5 to 20 cm from the eye (Nakatake, et. al., 1993; Romani, et. al., 1991; Strain et. al., 1990; Bichsel, et. al., 1988; Sims and Laratta, 1988). In smaller animals, such as the rat, the FEP may be collected from a restrained animal, utilizing LED's or ganzfeld domes (Herreros de Tejada, et. al., 1992; Deguchi, et. al., 1992), or from an unrestrained animal placed in a chamber that has three walls covered by mirrors and a fourth taken up by a strobe light stimulator (Boyes and Dyer, 1988, 1983b; Hetzler, et. al., 1988). Both recording methods result in similar wave forms. Caution should be taken to mask or muffle the click of the strobe when recording a FEP. The acoustic stimulus generates an auditory evoked response which may confound the data (Herr and Boyes, 1993).

Pattern Evoked Potential

The pattern evoked potential (PEP) is generated with stimuli identical to those used for the PERG. This manner of stimulation effectively reduces retinal activity elicited by intensity changes while increasing cortical responsiveness.

In contrast with the FEP, the first major peak of the PEP is a large positive inflection (P_1) at a latency of approximately 66 ms (figure 4B) (Boyes and Dyer, 1983a). The peak-to-peak amplitude of the P_2N_3 component of the waveform decreases with an increase in spatial frequency. Extrapolation to noise level at high spatial frequencies yields an estimate of visual acuity comparable to psychophysical estimates (Boyes and Dyer, 1983a). P_1N_3 amplitude increases with increasing spatial contrast, particularly at lower spatial frequencies (Boyes, et. al., 1985).

The generators of the PEP are found in the superficial layers of the visual cortex as well as in cortical regions outside of the primary visual cortex (Herr and Boyes, in press). Thalamocortical input is reflected by N_1. The initial positive inflection is generated in the supragranular layer (layer 3) of the primary visual cortex (Schroeder, et. al., 1991). The subsequent negative and positive peaks, N_2 and P_2, are likely generated by a combination of both local cortical processes and activity in extrastriate cortex (Schroeder, et. al., 1990).

Because the pattern elements are the critical components of the stimulus, precautions must be taken to control where the pattern is projected onto the retina, particularly with animals with retinal specialization for pattern vision. These animals, such as the cat, the rabbit, the dog and the primate, must be immobilized, either through behavioral or pharmacological means, for proper fixation and accommodation (Nakatake et. al., 1993; Bichsel et. al., 1988; Sims and Laratta, 1988; Ghilardi et. al., 1987). For rats, humane restraint of awake animals is adequate both because of their great depth of field (Green, et. al., 1980), making accommodation unnecessary, and their comparative lack of retinal specialization for acuity. Recording of the PEP from awake animals removes potential confounds introduced by anesthesia.

The VEP is well-represented in the toxicology literature for testing for disruption of the visual pathway (see Boyes, 1992, for review). Tests of different compounds within a class have produced very different results. The organometal triethyltin, for example, increased the latencies of FEP peaks (Dyer and Howell, 1982a, b) while methyl mercury reduced them (Dyer, et. al., 1978). Different organic solvents have also yielded different effects on the VEP. Acute exposure to toluene and p-xylene reduced FEP N_3 amplitudes (Dyer, et. al., 1988). Acute and chronic carbon disulfide exposure decreased amplitudes and increased latencies of FEP and PEP waveforms, though the increase in latency may have been secondary to hypothermia (Herr, et. al., 1992). Acute sulfolane exposure increased FEP but not PEP amplitudes relative to controls, and increased FEP latencies independent of hypothermia (Dyer, et. al., 1986). Organophosphates, formaldehyde, carbon dioxide, and ozone have also been shown to alter VEP responses in animals (Boyes and Dyer, 1988).

Direct anesthetic effects on the VEP along with possible interactions of test compounds and anesthetic agents have led to the development of techniques for recording from awake animals (Boyes and Dyer, 1983a). Comparisons of recordings of awake animals to animals dosed with urethane and ketamine showed significant decreases in the amplitudes of FEP negative components and increases in the amplitudes of the positive peaks as a result of anesthetic administration (Rigdon and Dyer, 1988; Dyer and Rigdon, 1987). The N_1 peak of the FEP appears to be somewhat resistant to the effects of chloralose, halothane, thiopental, and pentobarbital, though these anesthetics may change the amplitudes and latencies of other components (Bischel, et. al. 1988; Schwarz and Block, 1993). A comparison across studies of awake and pentobarbital- anesthetized rats suggested a slowing and diminution of the PEP due to the anesthesia, although other procedural factors may also have had an effect (Boyes and Dyer, 1983a; Onofrj, et. al., 1982).

The effects of anesthetics should be separated from the effects of changes in body temperature. Chloropent anesthesia accompanied by hypothermia led to an increase in FEP latency and complex changes in peak-to-peak amplitudes. When normal body temperature was maintained, the increase in FEP latencies was reduced, and amplitudes were not significantly different from normal (Dyer and Boyes, 1983). Similar results were obtained with chloral hydrate (Hetzler and Dyer, 1984).

CONCLUSION

A high percentage of chemicals with known neurotoxic effects adversely affect the sensory systems. In one sample of 764 compounds or compound classes, close to half were reported to produce sensory effects (Crofton and Sheets, 1989). Of these, 44% (148 compounds) produced adverse effects on the visual system. Boyes (1992) lists these compounds and the consequences of exposure on the visual system. The ubiquity of this problem has led the U.S.E.P.A. to issue proposed guidelines for using evoked potentials as measures of sensory neurotoxicity (Boyes, 1990).

The ERG, EOG, and VEP are valuable in characterizing the harmful effects of known and potential neurotoxicants on the visual system because each of these tests targets a different part of the visual pathway. They are especially useful because all three sets of techniques can be used in non-invasive assessment of the human visual system as well as in animal models, facilitating comparison between species.

Each animal mentioned in this review has merit for utilization in toxicology protocols. The pigmented rat, while sometimes criticized as an animal model for visual function, is well-suited for use in beginning toxicity studies. While there are obvious differences between the human and rat visual systems based mostly on diurnal versus nocturnal adaptations, the recorded ERG and VEP waveforms are similar between rats and humans, though individual peak latencies and amplitudes vary between species (Creel, 1973; Hudnell and Boyes, 1991). VEPs in rats and humans are comparably affected by pattern adaptation (Hudnell, et. al., 1990), and a mathematical approach has been derived that quantitatively relates rat and human spatial vision (Begninus, et. al., 1991). Pigmented rats are also an excellent model for the scotopic (i.e. rod) flash ERG; all of the features of the waveform which develop with increasing intensity in humans are also present in rat.

The use of the albino rat as an animal model for sensory testing is less defensible. Albino rats are highly susceptible to phototoxic degeneration of the outer nuclear layer as well as spontaneous retinal lesions (Heywood and Gopinath, 1990), making causal attribution of deterioration more difficult. Albinism has also been linked to a less densely myelinated optic nerve and projection abnormalities, such as a smaller proportion of uncrossed fibers at the chiasm (Vaegan and Burne, 1987). Exogenous compounds may bind with melanin within ocular tissues and thus may decrease toxicity by shielding other tissues from exposure or increase toxicity by causing greater concentrations of the material (Creel, 1984; Butler et. al. 1987; Menon et. al., 1991).

Physiologically, the latencies, threshold values, and amplitudes of PEP responses of albino and pigmented rats differ, with the patterned-response markedly worse in the albinos (Dyer and Swartzwelder, 1978; Boyes and Dyer, 1983a). FEP latencies are slower in albinos (Creel, 1984). The PERG can be recorded in pigmented rats but is unrecordable in albino rats (Vaegan and Burne, 1987).

Despite the differences between albino and pigmented species, however, both have similar spectral, temporal, and luminance sensitivities (Alpern, et. al. 1987) and ganglion cell density and distribution (Vaegan and Burne, 1987). Equivalent dark-adapted thresholds and low-level responses for the VEP and the ERG have been reported in both albino and pigmented strains (Herreros de Tejada, et. al., 1992; Green, et. al., 1991), though these results conflict with results from recordings from optic nerve and superior colliculus (Balkema, 1988). These physiologic and anatomic similarities allow limited inter-strain comparison to be performed, but where possible, pigmented strains are more appropriate as models of mammalian visual neurotoxicity.

Author AMG supported by USEPA cooperative agreement CR817643 with CEMLB, UNC-CH. The research in this article has been reviewed by the Health Effects Research Laboratory, U.S. Environmental Protection Agency, and approved for publication. Approval does not signify that the contents necessarily reflect the views and policies of the Agency nor does mention of trade names or commercial products constitute an endorsement or recommendation for use.

REFERENCES

Alpern, M., Fulton, A.B., and Baker, B.N. 1987. "Self-screening" of rhodopsin in rod outer segments. Vis. Res. 27: 1459-1470.

Arito, H., Tsuruta, H., and Oguri, M. 1988. Changes in sleep and wakefulness following single and repeated exposures to toluene vapor in rats. Toxicology 62: 76-80.

Bach, M., Gerling, J., and Geiger, K. 1992. Optic atrophy reduces the pattern-electroretinogram for both fine and coarse stimulus patterns. Clin. Vis. Sci. 7: 327-333.

Balkema, G.W. 1988. Elevated dark-adapted thresholds in albino rodents. Invest. Ophthal. Vis. Sci. 29: 544-549.

Bartel, P., Blom, M., Robinson, E. Van der Meyden, C., Sommers, DeK., and Becker, P. 1990. Effects of chlorpromazine on pattern and flash ERGs and VEPs compared to oxazepam and to placebo in normal subjects. Electroenc. Clin. Neurophys. 77: 330-339.

Benignus, V.A., Boyes, W.K., Hudnell, H.K., Frey, C.M., Svendsgaard, D.J. 1991. Quantitative methods for cross-species mapping (CSM). Neurosci. and Behav. Rev. 15: 165-171.

Berninger, T.A. and Arden, G.B. 1988. The pattern electroretinogram. Eye 2, suppl.: s257-s283.

Birch, D.G. 1989. Clinical electroretinography. Ophthal. Clinics of North America 2: 469-497.

Bichsel, P., Oliver, J., Coulter, D., and Brown, J. 1988. Recording of visual-evoked potentials in dogs with scalp electrodes. J. Vet. Int. Med. 2: 145-149.

Borel, L., and Lacour, M. 1992. Functional coupling of the stabilizing eye and head reflexes during horizontal and vertical linear motion in the cat. Exp. Brain Res. 91: 191-206.

Boyes, W.K. 1990. Proposed test guidelines for using sensory evoked potentials as measures of neurotoxicity. U.S.E.P.A. Document: EPA/600/x-90/166.

Boyes, W.K. 1992. Testing visual system toxicity using evoked potential technology, in R.L. Isaacson and K.F. Jenson, eds. The Vulnerable Brain and Environmental Risks, Volume 1. Plenum Press, New York.

Boyes, W.K., and Dyer, R.S. 1983a. Pattern reversal visual evoked potentials in awake rats. Br. Res. Bull. 10: 817-823.

Boyes, W.K., and Dyer, R.S. 1983b. Pattern reversal and flash evoked potentials following acute triethyltin exposure. Neurobehav. Toxicol. Teratol. 5: 571-577.

Boyes, W.K., and Dyer, R.S. 1984. Chlordimeform produces profound, selective, and transient changes in visual evoked potentials of the hooded rat. Exp. Neurology 86: 434-447.

Boyes, W.K., and Dyer, R.S. 1988. Visual evoked potentials as indicators of neurotoxicity. Office of Research and Development, U.S.E.P.A., Deliverable 2312A, Document number HER0653.

Boyes, W.K., Jenkins, D., and Dyer, R.S. 1985. Chlordimeform produces contrast-dependent changes in visual evoked potentials of the hooded rat. Exp. Neurol. 89: 434-449.

Boyes, W.K., Tandon, P., Barone, S., and Padilla, S. 1994. Effects of organophosphates on the visual system of rats. J. Appl. Tox. 14: 135-143.

Breton, M., Schueller, A.W., Lamb, T.D., and Pugh, E.N. 1993. Analysis of ERG a-wave amplification and kinetics in terms of the g-protein cascade of phototransduction. Inv. Ophthal. Vis. Sci. 35: 295-309.

Burchfield, D.J., Graham, E.M., Abrams, R.M., and Gerhardt, K.J. 1990. Cocaine alters behavioral states in the fetal sheep. Develop. Brain Res. 56: 41-45.

Bush, R.A. and Reme, C.E. 1992. Chronic lithium treatment induces reversible and irreversible changes in the rat ERG in vivo. Clin. Vis. Sci. 7: 393-401.

Butler, S.R., Ford, G.P., and Newbern, J.W. 1987. A study of the effects of vigabatrin on the central nervous system and retina of Sprague-Dawley and Lister-hooded rats. Toxicol. Pathol. 15: 143-148.

Chang, L.W., and Dyer, R. 1983. Trimethyltin induced pathology in sensory neurons. Neurobehav. Toxicol. Teratol. 5: 337-350.

Chuang, H.C., Kawano, S., Arai, M., Tsukada, T., Kita, M., Negi, A., and Honda, Y. The influence of argon laser panretinal photocoagulation on the rabbit ERG c-wave. Acta Ophthalmologica 70: 303-307.

Cideciyan, A. and Jacobson, S.G. 1994. Negative electroretinograms in retinitis pigmentosa. Inv. Ophthal. Vis. Sci. 34: 3253-3263.

Cillino, S., Guarneri, R., Guarneri, P., Pennica, C., Chichi, G., Piccoli, F., and Ponte, P. 1993. Electroretinographic Response in WAG/Rij rats after low-intensity cyclic light exposure. Ophthalmic Res. 25: 137-144.

Creel, D.J. 1973 Visually evoked responses in the rat, guinea pig, cat, monkey, and man. Exp. Neurol. 40: 351-366.

Creel, D.J. 1984. Albinism and evoked potentials: factors in the selection of infrahuman models to predicting the human response to neurotoxic agents. Neurobeh. Tox. and Terat. 6: 447-453.

Crofton, K.M., and Sheets, L.P. 1989. Evaluation of sensory system function using reflex modification of the startle response. J. Am. Coll. Toxicol. 8: 199-211.

Deguchi, K., Takeuchi, H., Miki, H., Yamada, A., Touge, T., Terada, S., and Nishioka, M. 1992. Electrophysiological follow-up of acute and chronic experimental allergic encephalomyelitis in the Lewis rat. Eur. Arch. Psychiatry Clin. Neurosci. 242: 1-5.

Dementi, B. 1994. Ocular effects of organophosphates: a historical perspective of Saku disease. J. Appl. Tox. 14: 119-129.

Domenici, L., Gravina, A., Berardi, N., and Maffei, L. 1991. Different effects of intracranial and intraorbital section of the optic nerve on the functional responses of rat retinal ganglion cells. Exp. Br. Res. 86: 579-584.

Drasdo, N., Cox, W., and Thompson, D.A. 1987a. The effects of image degradation on retinal illuminance and pattern responses to checkerboard stimuli. Doc. Ophthal. 66: 267-275.

Drasdo, N., Thompson, D.A., Thompson, C.M., and Cox, W. 1987b. Complementary components and local variations of the pattern electroretinogram. Inv. Ophthal. Vis. Sci. 28: 158-162.

Dyer, R.S. 1986. Interactions of behavior and neurophysiology. In Z. Annau (ed.) **Neurobehavioral Toxicology**. Johns Hopkins Univ. Press. pp. 193-213.

Dyer, R.S., Bercegeay, M.S., and Mayo, L.M. 1988 Acute exposures to p-xylene and toluene alter visual information processing. Neurotoxicol. and Teratol. 10: 147-153.

Dyer, R.S., and Boyes, W.K. 1983. Hypothermia and chloropent anesthesia differentially affect the flash evoked potentials of hooded rats. Brain Res. Bull. 10: 825-831.

Dyer, R.S., Boyes, W.K., and Hetzler, B.E. 1986. Acute sulfolane exposure produces temperature-independent and dependent changes in visual evoked potentials. Neurobehav. Toxicol. Teratol. 8: 687-693.

Dyer, R.S., Eccles, C.U., and Annau, Z. 1978. Evoked potential alterations following prenatal methyl mercury exposure. Pharmacol. Biochem. Behav. 8: 137-141.

Dyer, R.S. and Howell, W.E. 1982a. Acute triethyltin exposure: effects on the visual evoked potential and hippocampal afterdischarge. Neurobehav. Toxicol. Teratol. 4: 259-266.

Dyer, R.S. and Howell, W.E. 1982b. Triethyltin: ambient temperature alters visual system toxicity. Neurobehav. Toxicol. Teratol. 4: 267-271.

Dyer, R.S., and Rigdon G.C. 1987. Urethane affects the rat visual system at subanesthetic doses. Physiol. and Behav. 41: 327-330.

Dyer, R.S., and Swartzwelder, H.S. 1978. Sex and strain differences in the visual evoked potentials of albino and hooded rats. Pharmocol. Biochem. Behav. 9: 301-306.

el Azazi, M., and Wachtmeister, L. 1990. The postnatal development of the oscillatory potentials of the electroretinogram. I. Basic characteristics. Acta Ophtalmologica 68: 401-409.

el Azazi, M., and Wachtmeister, L. 1991a. The postnatal development of the oscillatory potentials of the electroretinogram. II. Photopic characteristics. Acta Ophtalmologica 69: 6-10.

19

el Azazi, M., and Wachtmeister, L. 1991b. The postnatal development of the oscillatory potentials of the electroretinogram. III. Scotopic characteristics. Acta Ophthalmologica 69: 505-510.

el Azazi, M., and Wachtmeister, L. 1992. The postnatal development of the oscillatory potentials of the electroretinogram. IV. Mesopic characteristics. Acta Ophthalmologica 70: 194-200.

Erny, B.C., Wexler, D.B., and Moore-Ede, M.C. 1985. Sleep-wake stages during the subjective night of the squirrel monkey. Physiology and Behav. 35: 189-194.

Finkelstein, M.A. and Gouras, P. 1969. Visual electrophysiology: an introduction to the ERG, EOG, ERP, and VER, in S.J.Fricker, ed., **Electrical Response of the Visual System (I.O.C. 914)**, pp. 857-881.

Fishman, G.A. 1990. The Electro-oculogram in retinal disorders. In Fishman, G.A., and Sokol, S. (eds.) **Electrophysiologic Testing in Disorders of the Retina, Optic Nerve, and Visual Pathway.** p.95. American Academy of Ophthalmology. San Francisco, C.A.

Flandrin, J.M., Courjon, J.H., Magnin, M., and Arzi, M. 1990. Horizontal optokinetic responses under stroboscopic illumination in cat, monkey, and man. Exp. Brain Res. 81: 59-69.

Fox, D.A. and Farber, D.B. 1988. Rods are selectively altered by lead: I. Electrophysiology and biochemistry. Exp. Eye Res. 46: 597-611.

Fox, D.A. and Katz, L.M. 1992. Developmental lead exposure selectively alters the scotopic ERG component of dark and light adaptation and increases rod calcium content. Vis. Res. 32: 249-255.

Fox, D.A., Katz, L.M., and Farber, D.B. 1991. Low level developmental lead exposure decreases the sensitivity, amplitude, and temporal resolution of rods. Neurotoxicol. 12: 641-654.

Fox, D.A. and Rubinstein, S.D. 1989. Age-related changes in retinal sensitivity, rhodopsin content and rod outer segment length in hooded rats following low-level lead exposure during development. Exp. Eye Res. 48: 237-249.

Ghilardi, M.F., Marx, M.S., Onofrj, M.C., Glover, A.A., and Bodis-Wollner, I. 1987. Scalp distribution of pattern visual evoked potentials in normal and hemianopic monkeys. Physiology and Behav. 41: 297-302.

Gitter, S., Pardo, A., Kariv, N., and Yinon, U. 1988. Enhanced electroretinogram in cats induced by exposure to mercury acetate. Toxicology 51: 67-76.

Gramoni, R. 1980. Retinal function of rats exposed to organomercurials. In Merigan, W.H., and Weiss, B. (eds.) **Neurotoxicity of the Visual System.** Raven Press, N.Y.

Grant, W.M. 1986. **Toxicology of the Eye, third edition.** Charles E. Thomas, Springfield, IL.

Graves, A., Green, D.G., and Fisher, L.J. 1985. Light exposure can reduce selectively or abolish the c-wave of the albino rat electroretinogram. Invest. Ophthal. Vis. Sci. 26: 388-393.

Green, D.G. 1973. Scotopic and photopic components of the rat electroretinogram. J. Physiol. 228. 781-797.

Green, D.G., Herreros de Tejada, P., and Glover, M.J. 1991. Are albino rats night blind? Invest. Ophthal. Vis. Sci. 32: 2366-2371.

Green, D.G., Powers, M.K., and Banks, M.S. 1980. Depth of focus, eye size, and visual acuity. Vis. Res. 20: 827-835.

Hawks, K.W., Bush, R.A., and Sieving, P.A. 1994. STR shows disproportionate loss compared to PII in RCS rat. Inv. Ophthal. Vis. Sci., suppl. 35: 2045.

Hawlina, M., and De Villiers, P.L.G. 1992. Light-emitting diodes and half-cell electrodes in experimental recording of electroretinogram c-wave. Doc. Ophthal. 81: 227-237.

Hendricks, J.C., Kovalski, R.J., and Kline, L.R. 1991. Phasic respiratory muscle patterns and sleep-disordered breathing during rapid eye movement sleep in the English bulldog. Am. Rev. Respir. Dis. 144: 1112-1120.

Herr, D.W. and Boyes, W.K., 1993. Potential confounding effects of strobe "clicks" in flash evoked potentials (FEPs) in rats. Toxicologist 13 (abstract): 216.

Herr, D.W. and Boyes, W.K., in press. Electrophysiological analysis of complex brain systems: sensory evoked potentials and their generators.

Herr, D.W., Boyes, W.K., and Dyer, R.S. 1991. Rat flash evoked potential peak N160 amplitude: Modulation by relative flash intensity. Physiol. Behav. 49: 355-365.

Herr, D.W., Dyer, R.S., and Boyes, W.K. 1992. Alterations in rat flash and pattern reversal evoked potentialsafter acute or repeated administration of carbon disulfide (CS_2). Fund. Appl. Toxicol. 18: 328-42.

Herreros de Tejada, P., Green, D.G., and Muñoz Tedo, C. 1992. Visual thresholds in albino and pigmented rats. Visual Neurosci. 9: 409-414.

Hess, R.F., and Baker, C.L. 1984. Human pattern-evoked electroretinogram. J. Neurophys.51: 939-951

Hetzler, B., and Dyer, R.S. 1984. Contribution of hypothermia to effects of chloral hydrate on flash evoked potentials of hooded rats. Pharmacol. Biochem. Behavior 21: 599-607.

Hetzler, B.E., Boyes, W.K., Creason, J.P., and Dyer, R.S. 1988. Temperature-dependent changes in visual evoked potentials of rats. Electroenc. Clin. Neurophys. 70: 137-154.

Hetzler, B.E., and Norris, L.K. 1988. Pentobarbital produces temperature-independent and dependent changes in the visual evoked potentials of rats. Annual Society for Neuroscience Abstracts, Toronto.

Heynen, H., Wachmeister, L., and van Norren, D. 1985. Origin of the oscillatory potentials in the primate retina. Vis. Res. 25: 1365.

Heywood, R., and Gopinath, C. 1990. Morphological assessment of visual dysfunction. Toxicol. Pathol. 18: 204-217.

Hodgkins, P.R., Morrell, A.J., Luff, A.J., Fetherston, T.J., and Good, P. 1992. Pigment epitheliopathy with serous detachment of the retina following intravenous iron dextran. Eye 6: 414-415.

Hood, D.C. and Birch, D.G. 1990. The a-wave of the human electroretinogram and rod receptor function. Invest. Ophthal. Vis. Sci. 31: 2070-2081.

Hood, D.C. and Birch, D.G. 1993a. Light adaptation of human rod receptors: the leading edge of the human a-wave and models of rod receptor activity. Vis. Res. 33: 1605-1618.

Hood, D.C. and Birch, D.G. 1993b. The human rod a-wave and phototransduction: interpreting the fit of the Lamb and Pugh model. Vis. Sci. and Applic. Tech. Digest (OSA).

Hubbard, N.P. and Naarendorp, F. 1994. Effects of dim background lights on the scotopic threshold response of the rat ERG. Inv. Ophthal. Vis. Sci., suppl. 35: 2047.

Hudnell, H.K. and Boyes, R. 1991. The comparability of rat and human visual-evoked potentials. Neurosci. Biobehav. Rev. 15: 159-164.

Hudnell, H.K., Boyes, W.K., and Otto, D.A. 1990. Rat and human visual -evoked potentials recorded under comparable conditions: a preliminary analysis to address the issue of predicting human neurotoxic effects from rat data. Neurotox. and Teratology 12: 391-398.

Imai, H., Miyata, M., Uga, S., and Ishikawa, S. 1983. Retinal degeneration in rats exposed to an organophosphate pesticide (fenthion). Environ. Res. 30: 453-465.

Imai, R. and Tanakamaru, Z. 1993. Visual dysfunction in aged Fischer 344 rats. J.Vet. Med. Sci. 55: 367-370.

Jarkman, S., Skoog, K., and Nilsson, S.E. 1985. The c-wave of the electroretinogram and the standing potential of the eye as highly sensitive measures of effects of low doses of trichloroethylene, methylchloroform, and halothane. Doc. Ophthal. 60: 375-382.

Johnson, M.A., and Massof, R.W. 1982. The photomyoclonic reflex: an artifact in the clinical electroretinogram. Br. J. Ophthal. 66: 368-378.

Kametani, H., and Kawamura, H. 1990. Alterations in acetylcholine release in the rat hippocampus during sleep-wakefulness detected by intracerebral dialysis. Life Sci. 47: 421-426.

Katz, L.M., and Fox, D.A. 1991. Prenatal ethanol exposure alters scotopic and photopic components of adult rat electroretinograms. Invest. Ophthal. Vis. Sci. 32: 2861-2872.

Kiyosawa, I., Aoki, M., Imamura, T., Naito, J., Saito, T.R., and Takahashi, K.W. 1993. Comparison of the gold wire electrode with cotton wick electrode for electroretinography in small laboratory animals. Exp. Anim. 42: 129-133.

Kommonen, B., Karhunen, U., and Raitta, C. 1988. Effects of thiopentone halothane-nitrous oxide anaesthesia compared to ketamine-xylazine anaesthesia on the dc recorded dog electroretinogram. Acta Vet. Scand. 29: 23-33.

Kovalzon, V.M., Obal, F.Jr., and Kalikhevich, V.N. 1986. [Peptidergic modulation of sleep: a comparative study of analogs of the peptide DSIP]. Zh. Evol. Biokhim. Fiziol. 22: 483-488.

Kraut, M.A., Arezzo, J.C., and Vaughan Jr., H.G. 1985. Intracortical generators of the flash VEP in monkeys. Electroenc. Clin. Neurophys. 62: 300-312.

Lachapelle, P., Benoit, J., Little, J.M., and Faubert, J. 1990. The diagnostic use of the second oscillatory potential in clinical electroretinography. Doc. Ophthal. 73: 327-336.

Lachapelle, P., and Blain, L. 1990. A new speculum electrode for electroretinography. J. Neurosci. Meth. 32: 245-249.

Larsby, B., Tham, R., Eriksson, B., and Odkvist, L.M. 1986. The effect of toluene on the vestibulo- and opto-oculomotor system in rats. Acta Otolaryngol. (Stockh.) 101: 422-428.

Maertins, T., Kroetlinger, F., Sander, E., Pauluhn, J., and Machemer, L. 1993. Electroretinographic assessment of early retinopathy in rats. Arch. Toxic. 67: 120-125.

Maffei, L., and Fiorentini, A. 1981. Electroretinographic responses to alternating gratings before and after section of the optic nerve. Science 211: 953-955.

Maffei, L., and Fiorentini, A. 1990. The pattern electroretinogram in animals and humans: physiological and clinical applications. In Cohen, B., and Bodis-Wollner, I. (eds.) **Vision and the Brain**. Raven Press, N.Y.

Mamelak, A.N., Quattrochi, J.J., and Hobson, J.A. 1991. Automated staging of sleep in cats using neural networks. Electroenceph. Clin. Neurophys. 79: 52-61.

Marini, G., Gritti, I., and Mancia, M. 1992. Enhancement of tonic and phasic events of rapid eye movement sleep following bilateral ibotenic acid injections into the centralis lateralis thalamic nucleus of cats. Neurosci. 48: 877-888.

Maruiwa, F., Kim, S.D., Nao-I, N., and Sawada, A. 1992. [Effects of metoclopramide, dopamine receptor blocker, on the EOG light peak]. Nippon Ganka Gakkai Zasshi 96: 375-380.

Massof, R.W., and Jones, A.E. 1972. Electroretinographic evidence for a photopic system in the rat. Vis. Res. 12: 1231-1239.

Menon, I.A., Trope, G.E., Basu, P.K., Wakeham, D.C., and Persad, S.D. 1989. Binding of tiomol to iris ciliary body and melanin: an in vitro model for assessing kinetics and efficacy of long acting anti-glaucoma drugs. J. Ocul. Pharmacol. 5: 313-324.

Millar, T.J., Vaegan, and Arora, A. 1989. Urethane as a sole general anesthetic in cats used for electroretinographic studies. Neurosci. Lett. 103: 108-112.

Mondelski, S. 1991. [Polish contribution to the electrophysiological studies in ophthalmology. I. Technology and animal studies]. Klin Oczna. 93: 94-96.

Mustonen, E. and Sulg, I. 1980. Electroretinography by skin electrodes and signal averaging method. Acta Ophthal. 58: 388-396.

Nakatake, N., Hori, A., Yasuhara, A., Naito, H., and Yasuhara, M. 1993. Oscillatory potentials of visual evoked potentials using source derivation techniques in rabbits. J. Neurolog. Sci. 114:144-151.

Nao-I, N, Kim, S., and Honda, Y. 1986. The normal c-wave amplitude in rabbits. Doc. Ophthal. 63: 121-130.

Narfstrom, K., Arden, G.B., and Nilsson, S.E.G. 1989. Retinal sensitivity in hereditary retinal degeneration in Abyssinian cats: electrophysiological similarities between cat and man. Br. J. Ophthal. 73: 516-521.

Onofrj, M., Bodis-Wollner, I., and Bobak, P. 1982. Pattern evoked potentials in the rat. Physiol. Behav. 28: 227-230.

Pall, H., Blake, D.R., Winyard, P., Lunec, J., Williams, A., Good, P.A., Kritzinger, E.E., Cornish, A., and Hider, R.C. 1989. Ocular toxicity of desferrioxamine- an example of copper promoted auto-oxidative damage? Br. J. Opthal. 73: 42-47.

Peachey, N.S., Alexander, K.R., Derlacki, D.J., Bobak, P., and Fishman, G.A. 1991. Effects of light adaptation on the response characteristics of human oscillatory potentials. Electroenc. Clin. Neurophys. 78: 27-34.

Peiffer, R.L., Armstrong, J.R., and Johnson, P.T. 1981. Animals in ophthalmic research concepts and methodologies. In Gay, W.I. (ed.) Methods of Animal Experimentation v. 6. Academic Press, New York, p. 206.

Penn, J.S., Thum, L.A., and Nash, M.I. 1989. Photoreceptor physiology in the rat is governed by the light environment. Exp. Eye Res. 49:205-215.

Peters, A.J., Abrams, R.M., Burchfield, D.J., and Gilmore, R.L. 1992. Seizures in a fetal lamb after cocaine exposure: a case report. Epilepsia 33:1001-1004.

Pivik, R.T., Bylsma, F.W., and Cooper, P.M. 1987. Variations in nuchal tonus following paradoxical sleep deprivation in the rabbit. Brain Res. 423: 196-202.

Rigdon, G.C., and Dyer, R.S. 1987. Ontogeny of flash-evoked potentials in unanesthetized rats. Int. J. Develop. Neurosci. 5: 447-454.

Rigdon, G.C., and Dyer, R.S. 1988. Ketamine alters rat flash evoked potentials. Pharmacol. Biochem. Behav. 30: 421-426.

Romani, A., Callieco, R., Bergamaschi, R., Versino, M., Cosi, V. 1991. Visual evoked potentials in the white New Zealand rabbit: source localization and normative aspects. Boll. Soc. It. Biol. Sper. 67: 601-607.

Rosner, M. Bobak, P., and Lam, T.L. 1993. Corneal electrode for recording electroretinograms in rats. Doc. Ophthal. 83: 175-180.

Rudolph, G. Wioland, N., Kempf., and Bonaventure, N. 1990. EOG and ERG modifications induced in the chicken eye after blockade of catecholamine and 5-hydroxytryptamine biosynthesis. Doc. Ophthal. 76: 47-53.

Rudolph, G., Wioland, N., Kempf, E., and Bonaventure, N. 1989. Electrooculographic study in the chicken after treatment with neurotoxin 6-hydroxydopamine. Doc. Ophthal. 72: 83-91.

Sandberg, M.A. 1994. Objective assessment of retinal function. In Albert, D.M., and Jakobiec, F.A. (eds.) **Principles and Practices of Ophthalmology: A Clinical Guide** W.B. Sanders Co. p 1195-1196.

Sandberg, M.A., Pawlyk, B.S., Crane, W.G., and Berson, E.L. 1988. Diurnal rhythm in the electroretinogram of the Royal College of Surgeons (RCS) pigmented rat. Exp. Eye Res. 46: 929-936.

Sato, T., Tadokoro, M., Kaba, H., Saito, H., Seto, K., and Takatsuji, H. 1993. Centrally administered ouabain aggravates central sleep apneas. J. Appl. Physiol. 74:545-548.

Schroeder, C.E., Givre, S.J., and Tenke, C.E. 1990. Extrast4riate contributions to surface VEP in the awake macaque. Inv. Ophthal. Vis. Sci. (suppl.) 31: 258.

Schroeder, C.E., Tenke, C.E., Givre, S.J., Arezzo, J.Z., and Vaughan, Jr., H.G. 1991. Striate cortical contribution to the surface-recorded pattern-reversal VEP in the alert monkey. Vis. Res. 31: 1143-1157.

Schwarz, M. and Block, F. 1993. Visual evoed potentials in the rat quinolinic acid model of Huntington's disease. Neurosci. Lett. 152: 81-83.

Sieving, P.A. 1991. Retinal ganglion cell loss does not abolish the scotopic threshold response (STR) of the cat and human ERG. Clin Vis. Sci 6: 149-158.

Sieving, P.A. and Bush, R.A. 1994. A proximal retinal component in the primate photopic ERG a-wave. Invest. Ophthal. Vis. Sci. 35: 635-645.

Sieving, P.A., Fishman, G.A., and Maggiano, J.M. 1978. Corneal wick electrode for recording bright flash electroretinograms and early receptor potentials. Arch. Ophthal. 96: 899-900.

Sieving P.A., Frishman, L.J., and Steinberg, R.H. 1986. Scotopic threshold response of proximal retina in cat. J. Neurophys. 56: 1049-1061.

Sieving, P.A. and Nino, C. 1988. Scotopic threshold response (STR) of the human electroretinogram. Inv. Ophthal. Vis. Sci. 29: 1608-1614.

Sieving, P.A. and Steinberg, R.H. 1987. Proximal retinal contribution to the intraretinal 8-Hz pattern ERG of the cat. J. Neurophys. 57: 104-120.

Sieving, P.A. and Wakabayashi, K. 1991. Comparison of rod threshold ERG from monkey, cat and human. Clin. Vis. Sci. 6: 171-179.

Sims, M.H., and Laratta, L.J. 1988. Visual-evoked potentials in cats, using a light-emitting diode stimulator. Am. J. Vet. Res. 49: 1876-1881.

Solomon, D. and Cohen, B. 1992. Stabilization of gaze during circular locomotion in light I. Compensatory head and eye nystagmus in the running monkey. J. Neurophys. 67: 1146-1158.

Stanford, M.R., Robbins, J., Kasp, E., and Dumonde, D.C. 1992. Passive administration of antibody against retinal S-antigen induces electroretinographic supernormality. Invest. Ophthal. Vis Sci. 33:30-35.

Steinberg, R.H., Frishman, L.J., and Sieving, P.A. 1991. Negative components of the electroretinogram from proximal retina and photoreceptor. Prog. in Retinal Res. 10: 121-160.

Steinberg, R.H., Linsenmeier, R.A., and Griff, E.R. 1983. Three light-evoked responses of the retinal pigment epithelium. Vis. Res. 23: 1315-1323.

Steinberg, R.H., Linsenmeier, R.A., and Griff, E.R. 1985. Retinal pigment epithelial contributions to the electroretinogram and electrooculogram. Prog. in Retinal Research 4: 33-66.

Strain, G.M., Jackson, R.M., and Tedford, B.L. 1990. Visual evoked potentials in the clinically normal dog. J. Vet. Int. Med. 4: 222-225.

Tashiro, C., Muranishi, R., Gomyo, I., Mashimo, T., Tomi, K., and Yoshiya, I. 1986. Electroretinogram as a possible monitor of anesthetic depth. Graefe's Arch. Clin. Exp. Ophthal. 224: 473-476.

Textorius, O., and Gottvall, E. 1992. The c-wave of the direct-current-recorded electroretinogram and the standing potential of the albino rabbit eye in response to repeated series of light stimuli of different intensities. Doc. Ophthal. 80: 91-103.

Thompson, D.A., and Drasdo, N. 1987. Computation of the luminance and pattern components of the bar pattern electroretinogram. Doc. Ophthal. 66: 233-244.

Tobimatsu, S., Celesia, G.G., Cone, S. and Gujrati, M. 1989. Electroretinograms to checkerboard pattern reversal in cats: physiological characteristics and effect of retrograde degeneration of ganglion cells. Electroenc. Clin. Neurophys. 73: 341-352.

Vaegan, Arora, A., Crewther, S.G., and Millar, T.J. 1990. The effect of various anaesthetics on the spatial tuning of two major wave peaks in the transient pattern electroretinogram of the cat: evidence for pattern and luminance components. Vis. Res. 30: 1401-1407.

Vaegan and Burne, J.A. 1987. Normal strobe electroretinograms without pattern electroretinograms in albino rats. Doc. Ophthal. 65: 113-124.

Wakabayashi, K., Geiser, J., and Sieving, P.A. 1988. Aspartate separation of the scotopic threshold response (STR) from the photoreceptor a-wave of the cat and monkey ERG. Inv. Ophthal. Vis. Sci. 29: 1615-1622.

Wasserschaff, M. and Schmidt, J.G.H. 1986. Electroretinographic responses to the addition of nitrous oxide to halothane in rats. Doc. Ophthal. 64: 347-354.

Wioland, N., Rudolph, G., and Bonaventure, N. 1990. Electrooculographic and electroretinographic study in the chicken after dopamine and haloperidol. Doc. Ophthal. 75: 175-180.

Wioland, N., and Bonaventure, N. 1985. Photopic c-wave in the chicken ERG: sensitivity to sodium azide, epinephrine, sodium iodate, barbiturates, and other general anesthetics. Doc. Ophthal. 60: 407-412.

Velazquez-Moctezuma, J., Shalauta, M., Gillin, J.C., and Shiromani, P. 1991. Cholinergic antagonists and REM sleep generation. Brain Res. 543: 175-179.

Yang, J., Xu, J., and Yang, S. 1990. [A simplified polygraphic method for studying sleep in the rat]. Hua Hsi I Ko Ta Hsueh Hsueh Pao. 21: 394-397.

Yoshikawa, H., Yoshida, M., and Hara, I. 1990. Electroretinographic changes induced by organophosphorus pesticides in rats. J. Tox. Sci. 15: 87-95.

Xi, L., Smith, C.A., Saupe, K.W., Henderson, K.S., and Dempsey, J.A. 1993. Effects of rapid-eye-movement sleep on the apneic threshold in dogs. J. Appl. Physiol. 75: 1129-1139.

RETINAL TOXICOLOGY STUDY
USING ELECTROPHYSIOLOGICAL METHODS
IN RABBITS

Yutaka Shirao and Kazuo Kawasaki

Department of Ophthalmology, Kanazawa University School of Medicine
13-1 Takara-machi, Kanazawa, Ishikawa 920, Japan

Intravitreal drug therapy has recently been recognized as a powerful therapeutic modality in clinical ophthalmology, because the blood-ocular barrier prevents intra-ocular penetration of most of systemically applied drugs. Since an excessive intravitreal dosage of any drug could easily be toxic to the eye, particularly to the retina, toxic overdoses should be strictly avoided in intravitreal drug therapy. Prior to clinical application, non-toxic dosage for intravitreal use must be tested first in animal experiments. Methods of examining retinal toxicity in animals include fundus examination, fluorescein fundus angiography, histological or histochemical examination and electrophysiological tests, which consist of the electroretinogram (ERG), the electro-oculogram (EOG) and the visual evoked potential (VEP). The VEP, of course, is not a response from the retina, but it is useful in retinal toxicology study in that the VEP often becomes abnormal in cases of retinal ganglion cell damage. Though the ERG evoked by pattern-reversal stimuli (P-ERG) is also supposed to contain responses from the retinal ganglion cells, the P-ERG needs a precise focusing of the stimulus pattern on the retina and therefore it is still difficult to record the P-ERG in animal experiments. These electrophysiological tests are sensitive, quantitative as well as non-destructive (*i.e.* repeatable).

The ERG has long been used in many retinal toxicology studies, where only the b-wave has been examined generally. However, the ERG consists of many other components, and some of them are more vulnerable to toxicity than the b-wave, as described below. Therefore, retinal toxicology studies using the ERG should deal with not only the b-wave but also other waves also. The present paper describes examples of multi-response analysis of the ERG in studying the retinal toxicity of antimicrobials.

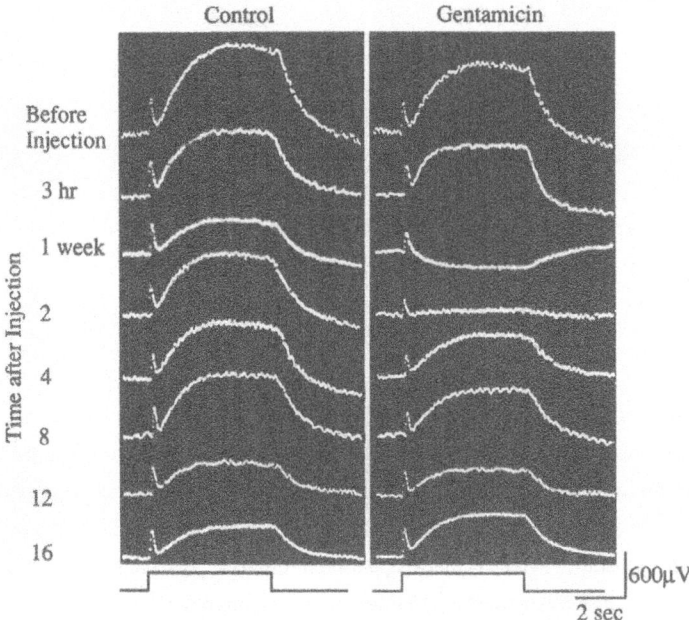

Figure 1. Effects of an intravitreal injection of 200 μg gentamicin on the ERG of a pigmented rabbit. The c-wave was abolished 1 to 2 weeks after gentamicin injection. The right and left columns show responses respectively from the antimicrobial-injected eye and the control fellow eye injected only with a vehicle in Figures 1 and 3. Stimulus intensity was 5 lux at the cornea. Rectangular traces at the bottom indicate the onset (upward deflection) and offset (downward deflection) of stimulus light in Figures 1, 2, 3 and 5. Direct-coupled amplification.

Albino and pigmented rabbits weighing 2-3 kg were used in accordance with the ARVO Statement on the Use of Animals in Ophthalmic and Vision Research. The methods of recording the ERG and the VEP were previously described[1]. The EOG is to record slow changes of the ocular standing potential, and is widely used in clinical ophthalmology. In animal experiments, however, the EOG is seldom used, because slow changes of the ocular standing potential can be recorded in immobilized animals with a use of non-polarizable electrodes and direct-coupled amplifiers in stead of EOG technique which requires constant saccadic eye movements.

First we studied gentamicin, one of aminoglycosides, which is known to have affinity with melanin in the retinal pigment epithelium (RPE). Gentamicin of 400 μg had once been recommended for an intravitreal injection in clinical use. However, reports on serious retinal damage caused by this amount of gentamicin frequently appeared thereafter. Figure 1 shows the ERG following an intravitreal injection of 200 μg gentamicin in a pigmented rabbit. The control fellow eye received the vehicle only (an intraocular infusion fluid for clinical surgeries, Opeguard® -MA, Senju Seiyaku; likewise hereafter in in-vivo experiments). The c-wave, which comes partly from the RPE, was completely abolished 1 to 2 weeks after gentamicin injection, while the b-wave was well preserved (Figure 1). Though the c-wave recovered to nearly normal 16 weeks later, the hyperosmolarity response, which originates solely in the RPE, was still abnormally large. The ocular fundus was hyperpigmented, and the fluorescein fundus angiogram revealed blocked hypofluorescence 16 weeks after 200 μg gentamicin injection.

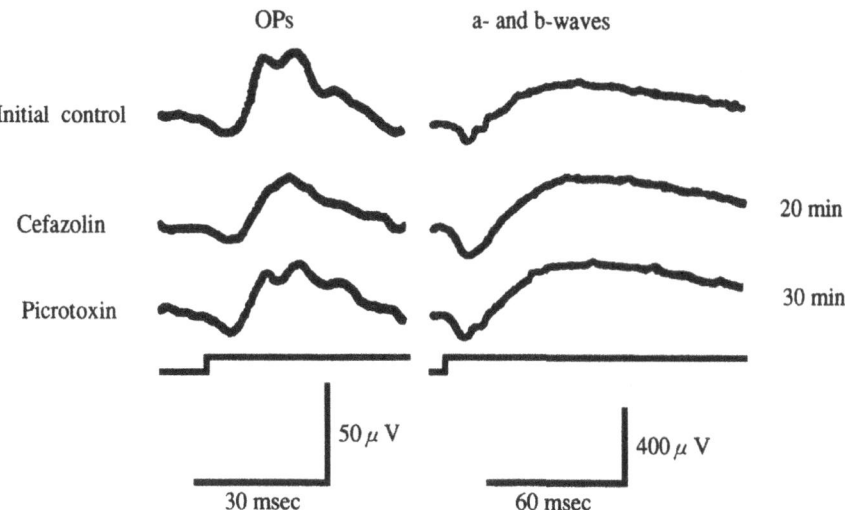

Figure 2.   Effects of an intravitreal injection of 1 mg cefazolin (CEZ) and an additional injection of 3 μg picrotoxin on the ERG of an albino rabbit. The oscillatory potentials were selectively suppressed by CEZ, and recovered after picrotoxin. Amplifier time constant was 3 msec in the left column and 2 sec in the right column. Stimulus intensity was 5×10^3 lux at the cornea.

An intravitreal injection of 200 μg sisomicin, which is also an aminoglycoside, irreversibly abolished the c-wave. The light rise, the hyperosmolarity response, the VEP and the retinal structure were severely damaged by 200 μg sisomicin. The responses related to the RPE, such as the c-wave, should be examined in studying toxic effects of chemicals with high melanin-affinity such as aminoglycosides.

An intravitreal injection of tobramicin or amikacin of 500 μg did not change any component of the ERG. Therefore, these aminoglycosides are less toxic than gentamicin or sisomicin. Intravitreal aminoglycosides are most toxic with sisomicin, next toxic with gentamicin and less toxic with tobramicin or amikacin by our electrophysiological study. This toxicity ranking coincides with the electron microscopic ranking[2].

ß-lactam antibiotics appear less toxic than aminoglycosides. For example, an intravitreal injection of none of 2 mg sulbenicillin, 1 mg cefazolin or 2 mg ceftazidime changed the b-wave. However, 1 mg cefazolin and 2 mg ceftazidime greatly suppressed the oscillatory potentials (Figure 2). Thus, the ERG component most sensitive to cefazolin and ceftazidime is the oscillatory potentials. If we had examined only the classical a- and b-waves, the non-toxic dose of these ß-lactams would have been over-estimated.

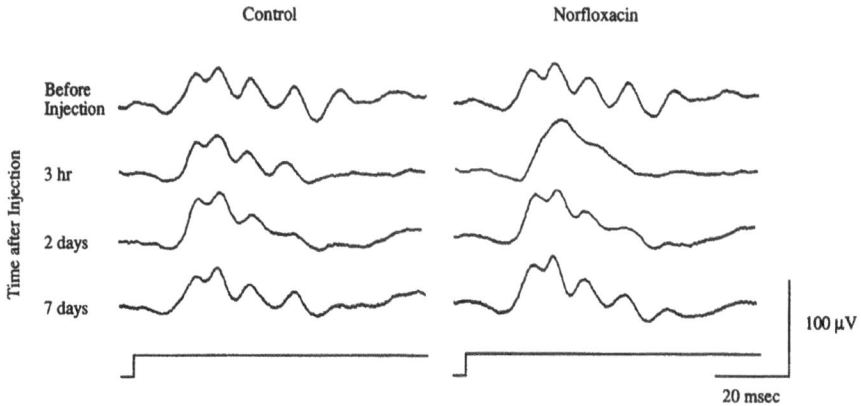

Figure 3. Effects of an intravitreal injection of 500 μg norfloxacin (NFLX) on the ERG of an albino rabbit. The oscillatory potentials were greatly suppressed in the NFLX-injected eye. Stimulus intensity was 5 x 10^3 lux at the cornea. Amplifier time constant was 3 msec.

Fluoroquinolones are promising antimicrobials with a broad spectrum. An intravitreal injection of 500 μg norfloxacin greatly suppressed the c-wave and the oscillatory potentials (Figure 3), leaving other ERG components virtually unchanged.

Melanin-affinity was reported for fluoroquinolones. Figure 4 shows the time course of lomefloxacin concentration in the ocular tissues after an intravitreal injection of 200 μg in pigmented and albino rabbits. Lomefloxacin concentration in the iris-ciliary body and retina-choroid was much higher in the pigmented rabbits than in the albino rabbits. Such difference between the pigmented and albino rabbits was absent in the ocular tissues without melanin such as the vitreous humor, the cornea and the lens.

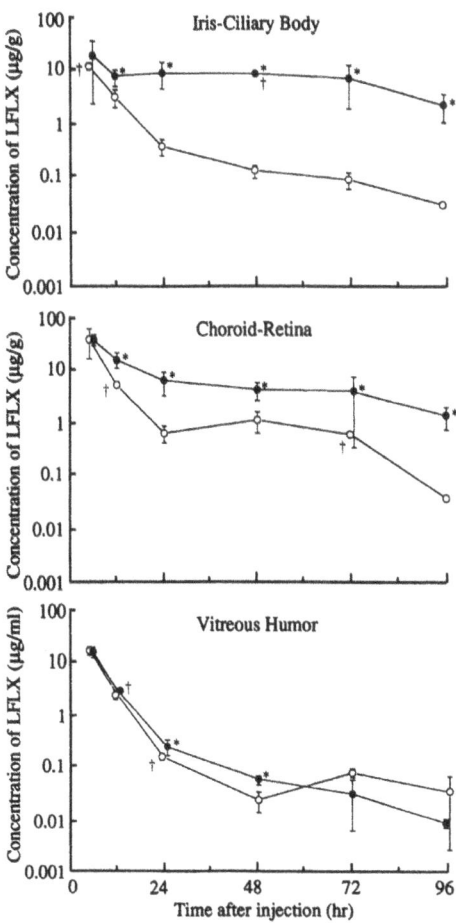

Figure 4. Concentration of lomefloxacin (LFLX) in the iris-ciliary body (upper graph), in the choroid-retina (middle graph) and in the vitreous humor (lower graph) of pigmented (filled circles) and albino (open circles) rabbits 6, 12, 24, 48, 72 and 96 hours after bilateral intravitreal injection of 200 μg LFLX. Each data point shows the mean +/- SD or the mean only. *, significantly higher (P<0.05) versus albino rabbit group. †, SD bars are smaller than the circles denoting the mean.

Recently, endogenous fungal endophthalmitis is drastically increasing, partially due to the wide-spread use of antibiotics, immunosuppressants and intravenous indwelling catheters. The concentration of fluconazole, an antifungal, in the vitreous and aqueous humor after an intravenous administration is as high as that in the serum. Thanks to the exceptionally high intraocular penetration of fluconazole, this drug need not be intravitreally injected to achieve a therapeutic intraocular concentration, though it has to be repeatedly administered to treat intraocular fungal infection. The b-wave, the c-wave, the oscillatory potentials and the VEP remained unchanged after fluconazole of 25 mg/kg/day was intravenously given for 7 days.

Viral endophthalmitis has become a major concern in AIDS management, and some of uveitis are shown to arise from viral origin (e.g. acute retinal necrosis). Intravitreal antiviral therapy is surely one of the crucial modalities. The b-wave, the c-wave, the oscillatory potentials and the VEP remained unchanged after 5 repetitive weekly (once a week) intravitreal injections of 200 μg ganciclovir.

BV ara U is a newly-developed antiviral drug particularly effective to varicella zoster virus. No changes in the b-wave, the c-wave or the oscillatory potentials were induced by an intravitreal injection of 100 μg BV area U or by intravitreal irrigation with 20 μg/ml BV ara U. The concentration of BV ara U after an oral administration was much lower in the vitreous than in the serum, which indicates that intraocular penetration of BV ara U is very poor. Furthermore, an enteral use of BV ara U in conjunction with some of antimetabolites reportedly causes serious systemic adverse effects. Therefore, a topical intraocular application of BV ara U is much preferable.

Most of retinal toxicology studies using the ERG examined only the b-wave, or simply described that "the ERG remained normal" or "the ERG became abnormal". As mentioned above, the ERG-waves other than the b-wave are more sensitive to some chemicals. In retinal toxicology study, one should examine not only the b-wave but also other responses, and should specify the response which he examined. Although the b-wave is the easiest to record among the ERG components, the oscillatory potentials and the a-wave are also readily recordable with a bright stimulus light such as commercially-available xenon flash. Among many electrical responses from the retina, presynaptic potentials (the early and late receptor potentials) are relatively insensitive to toxic agents. The early receptor potential, which is recordable only with an extremely intense stimulus light, is well known for its extreme resistance to toxic agents, and therefore is not useful as an index of retinal integrity. The a-wave, whose leading edge is composed of the late receptor potential, is also insensitive. If the early or late receptor potential of the retina is greatly suppressed or abolished, one should suspect a serious damage to the retina. In contrast, postsynaptic potentials, particularly polysynaptic potentials such as the oscillatory potentials, are very sensitive as shown above. Because rhythmic wavelets synchronous with the oscillatory potentials were reported to appear in intracellular responses from some of the amacrine cells[3], neuronal networks including postsynaptic neurones such as the amacrine cells and the interplexiform cells are supposed to be involved in the generation of the oscillatory potentials[4]. Since the oscillatory potentials are the only ERG component that reflect those inner retinal integrity, a quantitative analysis of the amplitudes and the peak latencies of each wavelet of the oscillatory potentials is strongly recommended. The present results that the oscillatory potentials were selectively deteriorated by some neurotoxic chemicals (Figures 2, 5) coincides with the inner-retinal neuronal origin of the oscillatory potentials. The oscillatory potentials are readily extractable with a use of a short amplification time constant or a digital filter; and easily displayed on a rapid-sweep, high-gain system.

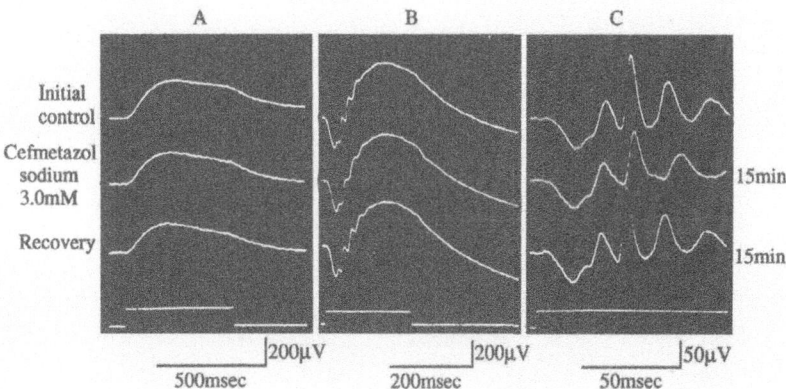

Figure 5. Effects of 3 mM cefmetazole (CMZ) on the ERG of the in-vitro eye-cup of an albino rabbit. The uppermost traces show responses during initial perfusion with a control solution (solutes, mM: NaCl ,119.50: KCl, 3.60: CaCl$_2$, 1.15: MgSO$_4$,1.06: glucose, 26.00: NaHCO$_3$, 25.10: NaH$_2$PO$_4$, 3.00). The second traces show responses during perfusion with the CMZ-containing solution (other constituents were the same as the control solution). The third traces show responses after the CMZ-containing solution was washed out by the control solution. CMZ at 3 mM concentration diminished the oscillatory potentials and prolonged their peak latencies, leaving the a- and b-waves virtually unchanged. Numerals at the right indicate the time (minutes) after onset of perfusion with the CMZ-containing solution or with the control solution. Stimulus intensity was 2.0 X 10^{-2} lux in A, and 3.3 X 10^2 lux in B and C. Direct-coupled amplification was used in A and B. The amplifier time constant was 3 msec in C.

The b-wave is an incidental response from the Müller cells originated by the postsynaptic neurones (probably the depolarizing bipolar cells) and is moderately sensitive to toxic agents. The abnormal b-wave alone, however, can not specify the site of retinal damage, because many kinds of retinal cells are involved in the generation of the b-wave.

The responses related to the RPE should be examined in studies on the toxic effects of chemicals with high affinity to melanin. In this respect, the c-wave should be examined, because the c-wave partly originates in the RPE as described below. Some chemicals greatly suppressed the c-wave, leaving other waves well preserved (Figure 1).

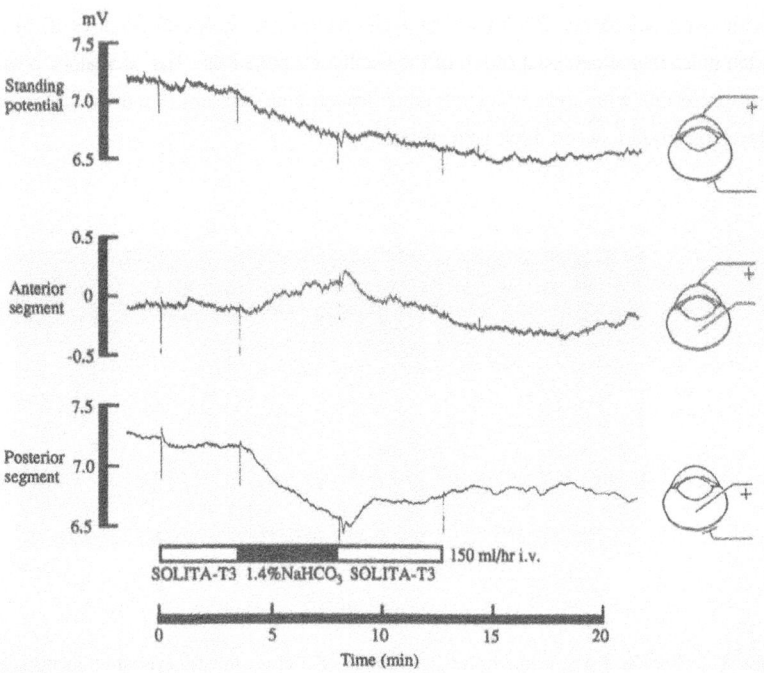

Figure 6 Bicarbonate response (a decrease in the ocular standing potential in response to bicarbonate) in an albino rabbit. An isotonic sodium bicarbonate solution was intravenously administered during the time indicated by a thick horizontal line. Direct-coupled amplification. No stimulus light.

The origin of the c-wave does not lie solely in the RPE. A response from the Müller cells (slow P III) is also involved in the c-wave. Furthermore, since the c-wave is a photically-evoked response, the c-wave depends also on the retinal photoreceptor cells. Therefore, the abnormal c-wave alone does not necessarily indicate RPE dysfunction. As far as we use photic stimuli, we could not exclude the influence of the photoreceptor cells. To by-pass this, we developed three kinds of responses from the RPE by non-photic stimuli. We found that an intravenous infusion of 7% sodium bicarbonate (Meylon®, Ohtsuka Seiyaku), Fructmanit® (a mixture of 12 % mannitol and 8 % fructose, Taiho Yakuhin, 1.33×10^3 mOsm) or acetazolamide (Diamox®, Lederlie) decreases the ocular standing potential, and designated these responses as the bicarbonate response, the hyperosmolarity response or the Diamox response, respectively. These responses are readily recordable in man by the conventional EOG technique[5] through a pair of electrodes placed on the inner and outer canthi in conjunction with a constant horizontal saccadic eye movements. We also confirmed in animal experiments that the above-mentioned agents directly alter the apical and/or basal membrane potentials of the RPE, resulting in a decrease in the ocular standing potential. Though in the monkey these responses are readily recordable with electrodes placed on the cornea and the back of the eye (or on the orbital margin), in the rabbit an electrode needs to be inserted into the vitreous cavity and referred to the back of the eye (or the upper orbital surface), because a response of the opposite polarity occurs from the anterior segment of the eye (presumably the iris-ciliary body) and masks the response from the RPE (Figure 6).

Table 1. ERG Components Vulnerable to Antimicrobials

Antinicrobial		Vulnerable Components of ERG
Sulbenicillin	(SBPC)	OPs & b-wave
Cefazolin	(CEZ)	OPs
Cefmetazole	(CMZ)	OPs
Ceftazidime	(CAZ)	OPs & b-wave
Flomoxef	(FMOX)	OPs & b-wave
Gentamicin	(G M)	c-wave & b-wave
Sisomicin	(SISO)	c-wave
Netilmicin	(SISO)	c-wave & b-wave
Amikacin	(AMK)	OPs & b-wave
Tobramycin	(TOB)	OPs & b-wave
Vancomycin	(VCM)	OPs & b-wave
Ofloxacin	(OFLX)	OPs
Lomefloxacin	(LFLX)	OPs
Norfloxacin	(NFLX)	OPs
Levofloxacin	(LVFX)	OPs
Ciprofloxacin	(CPFX)	OPs
Miconazole	(MCZ)	OPs & b-wave
Sorivudine	(BVaraU)	c-wave & b-wave
Ganciclovir	(DHPG)	OPs & b-wave

OPs : oscillatory potentials

The ERG from an excised eye-cup or an isolated retina is useful especially for studying the effects of chemicals at very precise concentrations by dissolving the chemicals in the perfusates. The a-wave, the b-wave and the oscillatory potentials are recordable from in-vitro preparations of even mammals for more than several hours[6] (Figure 5).

The most vulnerable component of the rabbit ERG is different among antimicrobials (Table 1), indicating the importance of the multi-response analysis of the ERG in the retinal toxicology study. Tables 2 and 3 summarize the non-toxic concentration of antimicrobials respectively for intravitreal single shot injection and intraocular irrigation during vitrectomy in man.

Table 2. Non-Toxic Doses (mg) for Intravitreal Injection

Aminoglycosides			Fluoroquinolones		
Gentamicin	(G M)	0.1	Ofloxacin	(OFLX)	0.2
Tobramycin	(TOB)	0.2	Lomefloxacin	(LFLX)	0.2
Amikacin	(AMK)	0.2~0.4	Norfloxacin	(NFLX)	0.05
Netilmicin	(NTL)	0.1~0.2	Ciprofloxacin	(CPFX)	0.1
			Antifungals		
β-Lactams			Miconazole	(MCZ)	0.03~0.05
Sulbenicillin	(SPBC)	2.0	Fluconazole	(FLCZ)	0.2
Cefazolin	(CEZ)	0.25	Antivirals		
Ceftazidime	(CAZ)	0.2~0.4	Ganciclovir	(DHPG)	0.1~0.2
Flomoxef	(FMOX)	0.2~0.4	Sorivudine	(BVaraU)	0.1
Glycopeptide			Steroid		
Vancomycin	(VCM)	1.0	Dexamethasone		0.1~0.2

Table 3. Non-Toxic Concentration (mg/ml) for Intravitreal Irrigation

Sulbenicillin	(SBPC)	0.2	Gentamicin	(G M)	0.01
Amikacin	(AMK)	0.02	Cefazolin	(CEZ)	0.05
Flomoxef	(FMOX)	0.05	Ceftazidime	(CAZ)	0.05
Ofloxacin	(OFLX)	0.02			
Miconazole	(MCZ)	0.01	Fluconazole	(FLCZ)	0.02
Aciclovir		0.04	Ganciclovir	(DHPG)	0.02
Dexamethasone		0.006			

ACKNOWLEDGMENTS

The data presented here were by Drs. J. Ohnogi, Y. Okayama, K. Mochizuki, Y. Segawa, M. Torisaki, K. Yamashita, K. Kitano, T. Sasaki, M. Komatsu, T. Tanahashi, T. Higashide, S.

Ohkubo and M. Ogata of Department of Ophthalmology, Kanazawa University School of Medicine.

REFERENCES

1. K. Mochizuki, M. Torisaki, M. Komatsu, T. Tanahashi, K. Ijichi and H. Machida, Retinal toxicity and ocular kinetics of 1-ß-D-arabinofuranosyl-E-5-(2-bromovinyl) uracil in rabbits, Graef Arch Clin Exp Ophthalmol. 232:503-508 (1994)

2. D. J. D'Amico, L. Caspers-Velu, J. Libert, E. Shanks, M. Shooen, L. A. Nanninen and K. R. Kenyon. Comparative toxicity of intravitreal aminoglycoside antibiotics. Am. J. Ophthalmol. 100: 264-275 (1985).

3. J. Toyoda, H. Hashimoto and K. Ohtsu. Bipolar-amacrine transmission in carp retina. Vision Res. 13:295-307 (1973)

4. C. Karwoski and K. Kawasaki. Oscillatory potentials. 125-128, in :Principle and Practice of Clinical Electrophysiology of Vision, J. R. Heckenlively and G. B. Arden, eds., Mosby Year Book, St. Louis (1991).

5. K. Kawasaki, J. Tanabe and K. Wakabayashi, Nonphotic standing potential responses: Hyperosmolarity, bicarbonate, and Diamox responses, 163-166, in: Principle and Practice of Clinical Electrophysiology of Vision, J. R. Heckenlively and G. B. Arden, eds., Mosby Year Book, St. Louis (1991)

6. K. Kawasaki, J. Ohnogi and Y. Okayama. Nontoxic concentration of amphotericin B for intravitreal use evaluated by in vitro ERG, Doc. Ophthalmol. 69:19-23 (1988)

ERG MEASUREMENTS IN THE DOG, CAT AND MONKEY
FOR TOXICOLOGY SPECIALLY TYPE OF ELECTRODE
AND ANESTHESIA FOR ERG RECORDINGS

Bernard Clerc[1] and Marie-José Sayn[2]

[1]Service d'Ophtalmologie
[2]Inra
Ecole Nationale Vétérinaire
7, avenue du Général de Gaulle
94704 Maisons-Alfort Cedex
France

INTRODUCTION

Differences of the retina in relationship to ERG in carnivores and primates

Electroretinograms in different species are related to the retinal structure and histology : prevalence of rods in nocturnal animals (rats), prevalence of cones in diurnal animals (squirrel) and the aspect of electroretinogram is related to the species.

The vasculature of the choroid and retina differs between species. In primates the arterial supply to the retina is via a central retinal artery. In other species with retinal vasculature the retinal arterial supply is via the short posterior ciliary arteries forming cilioretinal arteries. Various retinal patterns are present in mammals : holangiotic vasculature in primates, cats, dogs, rodents and cattle arises from the central retinal arteries or cilioretinal vessels and extends into the inner retinal layers throughout the retina ; merangiotic vasculature arises from cilioretinal vessels and radiates into the horizontal quadrants of the retina ; paurangiotic vessels are small and numerous and radiate only a small distance from the optic nerve into the retina ; the anangiotic pattern is a retina that lacks blood vessels. The relative contribution of the underlying choroid to retinal nutrition depends upon the extent of retinal vascularization. Animals with minimal retinal vascularization have thinner retinas facilitating diffusion of nutrients into and catabolism products from the choroid.

The density respectively of rods and cones differs also. Primates possess an area of specially high cone density in the retina called fovea centralis, which lacks rods and blood vessels. Dog and cats have a comparable area of increased cone density temporal to the optic disc named area centralis.

The Granit's works[1] drew the attention of researchers to the different kind of ERG : that of nocturnal animals (like the rat) of the E type and that of diurnal animal of the I type.

The response of I type retinas is characterized by large negative "a" wave and prominent off effects while E type retinas produce simple large "b" wave and prominent off effects. Retinas of the dog, cat and monkey have both rods and cones and show a mixed response however the cat is more "nocturnal" and the monkey a more diurnal animal. Use of different protocols allows the separation of cones and rods responses. These differences explain the variable susceptibility of species to a toxic agent, for instance the increased susceptibility of rats and mice to light injury compared to monkeys or dogs.

THE INTEREST OF ERG

Clinical interest

The aim of this report is to draw the frame of our activity which is partly similar to the interest in human ophthalmology and by this way to underline similarities that can be interesting in comparative ophthalmology. Toxicologists could have to evaluate the protective effect of new substances on the retina and the existence of animals models of human diseases. Information reprinted from Nick Millichamp[2] summarises these facts on a comparative ophthalmology basis.

Retinal degeneration occurs commonly in several laboratory species and man, although very rarely in any other primates. Retinal degeneration may be inherited, age or environment related, or due to nutritional deficiencies. These various etiologies should be recognized as potential causes of retinal atrophy in animals that will be used for any long-term toxicological studies. Inherited retinal degenerations occur in many breeds of dog, cats, rats, and mice. Inherited degenerations can primarily involve the retinal pigment epithelium (RPE) or the neural retina and may develop as disease in early postnatal life and progress rapidly or later in adult animals with slower progression. Most inherited retinal degenerations affect the rod photoreceptors initially and then progress to involve the cones and ultimately the remaining retinal neurons.

In man several different types of retinal dystrophy/degeneration have been reported. Some of these have an inherited basis, others are associated with other systemic and metabolic diseases.

In the dog and mouse various primary retinal degenerations involve the photoreceptors. Early-onset retinal degenerations (photoreceptor dysplasia) may vary between breeds or strains depending on the inheritance locus and biochemical defects involved. Where biochemical abnormalities are known in dogs and rodents they have been shown to involve the guanosine 3',5'-cyclic monophosphate (cGMP) phosphodiesterase involved in visual transduction (Aguirre[3]). Late-onset retinal degenerations in dogs, which are similar to some forms of inherited retinitis pigmentosa in man, involve the same gene locus in several different breeds. Abnormalities of photoreceptor membrane lipids have been detected in some poodles with late-onset retinal degeneration. Similar inherited retinal degenerations are also seen in the cat (Narfstrom[4]).

Retinal degeneration associated with a retinal pigment epithelial dystrophy is also seen in the dog. The diseased RPE accumulates lipopigment and the neural retina subsequently undergoes slow degeneration (Riis[5], Bedford[6]).

Photoreceptor dysplasia also occurs in mice. As in the dog, these are diseases seen in young animals with rapid progression. The best characterized are the rd and rds strains.

Retinal degenerations have also been reported in the rat. The best documented degeneration is seen in the RCS rat. The disease is a primary retinal pigment epitheliopathy. Failure of the RPE to phagocytize shed photoreceptor outer segments results in accumulation of membranous debris between retina and RPE and subsequent retinal atrophy in the early postnatal period. Retinal degenerations have occasionally been reported in other strains of rat that may not be inherited. Determination of the etiology of retinal degeneration in this species can be problematic since degenerations associated with old age and exposure to high light levels have also been reported.

Phototoxic retinal degeneration may also influence the interpretation of toxicologic studies in rodents. Rats and mice are particularly sensitive to light-induced retinal degeneration. In part this may be due to the prevalence of studies performed in albino strains of these species. Various other factors influencing the rate and severity of light-induced degeneration include : use of mydriatics, age (older animals are more susceptible), sex (females are more susceptible), environmental temperature (retinal degeneration proceeds more rapidly at higher temperatures), and maintenance of the animals under a continuous rather than cyclic lighting pattern.

Other retinal degenerations that may be confused with toxic reactions in the retina of laboratory species include nutritional retinal degeneration due to taurine deficiency in cats and vitamin E deficiency in dogs.

Toxicological interest in dog, cat and monkey

They are all used as models of human diseases or as models for toxicology studies involving the retina and consequently the ERG. The monkeys react in many aspects more like human than dogs and cats. In counterpart, monkeys are not easy to manipulate and for specific aspects dogs, cats or even rodents can also be good models and less expensive ones. The close similarities of monkey's eye with human eye has led to numerous studies of human drugs trials or physical injury (light-induced lesions, Sperling[7]). Retinal toxicity of systemic drugs like quinine have been performed in monkeys too. Retinal toxicity of drug injected in the vitreous (triaxone for instance) or used in the anterior segment surgery (viscoelastics) have been also tested in monkeys whose eye is very similar to the human one and damage to the retina is evaluated by ERG. Pharmacologic studies of drugs used in the treatment of human diseases, glaucoma for instance, are tried on macacus rhesus and this is probably a unique model for the pharmacologic study of antiglaucomatous drugs since the eye of carnivores, dogs and cats, differs notably from the human eye. ERG can be also helpful in these pharmacologic studies.

Dogs and cats can be used also, but the validity of this model must be checked every time as pointed out at the beginning of this paper. Eye structure and vascularization are different from those of man. When we make a review of recent literature on toxicology studies, we can observe that toxicity of intravitreal injected drugs on the retina are mainly studied in rabbits, but dogs and cats can also be used (Liverani[8]).

In conclusion, ERG studies for toxicology can be conducted on all these species. The choice depends on both scientific and economical considerations.

THE PRACTICE OF ERG IN DOG, CAT AND MONKEY

Restraint

Although records can be obtained from dogs without sedation we think that recording with appropriate sedative is preferable as it avoids most of the background noise.

Beagle dogs can be trained to ERG recordings but this is impossible with cats and monkeys.

General considerations. They are similar to those described by Whitacre and Ellis[9] for the human outpatients. Our toxicology animals (monkeys, dogs, cats) are often difficult to restraint and the stress provoked by the restraint can be more harmful than a "good sedation". What is the good sedative for ophthalmology and specifically for electroretinography ?

The ideal agent for tranquilization should be easy to administer and have a predictable and rapid onset. It should not produce respiratory depression or cardiac irregularities and its duration should be short. The airway and gag reflexes should remain unimpaired. The drug or its metabolites should not accumulate in the body, so that readministration should not have an effect longer than the initial dose. The agent should be reversible with a specific nontoxic antidote. There should be no effect on the ocular structures or function, e.g., eye position or movement, pupillary size or response, intraocular pressure or aqueous humor dynamics, or electrophysiological responses to retinal or visual cortical stimulation. The drug should have an analgesic effect, since many procedures are associated with discomfort.

At the present time no single drug, or combination of drugs, fulfills these criteria ; some are more suitable than others for certain ophthalmologic examinations or procedures.

At Maisons-Alfort, in the veterinary school, or in other laboratories, we had experienced some drugs but we have not found the ideal one.

We have selected a group of drugs used either for electrophysiology or by ophthalmologists in their practice.

Chemical restraint

- Thiopental.
General pharmacologic effects : barbiturates are general central nervous system depressants. At sedative or hypnotic doses they have little or no effect on heart rate or blood pressure. The respiratory rate is unaffected although apnea may occur following administration especially if the drug is given intravenously ; this apnea may compromise the airway. Laryngospasm may rarely occur. At subhypnotic doses following awaking from a hypnotic dose, barbiturates have a hyperesthetic effect. Thiopental is a short-acting barbiturate which may be administered intramuscularly, intravenously or rectally. The usual intramuscular dose is from 11 to 22 mg/kg and the intravenous dose from 10 to 15 mg/kg depending on the physical status of the patient and the concomitant use of other drugs and premedication. For the intramuscularly procedure, suitable in toxicology, it is recommended that a 5 % solution of the drug be given deep intramuscularly and away from the sciatic nerve. The injection can be painful. At least 15 minutes should elapse following administration before the effect of the first dose is judged insufficient by the absence of hypnosis, and a second dose (half of the first) is given. The usual time for the onset of hypnosis is 7 to 15 minutes, which is reduced if 1000 to 1500 units of hyaluronidase are added. The time for awaking is about 60 to 80 minutes following the onset of sleep and can be expected to be less if hyaluronidase is added. After awaking, the patient may remain drowsy for several hours and fall asleep again. Iccups and fasciculations may be less common with thiopental than with methohexital, but apnea may occur as commonly. Its intravenous administration should be avoided because of a higher incidence of apnea when the drug is administered by this route.

Usually, thiopental is used for induction of anesthesia during a long procedure and then the animal is intubated and placed under gas anesthesia with halothane. Halothane anesthesia is beyond our scope because it is used for long procedures which is not frequent in our usual laboratory procedures.

Ocular effects : the barbiturates affect both ERGs and VEPs. Knave and Persson[10] and Noell[11] found that a low dose of pentobarbital enhanced "a" and "b" wave amplitude ; this effect was greatest under moderate photopic conditions and least during complete dark adaptation when long duration stimuli were used. A high dose of pentobarbital increased the latency, decreased the slope and reduced the amplitude of the "b" wave.

Barbiturates also affect extraocular muscle motion with down rotation of the eye and mydriasis during phase II of anesthesia and myosis in phase III. Thus it is necessary to make a retrobulbar injection with saline to maintain the cornea in front of the eyelid opening. It has also an effect on the ocular motion and nystagmus is observed during phase II of anesthesia.

- Ketamine (Kommonen[12]) :
General pharmacologic effects : ketamine is an anesthetic agent which produces a

dissociated state in the cerebral cortex by blocking responses to environmental stimuli. It does not reliably produce analgesia or suppress movement. Ketamine has little effect in species with poorly developed cerebral cortices. It is used commonly in monkeys. The usual dose of ketamine to induce the cataleptic state characteristic of this agent is 1 to 2 mg/kg given intravenously over a period of at least one minute, or 5 to 10 mg/kg given intramuscularly. The onset of maximal drug effect occurs within less than one minute when the drug is given intravenously and 20 to 40 minutes when it is given intramuscularly. Additional doses of one-half the initial dose may be needed to induce or prolong anesthesia. The psychotropic effect of the drug persists several times longer than the anesthetic effects and patients will be confused for about one hour following intravenous administration and 2 to 3 hours following intramuscular administration.

Ketamine produces a mild increase in heart rate and systolic and diastolic blood pressure, but has generally been reported not to affect the respiratory rate. Because of laryngeal hyperreactivity, premedication with atropine or scopolamine is recommended, especially because salivation is increased by ketamine.

Ocular effects : Ketamine is known to cause seizure-like activity in electroencephalograms. Antal[13] observed ultrastructural changes in the inner segment of photoreceptors, the nuclear layers, the nerve fiber layer and Müller's cell layer following ketamine anesthesia of 60 minutes' duration. These changes almost completely regressed within three days. They were attributed to hypoxia occurring during an increase in electrical activity of the retina. Van Norren and Padmos[14] found that ketamine at a dose of 15 mg/kg did not affect dark adaptation of monkey cone ERGs. Kayama and Iwama[15] found that ketamine markedly enhanced the cortical evoked potentials produced by electrical stimulation of the optic chiasma in cats. It is generally used alone in monkeys. When associated with diazepam in dogs the results are not so satisfactory.

- Benzodiazepam :

General effects : All the benzodiazepines are cataractogenic. They have a depressant effect on the central nervous system and for this reason they are often used in veterinary medicine associated with ketamine. We have used Diazepam (Valium N.D.) given intramuscularly or intravenously associated with ketamine. The hypnotic effect is much longer than with ketamine alone (dosage : 0.25 - 0.5 mg/kg).

A commercial association of a benzodiazepine + one analog of ketamine (tiletamine) is available and often used in veterinary practice in France for small surgery and ERG recordings. It is named Zoletil N.D.used intravenously at the dosage of 5 mg/kg of tiletamine. It has a depressive effect on the respiration and induces excessive salivation that increase the effect of this depression.

Ocular effects : associations of ketamine or tiletamine + benzodiazepine have not effect on the eye position and the eye stays in place which facilitates the placement of electrodes.

- Medetomidine (Domitor (R)) :

General effects : it is a powerful a_2 adrenoreceptor agonist. It acts on the central nervous system, stimulating a_2 presynaptic receptors. As a result noradrenaline is blocked and the transmission of neuroimpulse is stopped. As a consequence, major effects of metomidine are sedation and analgesia. A unique feature is the possibility of stopping these effects with a specific antagonist atipemazole (Antisedan (R)) injected intramuscularly. Atipemazole has a greater affinity for a adrenoreceptors than medetomidine and reverse the action of medetomidine. We have tested it in ophthalmology specially for ERG recordings since the effect of sedation can be suppressed completely very quickly. This property is of special interest for outpatients.

After an initial arterial hypertension a decrease of arterial pressure is observed (around 10 %). Sinusal bradycardia is noted down to 30-40 beats/minute. This cardiac depression could be prevented by parasympatholytic like atropine (0.02 mg/kg), 10-15 minutes before the injection of medetomidine. Respiratory function is also depressed. Vomiting is quite frequently observed before the complete sedation. There is never vomiting during sedation.

Despite these adverse possible reactions, we have tested it for ERG recordings considering the total reversion of sedation after the procedure. We observed the following effects in the eye.

The ocular effects of medetomidine are moderate in the eye. In case of slight sedation (0.2 ml/10 kg), the animal keeps its lids open and the globe stays in the right position making placement of electrodes easy and retrobulbar injection unnecessary.

Modifications of ERG with Domitor are presented in the results. We observed a non significant increase of "a" and "b" latencies (see Table 3).

Though formerly studied in monkeys by Bodis-Wollner and al[16] we do not think that haloperidol is a very useful adjunct for chemical restraint of monkeys.

Preparation of the eye for ERG, PEV

Dogs, cats and monkeys receive systematically one drop of tropicamide onto the cornea at the time of premedication or 20 minutes prior to the sedation. Mydriasis is very important to obtain a good ERG, specially with sedated laboratory animals because the eyeballs can rotate downward during sedation and it becomes then impossible to record an ERG.

They usually do not receive topical anesthetic. It seems that the anesthetic does not produce a modification of the ERG.

Retrobulbar injection is used with the barbiturates, otherwise it is not useful. An injection of 2 ml of neurocaïne + hyaluronidase 250 UI is made. In the literature, injection of saline (2-6 ml) is recommended.

Methylcellulose or other contact medium is usually instilled onto the eye though it is not absolutely necessary with jet electrode. It is particularly useful with the scleral shell since curvature does not fit perfectly to the whole cornea. We use regularly jet electrodes but we have experience with other types of electrodes as described now.

Electrodes

Corneal electrodes. The eye of carnivores (conversely to primates) allows the use of large corneal electrodes. Many types of contact lenses have been developed and the most widely used in veterinary medicine were, until recently, scleral shells with different types of electrodes (silver loop, silver button) with conducting solution between cornea and shell. The response obtained with each type of lens is nearly the same if the lens is used properly.

Jet discardable electrodes. These small contact lenses have a thin ring of gold placed at the inner surface of the lense in contact with the cornea. They are very well tolerated and as they are very light, they stay on the cornea by capillarity. These electrodes are not very expensive and can be replaced easily. They are our favored electrodes for the dog now.

Needle or hook electrode. A needle or a flat metal hook which can be placed over the lower eyelid has also been used. It is quite confortable but the recordings are not as reliable as those obtained with other procedures. Perhaps, this instability arises from difficulty in keeping the electrode in a fixed position (Armington[17]).

Reference electrode. In recording the electroretinogram, voltage differences are measured between the cornea and some other part of the body. The corneal electrode is the active electrode and the other one is the reference electrode. The reference electrode, in dog and cat, is placed on the ear of the animal. Scarcity of fur in that area allows a good contact between skin and electrode. Needle electrode can be used also.

Polarization. When using silver electrodes, polarization occurs. Charges may build up on electrodes immersed in solutions causing a current to flow in the external circuit. These currents act as artefact signals which interfere with the electroretinogram. In extreme conditions, they will drive the recording equipment out of its operating range. Polarization problems may be reduced by depositing a layer of silver chloride upon the electrode surface. To chloride a silver electrode, thoroughly clean its surface and place it in an opaque non metallic container filled with 5 % sodium chloride solution (Armington[17]).

Electrodes in poor condition give rise to artefact pulses, baseline fluctuations and background noise.

Electrodes covered with gold like the jet electrodes do not have the same inconvenience and they also can be replaced easily.

ERG protocol

Until now, there is no standard protocol for all animals. Some protocols have been published for rodents and rabbits (Munguia et al.[18]) but none is generally accepted for dogs though some tentative protocoles have been proposed (Schaeppi and Liverani[19,20]). One standard protocol was adopted by I.S.C.E.V. for the human and published in 1989, revised in 1993. Some ophthalmologists are currently working on the establishment of a standard protocol for the dog (Narfström[4]). The aim of this protocol is testing for hereditary retinal diseases. We should need also a standard protocol for laboratory animal as the requirements might be different for toxicology studies. The use of adapted anesthesia for performing ERGs in dogs is probably one step for standardization and the establishment of a standard protocol remains one goal of further I.S.O.T. meetings.

If the parameters used for recording ERG are not precisely known, it is impossible to obtain accurate values for implicite time and amplitude of the waves. As an example, the illumination of the whole retina gives a higher amplitude for the waves. In Figure 1, we show the ERG of a young Siberian Husky with a cataract in one eye acting as a light diffuser.

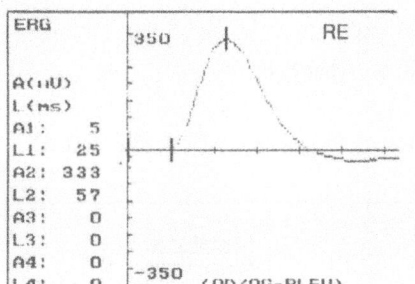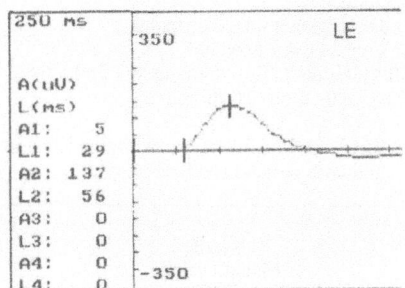

Figure 1. ERG (blue light) of a male Siberian husky dog of 6 months showing the same implicit time (± 1 ms) on both eyes but the presence of a cataract on the right eye acts as a light diffuser onto the retina. It shows the interest of fullfield stimulation (anesthesia medetomidine).

For instance also, Buist and Heywood[21], for the rhesus monkey, give the following values for "a" and "b" waves implicit times with white light with and without dark adaptation. "a" : 14.17 ± 0.75 ms to 19.25 ± 2.52 ms and for "b" : 36.75 ± 2.38 ms to 45.08 ± 3.78 ms.

These results show that numerical values are largely dependent on the recording technique. Each laboratory must have its own reference values according to his own protocol. Working in this direction, we made a study in our laboratory in Lyon and then in Maisons-Alfort with our post-graduate students (Molvot[22] and Kesseler[23]). The results of this study are presented below.

PERSONAL STUDY FOR ERG

We decided to study two factors influencing the ERG recording. One was the type of electrode used as many french veterinarians recommend the use of needle electrode set into the palpebra. The other factor studied was the type of anesthetic since we need an anesthesia for the ERG of many laboratory animals. Our model was the dog.

Use of needle or scleral shell electrodes

Material and methods (Experiment done with Molvot[20]). In veterinary medicine we have difficulties to find corneal electrodes fitting with the cornea since there are many variations of the cornea size and curvature according to the different breeds. For this reason, the use of subcutaneous needle electrodes was recommended by different authors. The needle in our protocol is inserted subcutaneously in the lateral canthus. Corneal electrodes are scleral shells of two different sizes placed on the cornea with a conducting medium (methylcellulose).

The stimulation is obtained by a group of twenty stimulations by a single flash of white light after dark adaptation of the dog during twenty minutes.

Recording is obtained from an ERG machine type Spectral produced by Sereme.

Comparison of different electrodes. Values of latencies and amplitudes of "a" and "b" waves were obtained with a Beagle population (20 beagles) at the Veterinary School of Lyon with the following conditions :
Spectral V.
Sedation : ketamine, diazepam
Scleral shells or needles
Stimulations : 20.   Intensity : 2500 lux at 10 cm, white light
Dark adaptation : 20 minutes.

Table 1.Results of recording of ERG in twenty Beagle dogs with needle electrode and with corneal shell electrode.

Needle Median values	Scleral shell Median values
"a" : latency : 12 ms amplitude : - 12 µV	"a" : latency : 14 ms amplitude : - 71 µV
"b" : latency : 34 ms amplitude : + 44 µV	"b" : latency : 36 ms amplitude : + 180 µV

These results show obviously that the type of electrode does not modifiy the implicit times but there is a considerable variation in the "a" and "b" wave amplitude. As the background noise remains the same, the risk of having artefacts masking the "a" wave (for instance) is not negligible. In conclusion, needle electrodes give recording with low amplitude and increase the risk of having waves masked by artefacts. For this reason, we recommend the use of scleral or corneal electrodes.

Type of anesthesia

The inhalation anesthesia is not practical for a toxicologist working on series of animals. We made a study of ERG under anesthesia obtained with diazepam-ketamine or demetomidine. Anesthetic drugs are used intramuscularly or intravenously for toxicology studies.

Material and methods. The dogs used were males and females from different breeds and ages seen at the Veterinary School for ERG examination. We used either diazepam (VALIUM N.D.) [0.1 - 0.2 mg/kg] + ketamine (IMALGENE N.D.) [0.25 - 0.50 mg/kg] or medetomidine (DOMITOR N.D.) [30 µg/kg] at the dosage recommended by the manufacturer after an atropine injection of 0.25 mg/kg, ten minutes before sedation. The electroretinograph is a Pantops model, produced by Alcon laboratory. The parameters were set as follows :

Table 2 : Standard ERG Pantops parameters

Amplification	
Gain x 1000	20
Filtrage	
Low frequency (Hz)	0.3
High frequency (Hz)	500
Reject (Hz)	50
Averaging	
Cycle duration (ms)	250
Stimulus/cycle	1/1
Cycles number	25
Artefact (%)	< 10
Flash	
Delay (ms)	0
Duration (ms)	10
On both eyes	
Filter colour	White, blue : 365 nm
Light intensity (lux)	maxi : 12 000 lux

The light was conducted to the eye using an optic fiber and the extremity of the fiber covered by a frosten glass set at 10 mm from the eye.

The corneal electrodes are jet electrodes placed on the cornea. The lids are sometimes maintained opened by one operator. The reference electrodes are silver ear ring maintained in contact with the skin with a conducting ointment. The neutral electrode is placed under the tongue of the animal.

ERG protocol. ERG was obtained from a group of twenty-five single flash of 10 ms, with white light and then with blue light after dark adaptation of 10 to 20 minutes.

Amplitude and implicit time for each response were determined. Implicit time is measured from the onset of light stimulus to the peak of "a" and "b" wave respectively "a" wave amplitude and "b" wave amplitude are measured from the baseline to the peak.

Results. The results give implicit times of "a" and "b" waves with both techniques. The amplitude of these waves was very variable and we do not calculate the median values of amplitude (see Tables 3 and 4).

The "a" and "b" waves are always observed and measured with white light. With the blue light, the "a" wave cannot be measured but the "b" wave is present. When we compare the results, we do not see any statistical difference between dogs anesthetized by ketamine-diazepam and dogs anesthetized with medetomidine.The amplitude of "a" and "b" waves was very variable and this variation is probably related to several factors : age, breed... but mainly to an insufficient standardization of dark adaptation. We should respect more strictly twenty minutes of dark adaptation in a future experiment. This factor is known to influence the amplitude of "a" and "b" waves.

Table 3 - Domitor N.D. Implicit times

| | Right eye | | | Left eye | | |
| | White | | Blue | White | | Blue |
wave	"a" wave	"b" wave	"b" wave	"a" wave	"b" wave	" b "
	14	31	45	15	30	42
	18	33	-	15	33	-
	18	49	-	16	39	64
	19	41	-	19	37	-
	16	32	58	15	32	59
	17	34	-	16	37	-
	13	33	-	13	34	-
	15	34	52	15	35	51
	15	33	56	14	30	53
	18	35	59	16	37	48
	15	32	51	13	29	46
	16	38	57	15	36	56
	16	35	54	15	33	51
	14	48	-	17	45	-
	18	34	56	18	34	55
	12	30	43	11	30	43
	16	33	55	15	33	53
Numb of ERG	17	17	11	17	17	12
Average	15.88	35.58	53.27	15.17	34.35	51.75
S.D.	1.90	5.32	4.93	1.82	3.87	6.15

Table 4 - Imalgène N.D. - Valium. implicit times

	Right eye			Left eye		
	White		Blue	White		Blue
wave	"a" wave	"b" wave	"b" wave	"a" wave	"b" wave	" b " wave
	11	30	46	13	33	49
	-	-	43	17	34	47
	11	32	41	-	-	-
	14	30	48	11	29	42
	11	33	-	-	-	-
	16	35	51	15	36	55
	13	33	48	12	30	39
	11	30	46	14	34	46
	14	30	46	15	31	52
Numb of ERG	8	8	8	7	7	7
Average	12.62	31.62	64.12	13.85	32.42	47.14
S.D.	1.79	1.79	2.89	1.88	2.32	5.11

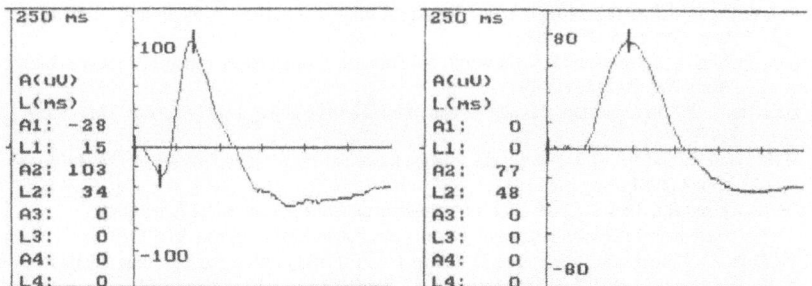

Figure 2. ERG of a dog (male Shitzu, 2 years) showing recording with jet electrodes on a dog anesthetized with medetomidine. "a" and "b" waves are clearly visible with implicit time and amplitude. Left figure : white light, right figure : blue light. The "a" wave is not visible in the right figure

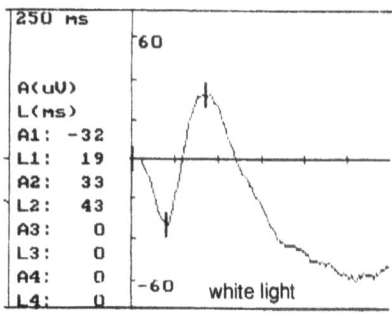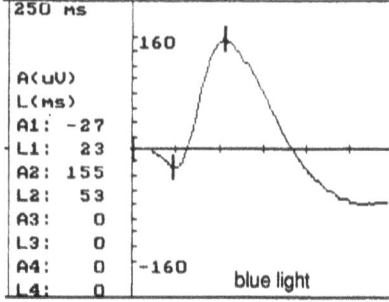

Figure 3. ERG (male european cat). It shows the pattern of "a" and "b" waves with white and blue light. The "a" wave is clearly visible, even in blue light (anesthesia medetomidine).

CONCLUSION

Hook or needle electrodes, very easy to use, allow an ERG recording but the amplitude of "a" and "b" wave is considerably reduced when compared to corneal electrodes.

Anesthesia or deep sedation is necessary for ERG recording. Ketamine is usually the recommended drug for the anesthesia of monkeys while ketamine + diazepam or medetomidine is recommended for dogs and cats.

REFERENCES

1. R. Granit. "The components of the retinal action potential in mammals and their relation to the discharge in the optic nerve," *J. Physiol., Lond.* 77:207 (1933).
2. N. Millichamp. "Factors affecting the interpretation of species differences in toxic responses of ocular tissues," *in*: "'Ophthalmic Toxicology," Chiou, Ravenpress, New-York (1992).
3. G. Aguirre and G. Acland. "ERG course," organized by the AREO Lyon, France. (1990)
4. K. Narfstrom, M. Willem and B.E. Andersson. "Hereditary retinal degeneration in the abyssinian cat : developmental studies using clinical electroretinography," *ISCEV Doc. Opht.* 69:111 (1988).
5. R.C. Riis and A.B. Siakotos. "Inherited lipid retinopathy within a dog breed," *Invest. Ophthalmol. Vis. Sci.* 30:308 (1989).
6. P.G. Bedford. "Retinal pigment epithelial dystrophy. A study of the disease in the Briard," *J. Small Anim. Pract.* 25:129 (1984).
7. H.G. Sperling, C. Johnson and R.S. Harwerth. "Differential spectral photic damage to primate cones," *Vision Res.* 20:1117 (1980).
8. F. Liverani. "Electroretinography as an indicator of toxic retinopathy in dogs," *Pharmac. Ther.* 5:599 (1979).
9. M.M. Whitacre and P.P. Ellis. "Outpatient sedation for ocular examination," *Survey of Ophthalmology* 28:643 (1984).
10. B. Knave and H.E. Persson. "The effect of barbiturate on retinal functions. I. Effects on the conventional electroretinogram of the sheep eye," *Acta Physiol. Scand.* 91:53 (1974).
11. W.K. Noell. "Discussion," *in*: Apter J.T., Pfeiffer C.C. : "Effect of hallucinogenic drugs on the electroretinogram," *Am. J. Ophthalmol.* 42:206 (1956).
12. B. Kommonen and C. Raitta. "Electroretinography in Labrador retrievers given Ketamine and Xylazine anesthesia," *Am. J. Vet. Res.* 48:1325 (1987).
13. M. Antal. "Ketamine-induced ultrastructural changes in the retina," *Albrecht von Graefes Arch. Klin. Ophthalmol.* 210:43 (1979).

14. D. Van Norren and P. Padmos. "Influence of anesthetics, ethyl alcohol, and Freon on dark adaptation on monkey cone ERG," *Invest. Ophthalmol. Vis. Sci.* 16:80 (1977).

15. Y. Kayama and K. Iwama. "The EEG evoked potentials and single-unit activity during ketamine anesthesia in cats," *Anesthesiology* 36:316 (1972)

16. I. Bodis-Wollner, M.S. Marx and M.F. Ghilardi. "Systemic haloperidol administration increases the amplitude of the light- and dark-adapted flash ERG in the monkey," *Clin. Vis. Sci.* 4:18-26 (1989).

17. J.C. Armington. "The electroretinogram," Academic Press, New-York, Ed. (1974)

18. D. Munguia, P. Svendsen and J. Heckenlively, C.A. Wiley, W.R. Freeman. "Standardization of the rabbit ERG for intraocular drug toxicology testing," ARVO, Sarasota, Florida, April-May 32:883 (1991).

19. U. Schaeppi and F. Liverani. "Procedures for routine clinical electroretinography (ERG) in dogs," *Agents and Actions* 7:347 (1977).

20. U. Schaeppi and F. Liverani. "Rod and cone component in the compound ERG of the beagle dog,"*Agents and Actions* 9:294 (1979).

21. D.P. Buist and R. Heywood. "A standardized procedure for electroretinographic examination of rhesus monkeys," *Lab. Anim. Sci.* 32:91 (1982).

22. J.L. Molvot. "Contribution à l'étude de l'électrorétinographie chez le chien : évaluation des techniques de stimulation et de recueil des signaux," Thèse Doct. Vét., Lyon (1990).

23. I. Kesseler. "Intérêt en clinique de l'électrorétinographie chez le chien (étude dans le cadre de la consultation spécialisée d'ophtalmologie de l'Ecole Vétérinaire de Lyon," Thèse Doct. Vet., Lyon (1993).

ELECTRORETINOGRAPHY IN THE NON-HUMAN PRIMATE

AS A STANDARDIZED METHOD IN TOXICOLOGY

Walter H. Bee, Rainhart Korte, and Friedhelm Vogel

HAZLETON DEUTSCHLAND GmbH
Kesselfeld 29
48163 Münster
Germany

ABSTRACT

Electroretinogram traces including the five standard responses were recorded from 80 cynomolgus monkeys (*Macaca fascicularis*) under general anesthesia. First, after 30 minutes of dark adaptation, the scotopic ERG was recorded by seven measurements with increasing flash intensity from the rod threshold up to the maximal response to the standard flash of 2.6 cds/m^2. A standard rod response was elicited with flashes 2.6 log units below the standard flash. The oscillatory potentials were then measured at 0.4 log units above the standard flash. At the onset of light adaptation and 10 minutes thereafter, 30 Hz flicker responses were obtained with the standard flash in presence of background illumination. For the next photopic electroretinogram, three red flash cone responses were recorded with increasing flash intensity. The final photopic trace to be recorded was the single flash cone response with the white standard flash. Beyond the requirements of the Standard for Clinical Electroretinography, electroretinograms were also recorded during the course of the dark adaptation at 4 minute intervals. The results of the recordings performed in accordance with the Standard for Clinical Electroretinography and of the dark adapted electroretinogram correspond very well with the results obtained in humans. Thus, the cynomolgus monkey has proved to be an excellent animal model for testing retinal (dys)functions in toxicity assessment.

Ocular Toxicology, Edited by I. Weisse *et al.*
Plenum Press, New York, 1995

INTRODUCTION

The retina is a complex neuronal structure that is very sensitive to the influence of drugs. Electroretinography permits an objective assessment of this influence on the function of the photoreceptors (rods, cones), neuronal cells (horizontal, bipolar, amacrine cells) and glia cells (Müller cells). Several types of electroretinograms (ERG) are available to differentiate between the responses of the various structures of the retina in response to light. The full-field ("Ganzfeld") ERG reflects the response of the entire retina. The Standard for Clinical Electroretinography (SCE), published by the International Society for the Clinical Electrophysiology of Vision (Marmor et al., 1989), proposes a minimum of five types of measurements in order to obtain international standardization for investigations in humans. On the basis of this guideline, a standardized method for ERG investigations was developed for the non-human primate.

In order to differentiate between the various structures, several types of ERGs can be performed (Figures 1 to 5). These reflect the electrical responses on flash stimulation under different adaptational conditions and can be recorded with a special contact lens from the cornea. A typical response includes an electronegative a-wave generated in the photoreceptors and an electropositive b-wave. The relationship between the intensity of the stimulus and the response amplitude (in μV) or the peak latency (in ms) can be expressed in a voltage vs. intensity or a time vs. intensity function (Figures 6 to 8). These functions are very sensitive to drug induced alterations. Thus, a functional defect is indicated early by a shift or compression of the curve. ERGs performed throughout dark adaptation (Figure 9) and those that elicit the oscillatory potentials and the flicker responses give further indications of possible effects on the function of certain structures. The work described below presents the experiences with the application of the international SCE supplemented with additional useful investigations, to 80 cynomolgus monkeys.

METHODS

Test system: 80 healthy captive-bred cynomolgus monkeys
(*Macaca fascicularis*)

Anesthesia: ketamine-HCl (Parke Davis)

Mydriasis: homatropine-HBr (Ursapharm)

Electrodes: corneal contact lens electrodes (Universo) with four small posts on the convex surface to keep the eyelids open, simultaneous bilateral recording; subdermal platin/iridium needles as reference and ground electrodes placed at the forehead and at the ear

Recording: signals were amplified, filtered, online averaged, saved on disc and displayed by a Compact Visual®(Nicolet); depending on the measured stimulus, up to 50 responses were averaged; in total, 23 single ERG measurements were taken in the following order:

- 7 scotopic recordings of increasing flash intensity from 0.643 mcds/m^2 to the standard flash (SF) at 2570 mcds/m^2
- 1 recording of the oscillatory potential at 6430 mcds/m^2
- 2 flicker ERG (30.1 Hz, SF) at the beginning and after 10 min of light adaptation with a rod saturating background illumination
- 3 red flash photopic recordings with flash intensities from 415 to 1038 mcds/m^2
- 1 white flash cone response with the SF
- 9 recordings over 32 minutes of dark adaptation with a constant stimulus of approximately 25 mcds/m^2

Stimulation: a full-field ("Ganzfeld") dome (Nicolet) illuminated by a xenon strobe;

flash intensity and background illumination determined before each session by a Gossen Mastersix Photometer;

flash intensity controlled by using the log scale of the computer and with neutral density filters (Kodak Wratten gelatine filter); Kodak Wratten No. 26 as red filter for the photopic recordings

Evaluation: peak latency and amplitude of each response were determined manually on the screen by setting a cursor on the peak concerned;

the respective values calculated automatically by the computer;

the amplitude of the waves measured from the baseline to the peak of the wave or, in presence of an a-wave, from the peak of the a-wave to the peak of the b-wave; the peak latency measured from the onset of the flash to the peak; in the case of the oscillatory potentials, latency measured from the onset of the flash to the second peak and the amplitude related to the following trough;

referring to the 30Hz flicker ERG, the second peak measured in relation to the preceding trough; results stored electronically for further evaluation

RESULTS

The results of the five standard responses recommended by the SCE are shown as means in table 1. Typical examples are depicted in figures 1 to 5; for comparison, respective data for humans (Jacobi et al., 1993) are given in square brackets in the table.

The responses of the cynomolgus monkey to the standard tests are similar to the responses of humans. Shape and latencies of the curves are highly comparable. Higher amplitudes (μV) in man can be explained by a bigger diameter and a larger surface of the eye which has an influence on the electric field and thus on the measured response.

Table 1. The results of the five standard responses recommended by the SCE as mean values of 80 cynomolgus monkeys; respective data for 20 humans are given in square brackets (human data from Jacobi et al, 1993)

Standard Response (recommended by SCE)	b-wave Amplitude (in μV)	b-wave Peak Latency (in ms)	Flash Intensity (mcds/m^2)	Adaptation Status
rod response	95 [223]	79 [80]	6.4	dark
maximal response	172 [424]	39 [39]	2570	dark
oscillatory potential	20 [79]	21.3 [23.8]	6430	dark
30 Hz flicker	66 [73]	46 [58]	2570	light
white flash cone response	84 [156]	27.5 [29.5]	2570	light

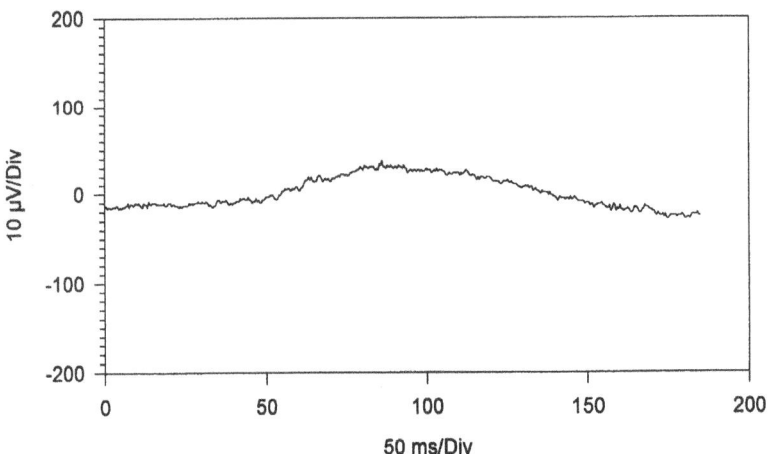

Figure 1. Rod response, elicited at 0.0064 cds/m^2 after 30 minutes of dark adaptation in a representative monkey

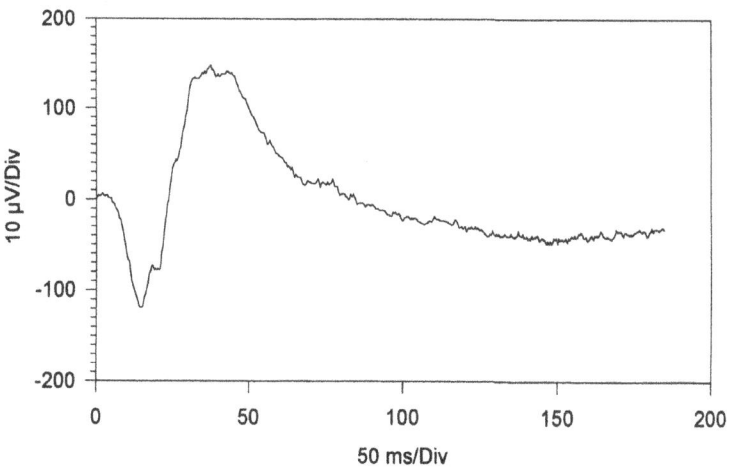

Figure 2. Maximal response, elicited at 2.57 cds/m^2 (standard flash) after 30 minutes of dark adaptation

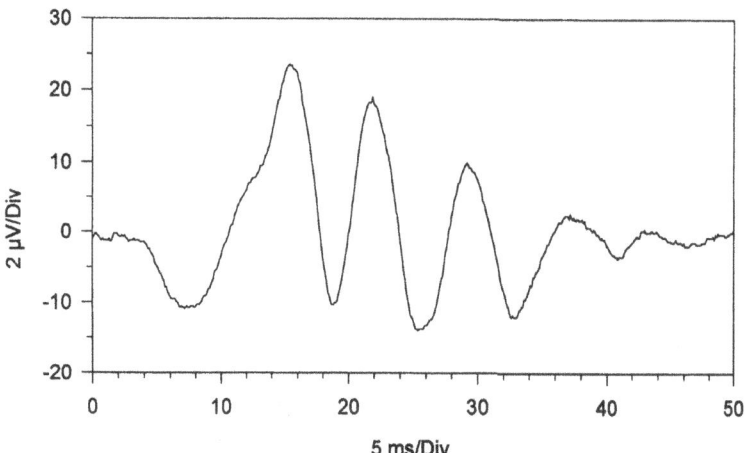

Figure 3. Oscillatory potentials, elicited at 6.43 cds/m^2 in the dark-adapted eye

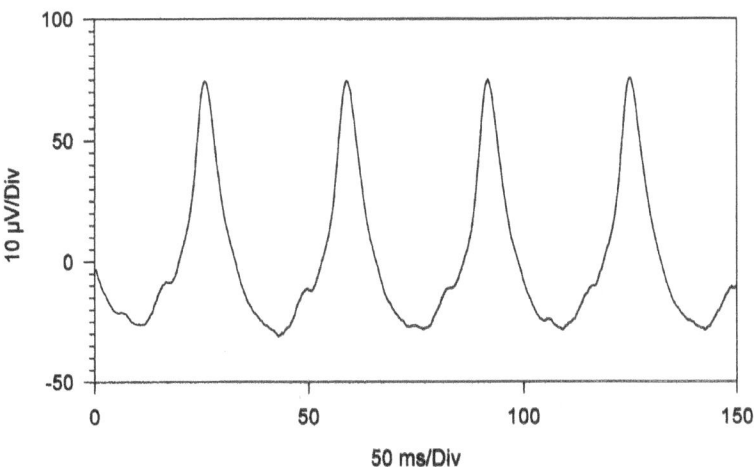

Figure 4. Flicker response (30 Hz), elicited at 2.57 cds/m^2 after 10 minutes of light adaptation

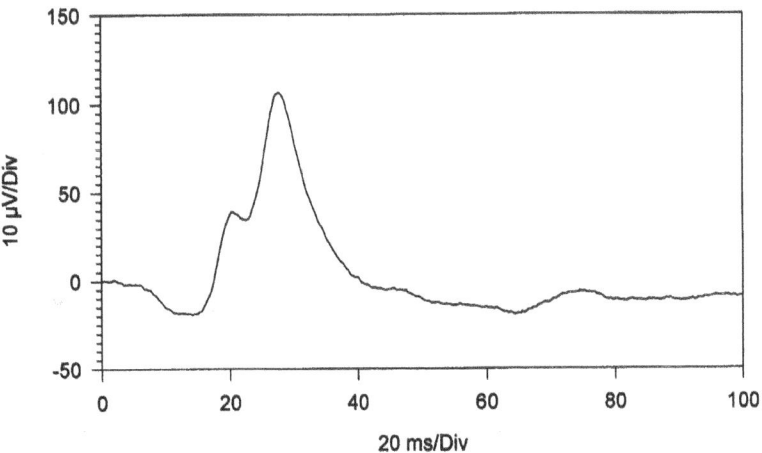

Figure 5. White flash cone response, elicited at 2.57 cds/m^2 in the light adapted eye

The five SCE responses were integrated into a larger protocol that included measurements of scotopic and photopic responses on stimuli below those used to elicit the maximum response or the white flash cone response. Figure 6 depicts the results of the scotopic b-wave voltage (amplitude) or time (peak latency) vs. log stimulus intensity functions. Curves of scotopic tests on 20 humans (Jacobi et al., 1993) are given in figure 7 for comparison. The sigmoid curve characterizes the amplitude as well as the latency function in the cynomolgus monkey and in humans.

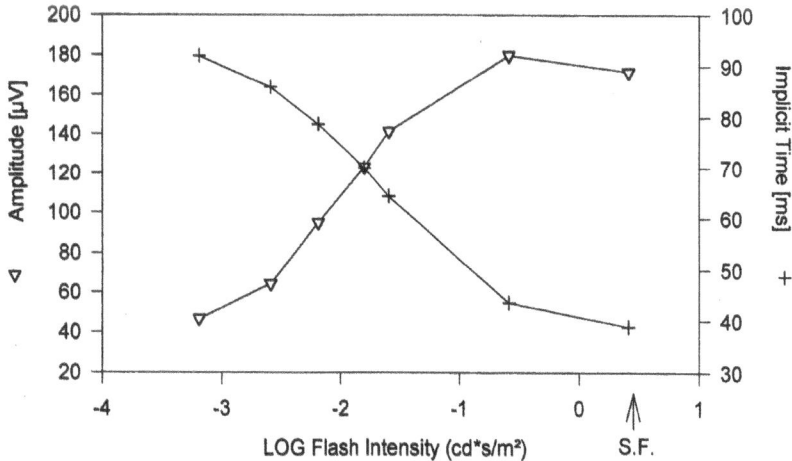

Figure 6. Response versus intensity function for b-wave amplitude and implicit time of the scotopic ERG in Cynomolgus monkeys. SF = standard flash at 2.57 cds/m^2

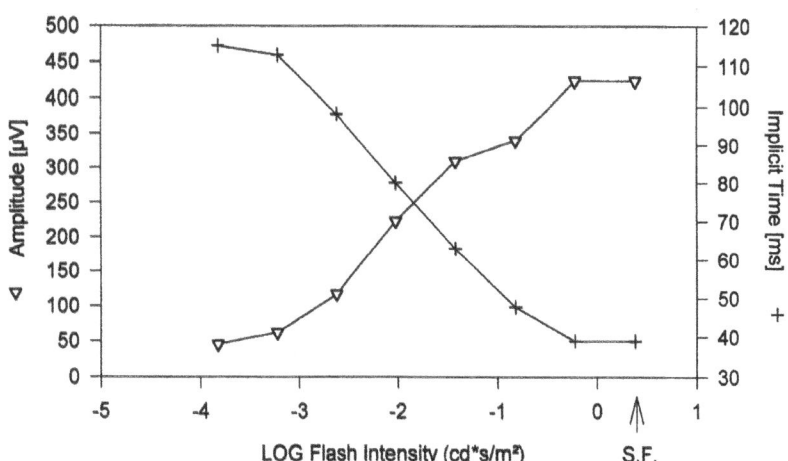

Figure 7. Response versus intensity function for b-wave amplitude and implicit time of the scotopic ERG in humans. SF = standard flash at 2.4 cds/m^2. Taken from Jacobi et al (1993)

The photopic log intensity functions are shown in figure 8. While the first three values used for this function represent cone responses on red flashes, the last one represents the white flash cone response. In contrast to the scotopic time vs. log intensity function, the intensity-response function of the cones' peak latency indicates a slight increase. This result is also known from studies on human retinal function (Jacobi et al., 1993).

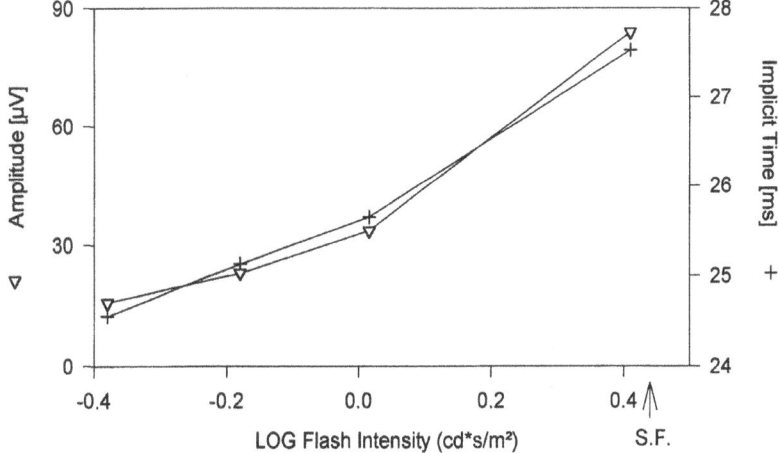

Figure 8. Response versus intensity function for b-wave amplitude and implicit time of the photopic ERG under rod-suppressing background illumination (25 cds/m^2). SF = standard flash at 2.57 cds/m^2.

The results of ERGs measured every 4 minutes throughout 32 minutes of dark adaptation with a dim white flash stimulus of constant intensity are shown in figure 9. Approximately 90 % saturation is reached after 16 minutes, which is also comparable to humans.

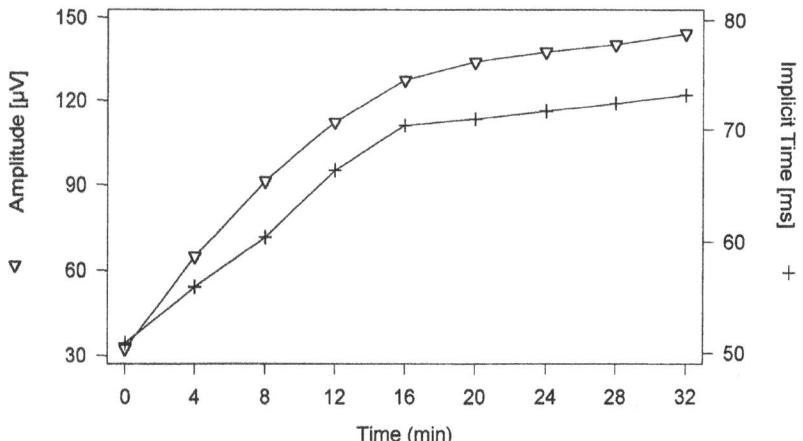

Figure 9. Response versus time functions or b-wave amplitude and implicit time throughout dark-adaptation elicited at 0.025 cds/m^2

CONCLUSION

The results of the recordings performed in accordance with the SCE and of the ERG covering the dark adaptation correspond very well with the results obtained in humans. Thus, the cynomolgus monkey has proved to be an excellent animal model for the test of retinal functions in toxicity assessment.

REFERENCES

Jacobi, P., Miliczek, K.-D., and Zrenner, E., 1993, Experiences with the international standard for clinical electroretinography: normative values for clinical practice, inter- and intraindividual variations, *Doc Ophthalmol* 85:95-114.

Marmor, M.F., Arden, G.B., Nilsson, S.E.G., and Zrenner, E., 1989, Standard for clinical electroretinography, *Arch Ophthal* 107:816-819.

EFFECTS OF CLINDAMYCIN ON NEURAL FUNCTION IN THE ISOLATED PERFUSED VERTEBRATE RETINA

Peter Walter,[1] Christoph Lüke,[2] and Werner Sickel[2]

[1]Department of Ophthalmology
[2]Institute of Neurophysiology
University of Cologne
Joseph Stelzmann Str.9
D-50931 Cologne
Germany

INTRODUCTION

The application of antibiotics during vitrectomy has become an established technique in treatment of bacterial endophthalmitis. During surgery antibiotics are used in the vitreous replacement fluid and as an intraocular injection at the end of the surgical procedure. A number of morphological and electrophysiological studies have been performed to evaluate non-toxic dosages of the antibiotics. Testing retinal toxicity of a substance being directly injected into the vitreous poses a main problem: the distribution of the drug on the retinal surface may be not homogenous due to inhomgenities of the vitreal structure. As a consequence different retinal areas may be exposed to different concentrations of the drug. Thus may lead to confusing results in retinal toxicity testing. It has been suggested to perform these tests in the vitrectomized eye in order to better model the situation during vitrectomy.

Beside the in-vivo tests an electrophysiological in-vitro technique for fast screening of retinal toxicity in higher vertebrates is available. The isolated perfused vertebrate retina method was described by Lippmann and Sickel[1] in 1959. With this technique it is possible to maintain e.g. bovine retina in a functioning state over several hours as indicated by a normal electroretinogram (ERG) after light stimulation. The physiological state can be affected by application of potentially toxic substances in precise known concentrations to the perfusate. The ERG before, during, and after perfusation with the toxic agent serves as an indicator of the integrity or non-integrity of the photoreceptors, the first retinal synapse, and the postsynaptic bipolar layer with its interaction with the retinal glial cells.

Clindamycin is one of the antibiotics used in our department during vitrectomy for bacterial endophthalmitis. Previously performed studies disclosed a maximum non-toxic dose of 10 µg/ml in human[2] and rabbit eyes[3]. Clindamycin is available in a solution

Ocular Toxicology, Edited by I. Weisse *et al.*
Plenum Press, New York, 1995

63

containing Benzyl Alcohol (Sobelin ®). We studied the effects of Clindamycin/Benzyl Alcohol preparations on the electroretinogram in the isolated perfused bovine retina.

MATERIAL AND METHODS

Under dim red light freshly enucleated bovine eyes were opened equatorially and the vitreous was removed. Scleral-choroid-retina blocks were trimmed to the size of the perfusing chamber using a 7-mm trepan. In a bath containing the perfusing medium the retina was isolated from the underlying pigment epithelium. The retina was mounted on the core of the perfusing chamber which allows also for recording of the transretinal potential by two ringlike Ag-AgCl electrodes on each side of the retina. The chamber was installed in an electrically, optically, and thermically isolated device. The perfusion velocity was controlled with a roller-pump and usually being set to 1 ml/min. The temperature was set to 30°C. The perfusate was preequlibrated with oxygen. The retina was stimulated in intervals of five minutes with white flashes. The flash intensity was set to 6.3 mlxs and a duration of 1 second using a photo shutter and calibrated neutral density filters. The ERG was amplified 10000 fold (bandpass between 0.1 and 300 Hz). Single responses proved to be stable and noiseless enough, so that neither an artifact rejection system nor an averager were necessary for signal acquisition. The signal was AD converted, analyzed, stored and printed using a PC based signal acquisition and analysis system.

The retina was initially perfused with the normal perfusate (NaCl 120, KCl 2, $MgCl_2$ 0.1, $CaCl_2$ 0.15, NaH_2PO_4 1.5, Na_2HPO_4 13.5, and glucose 5; concentrations given in mMol/l.) and stimulated repeatedly until the b-waves showed a steady-state with a standard deviation of less then 10 % in amplitude. Then the perfusate was changed to the Clindamycin containing medium and responses were recorded in five minutes intervals for 45 minutes. Then the retina was reperfused with standard solution and the responses to the standardized flashes were recorded.

The b-wave amplitude was measured from the trough of the a-wave (inital negative deflection) to the peak of the b-wave. The b-wave reduction was calculated as $1-b_c/b$ where „b_c“ is the b-wave amplitude at the end of the Clindamycin perfusion phase and „b“ is the b-wave amplitude prior to the Clindamycin perfusing phase. Clindamycin was added to the perfusate in the following concentrations: 0.1, 0.3, 1, 3, and 10 mMol/l. Because the available Clindamycin preparation contains a certain amount of Benzyl Alcohol we also investigated the effects of Benzyl Alcohol on the ERG of the isolated perfused bovine retina using concentrations between 0.1 and 10 mMol/l.

RESULTS

Recording Conditions

A preliminary series of experiments showed that the amplitude of the b-wave was sensitive to temperature. The maximum and most stable b-wave amplitudes were found with a surrounding temperature of 30°C.

Oxygen supply may also affect retinal function. The perfusing medium was saturated with oxygen by bubbling the gas into the solution. Procedures were compared when the gas was inflated throughout the experiment with techniques when the bubbling was stopped prior to the recording session. The b-wave amplitudes were not significantly different in both groups. However, the results were significantly better when compared to a solution just saturated with room air oxygen. Therefore the prebubbling method was used throughout the experiments described in the following.

Clindamycin/Benzyl Alcohol (Sobelin ®)

A Clindamycin concentration of 0.1 mMol/l did not affect the b-wave of the electroretinogram during 45 minutes of perfusion. With higher concentrations of Clindamycin the b-wave was found to be reduced. After 20 minutes a steady state could be reached (Figure 1). The b-wave reduction correlated with the concentration of Clindamycin (Figure 2). During reperfusion with normal perfusate the b-wave showed a slow, but nearly complete recovery.

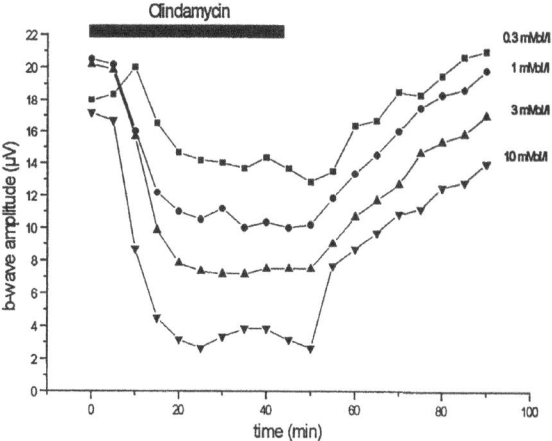

Figure 1. B-wave amplitude of the isolated perfused bovine retina during and after perfusation with Clindamycin containing medium. The Clindamycin concentrations are indicated.

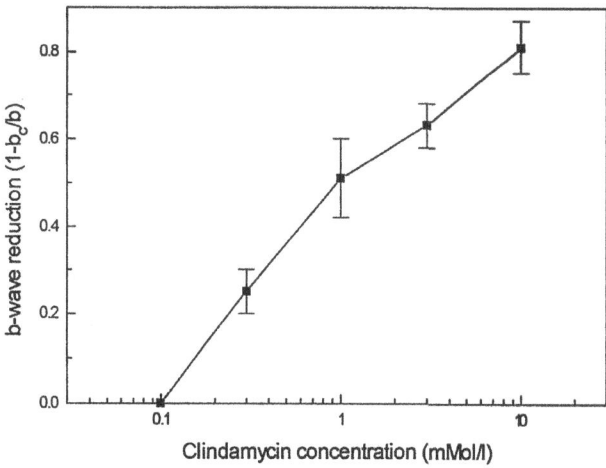

Figure 2. Dose-Response-Curve of Clindamycin induced b-wave reduction in the isolated perfused bovine retina. Averages ± standard deviation.

Benzyl Alcohol

Benzyl Alcohol in concentrations of 0.3 and 1 mMol/l did not affect the ERG b-wave. However, higher concentrations disclosed a relatively fast reversible reduction of the b-wave (Figure 3). The b-wave recovery was significantly faster when compared to the recovery in the Sobelin ® series. A Sobelin ® solution with 1 mMol/l Clindamycin contains about 0.3 mMol/l Benzyl Alcohol. Figure 4 shows the Benzyl Alcohol related b-wave reduction in Clindamycin/Benzyl Alcohol preparations.

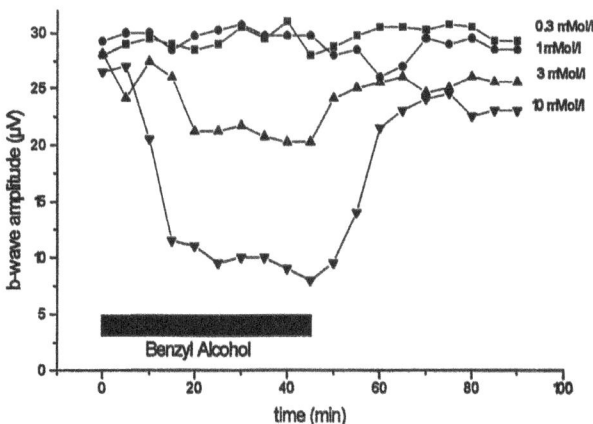

Figure 3. Effects of different concentrations of Benzyl Alcohol in the perfusate on the b-wave of the ERG of the isolated perfused bovine retina.

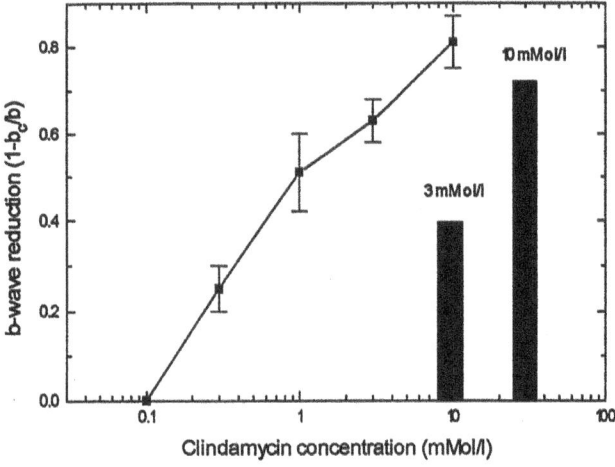

Figure 4. B-wave reduction by application of Clindamycin / Benzyl Alcohol preparation (Sobelin ®, line) and by application of Benzyl Alcohol (bars) in the concentrations indicated. Note that half of the effect at 10 mMol/l Clindamycin is due its Benzyl Alcohol content.

CONCLUSIONS

Using the isolated perfused vertebrate retina technique effects of potentially toxic substances on the photoreceptors, the first retinal synapse and the interaction between the bipolar layer and the retinal glial cells can be monitored over hours. Each parameter of the experimental setup is adjustable and can be controlled. One advantage of the technique is that the concentration of the substance being tested is precisely known. From ERG recordings information can be drawn concerning retinal metabolism under the acute perfusation with the toxic agent[4,5].

The experiments presented here revealed toxic effects of Clindamycin / Benzyl Alcohol in concentrations higher then 0.1 mMol/l i.e. 50 µg/ml Clindamycin. This concentration is about five times higher then currently used for vitrectomy[2]. Stainer et al.[3] reported about even extinguished ERGs in rabbits with 0.1 mMol/l. These differences may be explained with species differences and can not be confirmed in bovine retina.

The Benzyl Alcohol portion of the Clindamycin preparation is non-toxic in the concentrations used for vitrectomy. With higher concentrations its effect is about half of the b-wave reduction induced by Clindamycin / Benzyl Alcohol. The b-wave recovery was faster after Benzyl Alcohol when compared to the Clindamycin / Benzyl Alcohol preparation, suggesting a different mechanism of toxic action of both substances on the outer retina.

REFERENCES

1. H.G.Lippmann and W.Sickel, Die isolierte Netzhaut als Praeparat fuer objektiv-sinnesphysiologische und stoffwechsel-analytische Untersuchungen, Pfluegers Arch ges Physiol, 270:30 (1959).
2. G.A.Peyman and J.A.Schulman, Intravitreal drug therapy, Jpn J Ophthalmol 33:392 (1989).
3. G.A.Stainer, G.A.Peyman, H.Meisels, and G.Fishman, Toxicity of selected antibiotics in vitreous replacement fluid, Ann Ophthalmol, 9(5):615(1977).
4. W.Sickel, The isolated retina maintained in a circulating medium; combined optical and electrical investigations of metabolic aspects of generation of the electroretinogram, in: „Clinical Electroretinography," H.M.Burian and J.H.Jacobson, eds., Oxford Pergamon Press, pp. 115-124 (1966).
5. W.Sickel, Retinal metabolism in dark and light, in: „Handbook of Sensory Physiology Vol. VII/2," M.G.F.Fuortes, ed., Springer Berlin, Heidelberg, New York. pp. 667-727(1972).

DETERMINATION OF THE EFFECT OF KETAMINE, THIOPENTAL AND HALOTHANE ON THE OCULAR ELECTRORETINOGRAPHIC EXAMINATION OF THE BEAGLE DOG TO DEFINE PROTOCOLS TO BE USED IN DOGS, MONKEYS AND MICROPIGS

Olivier Loget[1] and Gérard Saint-Macary[2]

[1]Pharmakon Europe
Domaine des Oncins - BP 0118
69593 L'Arbresle Cédex
France

[2]Synthélabo Recherche
Département d'Etude sur la Sécurité du Médicament
2-8 Route de Rouen
78840 Gargenville
France

SUMMARY

A preliminary study performed on anesthetized beagle dogs permitted definition of a protocol for electrophysiological examinations. This first protocol included dark adaptation and specific stimulation of cones (red flashes) and rods (blue flashes).

As the less variable and therefore most interpretable values were latencies and not amplitudes, and as dark adaptation only increases amplitude, it was decided to perform further routine examinations without dark adaptation.

It was also decided not to evaluate systematically differential receptor function in further routine studies. Therefore, most of the records were obtained using only polychromatic light (white flashes).

A subsequent study was performed in order to compare the influence of different types of anesthetics on two of the main electroretinogram waves in the beagle dog and showed good homogeneity of values for each kind of anesthetic and a trend to variable increases in latencies depending on the anesthetic. It was found that results could be easily obtained in conscious dogs.

Consequently, it was decided to perform further examination without anesthesia in beagle dogs and, where possible, in other species such as micropigs. It is not possible to perform electroretinographic records in conscious animals for species such as primates. In this case, it was decided to anesthetize the animals, using ketamine, which was the drug which produced the least marked increase in the wave latencies in the beagle dog.

This survey is illustrated by records performed on normal eyes of beagle dogs, cynomolgus macaques and Yucatan micropigs and by some spontaneous or induced pathological changes.

INTRODUCTION

Ocular electrophysiological changes induced by anesthetics have been reported in laboratory animals. Granit[17] has shown that ether inhalation markedly decreased the amplitude of the visual evoked potentials (VEP). The amplitude of the electroretinogram (ERG) is known to decrease with anesthesia[4, 15, 24, 25, 26, 38, 40, 48].

In our experiments, we have tried to detect if ketamine[20, 25, 26, 27, 43], thiopental[26] or halothane[7, 14, 23, 26, 47, 49, 50] induced an increase in two of the main ERG wave latencies in the beagle dog and to determine if there are statistical differences. The results showed good homogeneity of values for each kind of anesthetic and a trend to variable increases in latencies depending on the anesthetic. As results could be easily obtained in conscious dogs, further examinations were therefore performed without anesthesia in beagle dogs and, where possible, in other species such as micropigs. ERG's can generally not be recorded in conscious primates. Consequently, it was decided to anesthetize these animals, using ketamine, which was the drug which produced the least marked increase in the wave latencies in the beagle dog.

MATERIAL AND METHODS

The study was carried out on ten female beagle dogs and in eighteen cynomolgus monkeys (9 males and 9 females). Four Yucatan micropigs were also examined. The animals were housed singly in an air-conditioned, protected building with a 12 hour light (artificial)/12 hour dark lighting cycle (dogs and micropigs in pens and monkeys in cages). The animals were fed with pelleted commercial diet and received mains water *ad libitum* via an automatic watering system.

All the animals underwent ophthalmoscopic, slit-lamp and electroretinographic examinations to ensure that they were free from pathological disorders. Ophthalmoscopic and slit-lamp examinations were carried out on conscious dogs and micropigs and on ketamine anesthetized monkeys. In dogs, the ERG's were recorded in the first instance under ketamine anesthesia. This preliminary study performed on anesthetized beagle dogs permitted definition of a protocol for electrophysiological examinations. This first protocol included dark adaptation and specific stimulation of cones (red flashes) and rods (blue flashes) as follows.

The ERG's were recorded after a period of dark adaptation lasting 30 minutes. At the beginning of this period and again 15 minutes later a mydriatic agent (tropicamide Mydriaticum) was instilled into the eyes. We decided to adopt a 30 minutes dark adaptation period in order to have less variation in wave amplitudes[39]. However, due to the kind of stimulator which was used, the less variable and therefore most interpretable values were latencies and not amplitudes. Consequently, it was decided to measure latencies only.

At the end of the dark adaptation period, 32 consecutive stimulations were performed. Each flash lasted 10,000 μs at an intensity of two lux. Flashes occurred at a frequency of 3 Hz. The light source was placed at 20 cm from the eyes when white light was used, at 10 cm with blue light and at 20 cm with red light. Each final plot was obtained after averaging the results of the 32 plots obtained for the 250 ms following the light flashes. The latencies of the "a" and "b" waves were recorded. The first 32 stimulations were performed using white light. Thereafter, the same stimulation protocol was followed using successively blue and red filters. In order to simplify the protocol for use in routine toxicology studies, we started with white light stimulation. If no change is seen with white light, the use of coloured light could be considered unnecessary. If changes were seen with the white light, then stimulation with blue or red light could be used to determine which photoreceptors were involved.

The measurement was performed on two occasions on conscious dogs and on one occasion each under ketamine or thiopental anesthesia. Only two animals were anesthetized by halothane inhalation (on two occasions).

For statistical analysis, the latencies measured on conscious dogs were averaged for each eye in order to obtain the same number of data points as for the ketamine and thiopental anesthetic trials. Statistical analysis was performed using the Fischer test.

RESULTS

Slit-lamp and ophthalmoscopic examinations

The animals were examined during the week before the first anesthesia. No corneal deposits were observed in any of the animals and no opacities capable of modifying the quantity of light received on the retina were detected in the lens, except in one male cynomolgus monkey which presented a bilateral cataract. Consequently, this animal was not retained for the study.

One of the ten dogs presented a chorioretinitis of the right eye. Consequently, the left eye only was studied for this female.

Electroretinograms in dogs

Normal eyes (Figure 1). The latencies of both "a" and "b" waves, measured on two occasions, remained essentially constant in anesthetized and conscious dogs.

The mean results obtained in conscious dogs and in ketamine and thiopental anesthetized dogs were as follows:

Conscious dogs (38 values) :
    "a" wave = 19.2 ms (standard deviation = 1.1 ms),
    "b" wave = 41.1 ms (standard deviation = 3.1 ms),

Ketamine anesthetized dogs (19 values) :
    "a" wave = 21.0 ms (standard deviation = 2.9 ms),
    "b" wave = 42.6 ms (standard deviation = 3.7 ms),

Thiopental anesthetized dogs (19 values) :
    "a" wave = 19.6 ms (standard deviation = 1.6 ms),
    "b" wave = 48.0 ms (standard deviation = 4.6 ms),

Halothane anesthetized dogs (6 values) :
    "a" wave = 21.0 ms (standard deviation = 3.3 ms),
    "b" wave = 47.2 ms (standard deviation = 6.5 ms).

Halothane[7, 14, 23, 26, 47, 49, 50] seems to markedly increase the "a" and "b" wave latencies. However, only two animals were examined under halothane anesthesia. Moreover, one of these dogs was the female with an unilateral chorioretinitis. Although ERG's were recorded at two different occasions, only 6 values were obtained for each wave and these results were therefore not used in the statistical comparison.

The Fisher test showed statistically significant differences in "a" wave latencies between conscious and ketamine anesthetized animals and in "b"wave latencies between conscious and ketamine and thiopental anesthetized animals[20, 25, 26, 27, 43]. Although differences only involved the "b" wave with thiopental, ketamine was considered to be a better choice because it had a less marked effect on the "b" wave.

It was found that results could be easily obtained in conscious dogs. Consequently, it was decided to perform further examination without anesthesia in beagle dogs and, where possible, in other species such as micropigs. It is not possible to perform electroretinographic recordings in conscious animals for species such as primates. In this case, it was decided to anesthetize the animals, using ketamine, which was the drug which produced the least marked increase in the wave latencies in the beagle dog.

Spontaneous ocular pathological changes. In the female beagle dog with an unilateral chorioretinitis[2, 31, 32, 33, 36], the ERG amplitudes were markedly reduced in this eye and the VEP's were absent. However, the ERG wave latencies were similar to those observed in the other eye of this dog and in other dogs.

Electroretinograms in Monkeys

Normal eyes (Figure 1). In cynomolgus monkeys, the ERG's were less rounded with sharper peaks than in dogs and the "a" wave was often, but not always, separated into two waves[21, 39]: "a_1" (photopic) and "a_2" (scotopic)[3]. The scotopic "a" wave was always seen, even with the red filter. The photopic "a" wave was only occasionnally seen, even with the blue filter.
Amplitudes were more homogenous than in dogs. However, qualitative estimation is probably normally sufficient for routine toxicology studies.

Nine males and eight females were examined twice after ketamine anesthesia and one female was examined once after ketamine anesthesia and once unanesthetized. Using the 70 ERG's performed after ketamine anesthesia, we obtained mean latency values as follows :

In females :
    "a_1" wave (only 26 values)   = 14.6 ms (standard deviation = 2.80 ms),
    "a_2" wave (34 values)   = 23.4 ms (standard deviation = 3.00 ms),
    "b"   wave (34 values)   = 45.5 ms (standard deviation = 4.40 ms),

In males :
    "a_1" wave (only 26 values)   = 16.6 ms (standard deviation = 0.11 ms),
    "a_2" wave (34 values)   = 23.7 ms (standard deviation =1.80 ms),
    "b"   wave (34 values)   = 44.9 ms (standard deviation = 3.30 ms),

Both sexes combined :
    "a_1" wave (only 37 values)   = 15.2 ms (standard deviation = 2.70 ms),
    "a_2" wave (36 values)   = 23.5 ms (standard deviation = 2.40 ms),
    "b"   wave (36 values)   = 45.2 ms (standard deviation = 3.90 ms).

One female macaque was born at the testing facility and was therefore tame. Consequently, it was possible to examine this animal without any anasthesia as well as with ketamine anesthesia. In this monkey, the waves seemed to occur slightly later in conscious animal than with anasthesia. However, the significance of this finding, in one animal is obviously doubtful.

Spontaneous ocular pathological changes. ERG's recorded in the cynomolgus macaque with bilateral cataract were normal[10, 46] and confirmed that the retina was unaffected.

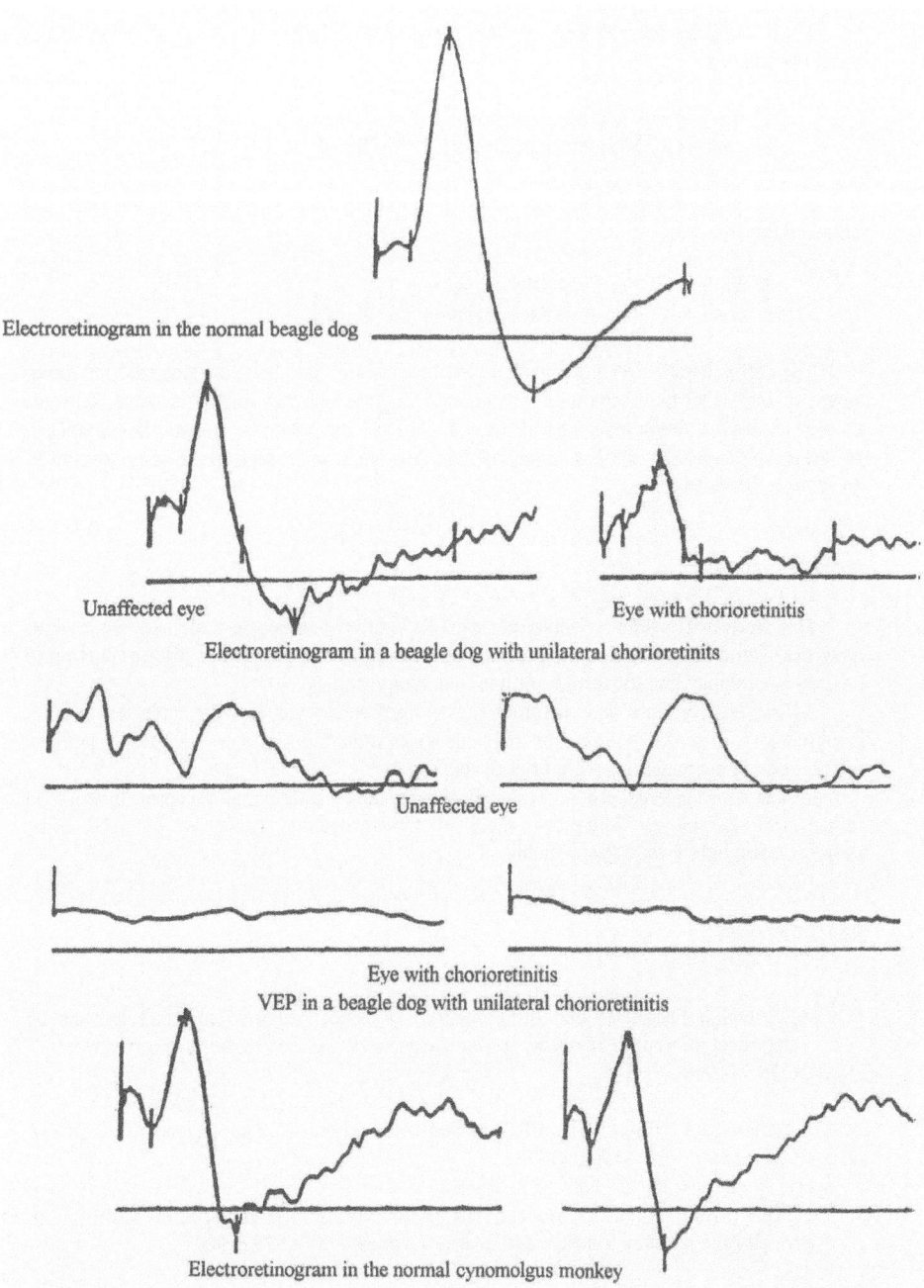

Electroretinogram in the normal beagle dog

Unaffected eye   Eye with chorioretinitis
Electroretinogram in a beagle dog with unilateral chorioretinits

Unaffected eye

Eye with chorioretinitis
VEP in a beagle dog with unilateral chorioretinitis

Electroretinogram in the normal cynomolgus monkey

Figure 1. Survey of ERG and VEP records from normal and diseased dog eyes and normal monkey eyes.

73

Electroretinograms in Micropigs

ERG's recorded in Yucatan micropigs were very close to those of dogs.

Four conscious animals were studied. Using these 8 ERG's, we obtained mean latency values as follows :

"a" wave = 21.3 ms (standard deviation = 1.70 ms),
"b" wave = 37.8 ms (standard deviation = 3.28 ms).

J.F. Charlin[7] studied fourteen Yucatan micropigs using halothane anesthesia and obtained the following values:

"a" wave = 17.7 ms (standard deviation = 4.27 ms),
"b" wave = 42.3 ms (standard deviation = 4.90 ms).

The comparison of results obtained in conscious and halothane anesthetized micropigs seems to show that halothane tends to decrease "a" wave latency and to increase "b" wave latency. However, the number of animals was not high enough to be statistically significant. In any case, as ERG's are easily recorded in conscious micropigs, there is no reason to anesthetize these animals.

CONCLUSION

This study was useful to obtain normal ERG patterns in beagle dogs and cynomolgus monkeys. Some recordings were performed on micropigs, but not yet in sufficient number to be used as baseline data for further routine toxicology studies.

As the less variable and therefore most interpretable values were latencies and not amplitudes, and as dark adaptation only increases amplitude, it was decided to perform further routine examinations without dark adaptation.

It was also decided not to systematically evaluate differential receptor function in further routine studies. Therefore, most of the recordings could be obtained using polychromatic light (white flashes) only.

REFERENCES

1. G.M. Acland, Diagnosis and differentiation of retinal diseases in small animals by electroretinography, *Seminars in veterinary medicine and surgery (small animal).* 3 (1):15 (1988).

2. G. Aguirre, L.F. Rubin, The ERG in dog with inherited cone degeneration, *Invest. Ophthalmol. Vis.* 14:840 (1975).

3. D.A. Baylor, B.J. Nunn, J.L. Scnapf, The photocurrent, noise and spectral sensitivity of rods of the monkey Macaca fascicularis, *J. Physiol.* 357:575 (1984).

4. C.H. Brown, D.G. Green, Rod saturation in b wave of the rat-electroretinogram under two different anaesthetics, *Vision Res.* 24:87 (1984).

5. D.L. Bruce, M.J. Bach, Effects of three anaesthetic gases on behavioural performance of volonteers, *Br. J. anaesth.* 48:871 (1976).

6. D.P. Buist, R. Heywood, A standardized procedure for electroretinographic examination of Rhesus monkeys (Macaca mulatta), *Lab. Animal Sci.* 32 (1):595 (1982).

7. J.F. Charlin, Etude expérimentale chez le microporc d'un substitut du vitré : le collagène IV humain placentaire, *Thèse de Doctorat de Sciences Médicales présentée à la Faculté de Médecine de l'Université de Rouen* (1991).

8. J.P. Chevaleraud, Explorations électrophysiologiques sensorielles, *in*: "Encycl. Méd. Chir., Ophtalmologie, 21046 A10", 12, Paris (1982).

9. J.P. Chevaleraud, Les explorations électrophysiologiques, *Revue Chibret.* 101:25 (1982).

10. J.P. Chevaleraud, Intérêt pronostique de l'ERG dans la chirurgie de la cataracte, *Bull. Soc. Ophtalmol. Fr.* 72:11 (1972).

11. J.P. Chevaleraud, Phénomènes électriques rétiniens, *in*: "Encycl. Méd. Chir., Ophtalmologie, 21027 A10", 9, Paris (1980).

12. J.J. Coulon, L'électrophysiologie sensorielle oculaire, ses fondements, son intérêt, ses indications, Laboratoires Chauvin-Blache (1983).

13. J. Fine, J. Weismann, S.C. Finestone, Side effects after ketamine anaesthesia: transient blindness, *Anaest. Analg.* 53:72 (1974).

14. E.A. Gall, Report of the pathology panel: National halothane study, *Anaesthesology.* 29:233 (1968)

15. B.G. Gerritsen, The effect of anaesthetics on the electroretinogram and the visually evoked response in the rabbit, *Doc. Ophthalmol.* 29:289 (1971).

16. P. Gouras, ERG: some basis principles. *Invest. Ophthalmol. Vis. Sci.* 9:557 (1970).

17. R. Granit, The components of the retinal action potential in mammals and their relation to the discharge of the optic nerve. J. Physiol. (London). 77:207 (1933).

18. G.G. Gum, Electrophysiology in veterinary ophthalmology, Vet. Clinics N.A.V. 10 (2):437 (1980).

19. JC. Hache, P. François, Une tentative de classification des altérations électrorétinographiques. *Bull. Soc. Ophthalmol. Fr.* 6:745 (1976).

20. S.C. Haskins, T.B. Farver, J.D. Patz, Ketamine in dogs, *Amer. J. Vet. Res.* 47:636 (1986).

21. H.E. Henkes, Differenciation and evaluation of rod and cone syst. responses in the human electroretinogram, *Ophthalmologica.* 135:138 (1959).

22. D.R. Howard; W.F. Keller, G.L. Blanchard, Clinical electroretinography : a protocol for testing the retina, *J.A.A.H.A.* 9:219 (1973).

23. S. Jarkmann, K.O. Skoog, S.E.G. Nilsson, The c wave of the electroretinogram and the standing potential of the eye as highly sensitive measures of effects of low doses of trichloroethylene, methylchloroform, and halothane, *Doc. Ophthalmol.* 60:375 (1985).

24. B. Knave, H.E. Persson, The effect of barbiturate on retinal functions III. The c wave of the electroretinogram and the standing potential of the sheep eye, *ACTA Physiolo. Scand.* 91:180 (1974).

25. B. .Kommonen, The DC recorded electroretinogram in ketamine-medetomidine anaesthesia, *ACTA vet. scand.* 29:35 (1988).

26. B. Kommonen, U. Karhunhen, C. Raitta, Effects of thiopentone halothane-nitrous oxide anaesthesia compared to ketamine-xylazine on the DC recorded dog electroretinogram, *ACTA vet. scand.* 29 (1):23 (1988).

27. B. Kommonen, C. Raitta, Electroretinography in Labradors retrievers given ketamine-xylazine anaesthesia. *Am. J. Vet. Res.* 48 (9):125 (1987).

28. G.H.M. van Lith, Quantitative evaluation of the electroretinogram, *Ophthalmologica, Basel.* 182:218 (1981).

29. V. Logeais, L'électrorétinographie: principe, matériel et application chez le chien, Th. Med. Vet, Nantes (1986).

30. O. Loget, L'électrophysiologie sensorielle oculaire chez les animaux de laboratoire. Th. Med. Vet, Nantes (1990).

31. H. Parry, Degeneration of the dog retina : I, *Br J. Ophthalmol.* 37:487 (1953).

32. H. Parry, Degeneration of the dog retina : II, *Br J. Ophthalmol.* 38:653 (1954).

33. H. Parry, Degeneration of the dog retina : III, *Br J. Ophthalmol.* 39:29 (1955).

34. H. Parry, K. Tansley, L.C. Thomson, The ERG in normal dog, *J. Physiol.* 115:47 (1951).

35. H. Parry, K. Tansley, L.C. Thomson, The ERG in the dog, *J. Physiol.* 120:28 (1951).

36. H. Parry, K. Tansley, L.C. Thomson, ERG during the development of hereditary retinal degeneration in the dog, *Br.- J. Ophthalmol.* 39:349 (1955).

37. G. Perdriel, Les indications actuelles de l'électrorétinographie. *Clin. Ophthalmol.* 1:31 (1968).

38. C. Raitta, V. Karhunen, A.M. Seppalaienen, M. Naukarinen, Changes in the electroretinogram and visual evoked potential during anaesthesia, *Graefes Arch. Klin. Exp. Ophthalmol.* 221:139 (1979).

39. J. Real Brunette, G. Lafond, ERG responses of rods and cones during dark adaptation, *Canad. J. Ophthalm.* 13:186 (1978).

40. M. Roze, Valeur de l'électrorétinographie en ophtalomogie canine, *Pratique médicale et chirurgicale de l'animal de compagnie.* 2:98 (1987).

41. L.F. Rubin, Clinical electroretinography in dogs. *J.A.V.M.A.* 151 (11):1456 (1967).

42. H. Sarauh, Y. Grall, J. Keller, B. Nou, J.J. Bertrand, Intérêt clinique de l'étude des ERG, *Ann. Oculist (Paris).* 207 (3):201 (1974).

43. D. Sasovets, Ketamine hydrochloride: an effective general anaesthetic for use in electroretinography. *Ann. Ophthalmol.* 10:1510 (1978).

44. S. Sato, S. Sugimoto, T. Ando, H. Miyajima, S. Chiba, A procedure for recording ERG and VEP in conscious dogs, *J. Pharm. Meth.* 8:173 (1982).

45. U. Schaeppi, F. Liverani, Procedure for routine electroretinography (ERG) in dogs, *Agents and actions.* 7 (3):347 (1977).

46. R. Sicault, L'ERG dans les opacités des milieux, *Revue Chibret.* 60:31 (1969).

47. A. Stute, J.G.H. Schmidt, E. Xeber, On the effect of urethane and halothane on the ERG of rats. *Docum. Ophthal. Proc. Ser.* 15:13 (1877).

48. C. Tashiro, A. Muranishi, I. Gomyo, T. Mashimo, K. Tomi, I. Yoshiya, Electroretinogram as a possible monitor of anaesthetic depth. *Graefe's Arch. Clin. Exp. Ophthalmol.* 224:473 (1986).

49. M. Wasserschaff, J.G.H. Schmidt, Electroretinographic response to the addition of nitrous oxide to halothane in rats, *Doc. Ophthal.* 64:347 (1986).

50. A. Wirth, G. Tota, A. Vagelli, The effect of fluothan anaesthesia on the electroretinogram of the rabbit, *in*: "7th ISERG Symph. Istanbul". 289:292 (1969).

EXPERIMENTAL STUDY OF THE RETINAL TOXICITY OF IRON AFTER VITREOUS HEMORRHAGE

Wei-Jia Nie and Xiao-Fang Zhang

Department of Ophthalmology
First Teaching Hospital
Henan Medical University
Zhengzhou 450052, Henan
P.R. China

INTRODUCTION

Vitreous hemorrhage is a frequent complication of several ocular diseases. It is known that the ocular toxicity of iron has been demonstrated.[1,2] Since a significant amount of iron is stored in erythrocytes, iron released by breakdown of red cells after vitreous hemorrhage could be a potential source of toxicity for the retina. To determine the toxic effect of vitreous hemorrhage on retina, the concentration of iron in intraocular fluids and the morphological change of the retina and ERGs were investigated experimentally.

MATERIALS AND METHODS

New Zealand white rabbits (2-2.5 Kg) were anesthetized with an intravenously administered 3% sodium pentobarbital (30 mg/Kg of body weight). Both eyes of each rabbit were dilated with 1% cyclopentolate and 10% phenylephrine. Using a 28-gauge needle on a 1.0 ml syringe, 0.2 ml of aqueous humor was removed bilateraly. The vitreous of the left eye was injected with 0.2 ml of whole blood from the ear vein at the pars plana in the supperior temporal quadrant. The right eye received 0.2 ml of sterile normal saline. We monitored intraocular pressures by Shiøtz tonometry immediately after each injection.

Group 1: Both eyes from each animal were enucleated immediately after death and aspirated intraocular fluids that the iron was determined with AAS (atomic absorption spectrophotometer) as previously decribed.[3]

Group 2: Both eyes from each, animal were enucleated immediately after death and placed directly into 2.5% glutaraldehyde in phosphate buffer (pH 7.4) for transmission electron microscopy.

Group 3: ERGs were performed after the retina being examined with B-scan before injection and at 2, 7, 14 and 28 days after injection.

RESULTS

Changes of iron concentration in aqueous and vitreous humor were followed at different intervals. The iron concentration of the aqueous and vitreous humor was elevated at 2 days, increased to a peak level at 7 days and then decreased until 28 days that the level indicates significantly different from control eyes (Table 1).

Table 1. The Fe concentration of intraocular fluids.

Samples	Time (day)	No.	Fe concentration[1] (mean $\pm$ SE, ug/ml)
Aqueous	2	6	0.252 ± 0.024
Humor	7	6	0.068 ± 0.085
	14	6	0.250 ± 0.654
	28	6	0.283 ± 0.142
Vitreous	2	6	1.136 ± 0.043
	7	6	2.846 ± 0.254
	14	6	1.115 ± 0.083
	28	6	0.788 ± 0.068

[1]Fe concentration of the left eye minus Fe concentration of the right eye in each rabbit. Fe concentration indicates significant different ($P < 0.05$) from control eye at 2, 7, 14 and 28 days.

The eye enucleated at 2 days after injection displayed that no retinal changes were evident. The eye enucleated at 7 days showed macrophage containing numerous ingested erythrocytes, mitochondrion vacuoles degeneration of the inner segment and lameller disruption of the outer segment of photoreceptor cells. Degenerative changes of the inner and outer segments become more serious (Figure 1-3).

The ERG of the left eyes at 7 days showed greatly decreased a-wave and b-wave after injection. Blood-injected eyes had marked reduced a-wave and b-wave at 28 days after injection. It is found that reduction in a-wave exceeded the decrease in b-wave (Figure 4).

DISCUSSION

Under normal physiological condition, intraocular fluids have Fe-binding proteins with high affinity for Fe and unsaturated capacity. The residual binding capacity is useful for scavenging Fe, which arises from red blood cell death. During vitreous hemorrhage, our experiment indicated that concentration of iron in intraocular fluids exceed Fe-binding proteins with affinity for Fe. Iron can catalyze the formation of tissue damaging radicals, that can lead to peroxidation of lipids and other cellar macromolecules.[4] Because photoreceptor outer and inner segments are rich in polyunsaturated fatty acids, they are susceptible to lipid oxidation, the peroxidation of lipids resulted in retinal damage.

Doly[5] had shown that red blood cells are lysed in the vitreous medium, hemoglobin are broken down and iron released migrates from the vitreous to the retina. It is also demonstrated that hemoglobinic iron has a significant toxicity on the retina. We also confirm this fact.

The ERG changes correlated well with histologically evident damage. These changes were not due to the effect of the opaque blood because the ERG did not recover after vitrectomy.[6] Thus, ERG may be significant in demonstrating a blood-induced toxic effect on the retina.

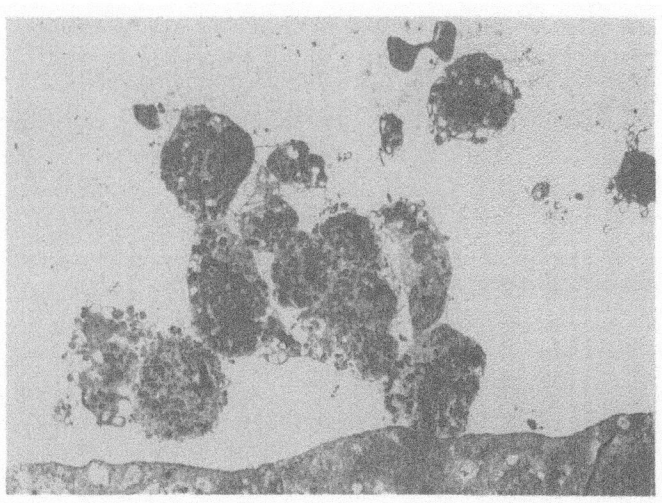

Figure 1. Macrophage containing numerous injested erythrocytes 7 days after injection (x1000).

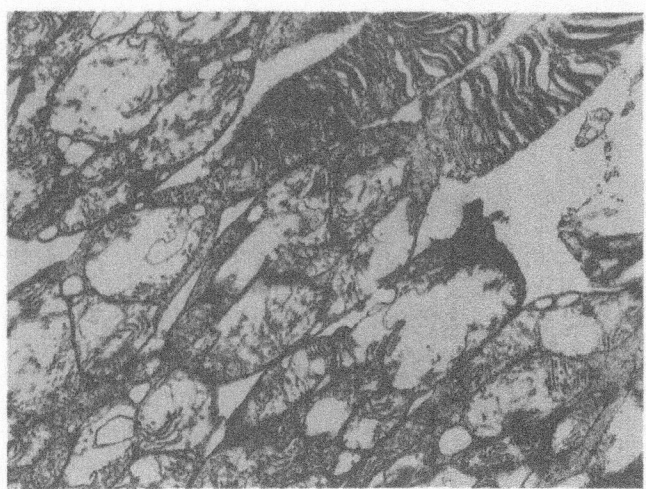

Figure 2. The retina showing lamellar disruption of outer segment and vacuolar degeneration of inner segment of the photoreceptor cells, 14 days after injection (x5000).

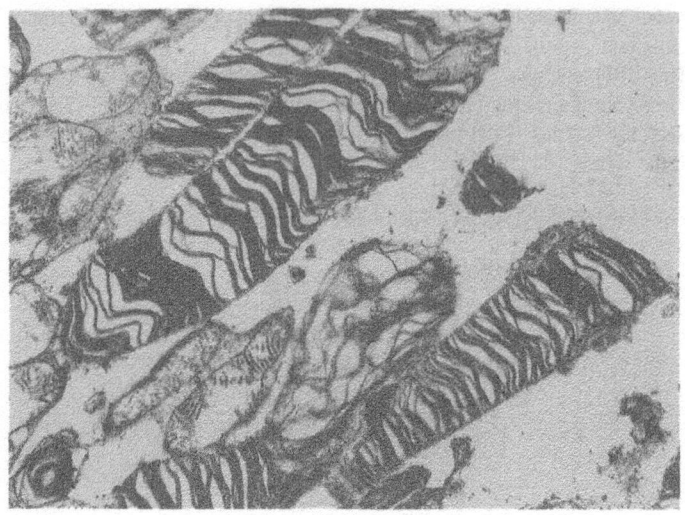

Figure 3. The retina showing lamellar disruption of outer segment and vacuolar degeneration of inner segment of the photoreceptor cells, 28 days after injection (x7500).

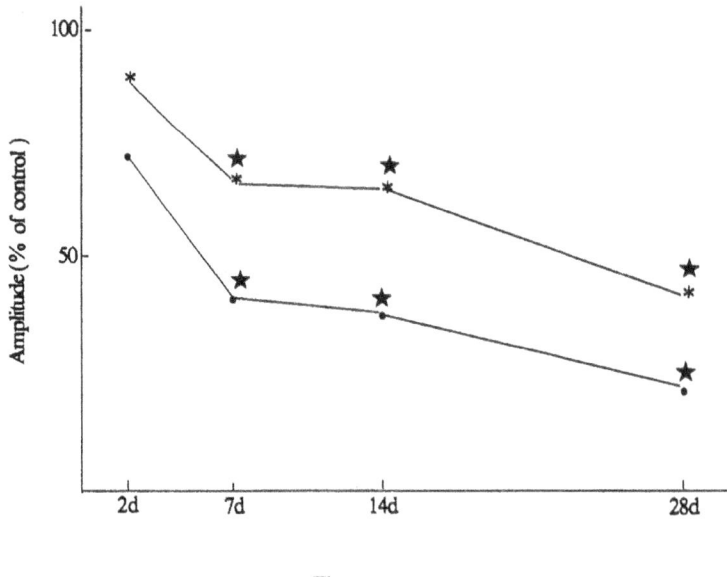

Figure 4. Changes in amplitude in the a-wave (●—●) and the b-wave (*— *). Each point is the mean of six rabbits. Star (★) indicates significantly different (P < 0.05) from ERG before injection.

REFERENCES

1.   P.A. Cibis and T. Yamashita, Experimental aspects of ocular sideresis and hemosiderosis, *Am J Ophthalmol.* 48:465(1959).

2.   L. Masciulli, D.R. Anderson and S. Charles, Experimental ocular sidersis in the squirrel monkey, *Am J Ophthahnol.* 74:638(1972).

3.   W.J. Nie, X.F. Zhang and L. Wang, Method for determination of iron in intraocular fluids with the graphite furnace, *J Henan Med Univ.* 29:77(1994).

4.   J.M.C. Gutteridge, Tissue damage by oxd-radicals: the possible involvement of iron and copper complexs, *Med Biol.* 62:101(1984).

5.   M. Doly, B. Bonhomme and J.C. Vennat, Experimental study of the retinal toxicity of hemoglobinic iron, *Ophthalmic Res.* 18:21(1986).

6.   E.G. Buckley, J.A. Salisbury and R. Machemer, Is blood toxicity to the retina reversible, *Surg Forum.* 31:490(1980).

RETINAL TOLERANCE OF INTRAVITREAL LOW-MOLECULAR-WEIGHT HEPARIN, COLCHICINE OR INTERFERON β DETERMINED BY EYE-CUP ERG IN ALBINO RABBITS

Yohko Yamashita, Kiyofumi Mochizuki, Hiroyuki Sakai,
Makoto Torisaki and Jhoji Tanabe

Department of Ophthalmology,
Kanazawa University School of Medicine
13-1 Takara-machi, Kanazawa, 920 Japan

ABSTRACT

We investigated the effects of the following drugs on the eye-cup electroretinogram in albino rabbits: low-molecular-weight heparin to treat inflammation, colchicine to prevent postoperative cellular proliferation in the vitreous cavity and interferon β for antiviral treatment . The a- and b-waves and the oscillatory potentials were unchanged during perfusion with 5 and 20 IU/ml low-molecular-weight heparin, 25 and 50 µg/ml colchicine or 5,000 and 10,000 IU/ml interferon β. Potential clinical intravitreal use of low-molecular-weight heparin and interferon β was suggested, respectively, for prophylaxis of postoperative intraocular fibrin reactions and proliferative vitreoretinopathy, and to treat viral retinitis.

INTRODUCTION

Despite the recent development of microsurgical techniques, intraocular surgery can still fail because of postoperative complications, such as fibrin formation and proliferative vitreoretinopathy (PVR). Fibrin formation tends to be more severe in eyes with increased vascular permeability after vitrectomy in endophthalmitis, proliferative diabetic retinopathy or PVR. Fibrin, the end product of the blood coagulation cascade, is formed by the conversion of fibrinogen to fibrin with thrombin. A family of heparin-related compounds affects intraocular coagulation and cellular activities, and may be potentially useful to treat patients undergoing vitreoretinal surgery. PVR is characterized by the formation of cellular membranes both on the retinal surface and in the vitreous. Colchicine is a potent inhibitor of retinal pigment epithelium (RPE) cell, astrocyte and fibroblast migration that acts by stopping microtubular metabolism[1]. Intravitreal colchicine has been evaluated to determine its ability to prevent cellular proliferation in the vitreous[2]. Intraocular drug therapy can also be useful to treat viral retinitis such as acute retinal necrosis, herpes simplex viral retinitis and cytomegalovirus retinitis. Interferon has been used to treat intraocular viral infection[3] and intraocular neoplasms[4,5]. In the present study, we investigated the retinal effects of three compounds, low-molecular-weight heparin, colchicine and interferon β, by the eye-cup electroretinography in albino rabbits, and evaluated the potential for intravitreal use of these drugs.

MATERIALS AND METHODS

Low-molecular-weight heparin (Fragmin®, Kissei Pharmaceutical Co., Ltd., Matsumoto, Japan), colchicine (Sigma Chemical Co., St. Louis, MO, USA) and interferon β (Feron®, Toray Industries, Inc., Tokyo, Japan) were used.

One eye each of 30 albino rabbits weighing 2.0 - 3.5 kg was used. After general anesthesia was induced by an intramuscular injection of 50 mg ketamine hydrochloride, the eyes were enucleated after dark adaptation longer than 24 hours. The posterior half of the eye-cup, including the retina, the choroid and the sclera, was mounted between two chambers, the volume of which was 100 ml, and perfused at 25 ml/min with a control solution (Nagayama's solution: 119.50 mM NaCl, 3.60 mM KCl, 1.15 mM $CaCl_2$, 1.06 mM $MgSO_4$, 26.00 mM glucose, 25.10 mM $NaHCO_3$ and 3.00 mM NaH_2PO_4). The temperature and pH of the perfusing solution were maintained at 31 ± 1 °C and 8.0-8.1, respectively. The electroretinogram (ERG) was recorded by a pair of Ag-AgCl electrodes (NS-type, Nihon Kohden, Tokyo, Japan) placed in the two chambers. The a- and b-waves and the oscillatory potentials (OPs) of the ERG were evoked by a rectangular stimulus light of 3.5×10^2 lux at the retina with a 200-msec duration. The ERG was amplified by an alternating current amplifier (Polygraph type 366, Nihondenki San-Ei, Tokyo, Japan) with a time constant of 0.3 second for the a- and b-waves and 0.003 second for the OPs. A control ERG was recorded after dark adaptation of 30 minutes during perfusion of the control solution, followed by 15 minutes of perfusion of test solutions containing 5 and 20 IU/ml of low-molecular-weight heparin, 25 and 50 μg/ml colchicine, or 5,000 and 10,000 IU/ml of interferon β. Five eyes were used with each concentration. The drug-treated eye-cup then was perfused with the control solution for 30 minutes before the final control ERG was recorded to evaluate the reversibility of the ERG changes.

The amplitude and peak latency of the a- and b-waves and the OPs were expressed as the percentage of the control ERG values during the initial perfusion of the control solution. Statistical analysis of the ERG changes was done with the Student's t -test (paired), with $p < 0.05$ indicating a significant difference.

RESULTS

1. Low-molecular-weight heparin

Similar results were obtained in each of the five eyes with either concentration. The amplitude and peak latency of the a- and b-waves and the OPs were not significantly changed by perfusing the eye-cups with 5 or 20 IU/ml concentrations of low-molecular-weight heparin (Figs. 1 and 2).

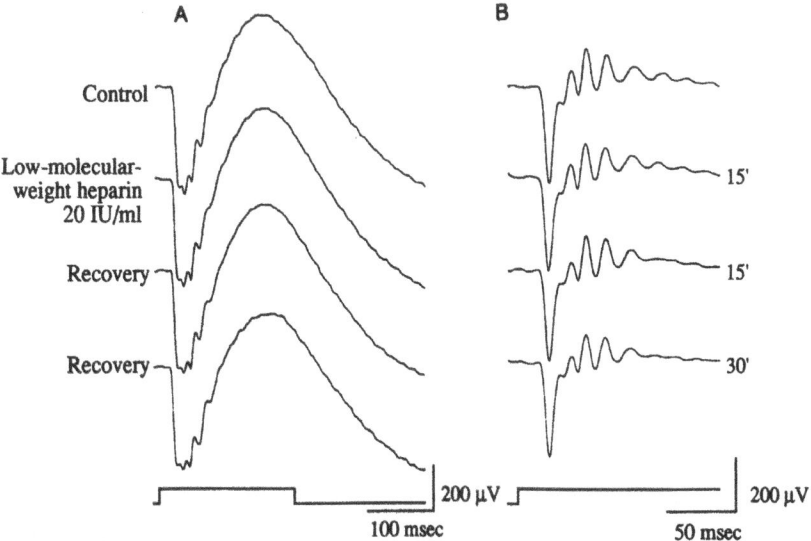

Figure 1. Effects of 20 IU/ml low-molecular-weight heparin on the eye-cup ERG of the albino rabbit. The uppermost tracing shows responses during the initial perfusion with the control solution (Nagayama's solution). The second tracing from the top shows responses during perfusion with a solution containing low-molecular-weight heparin. The third and fourth tracings show responses after low-molecular-weight heparin was washed out by perfusion with Nagayama's solution. Numerals on the right indicate the time (minutes) after onset of perfusion with Nagayama's solution or a solution containing low-molecular-weight heparin. The amplifier time constants were 0.3 second in A and 0.003 second in B.

2. Colchicine

Similar results were obtained in each of the five eyes with either concentration. The amplitude and peak latency of the a- and b-waves and the OPs of the eye-cup ERG were not significantly changed by perfusing 25 or 50 μg/ml colchicine (Fig. 3).

3. Interferon β

Similar results were obtained in each of the five eyes with either concentration. No significant changes were observed in the amplitude or peak latency of the a- and b-waves or the OPs of the ERG during perfusion with 5,000 or 10,000 IU/ml interferon β (Fig. 4).

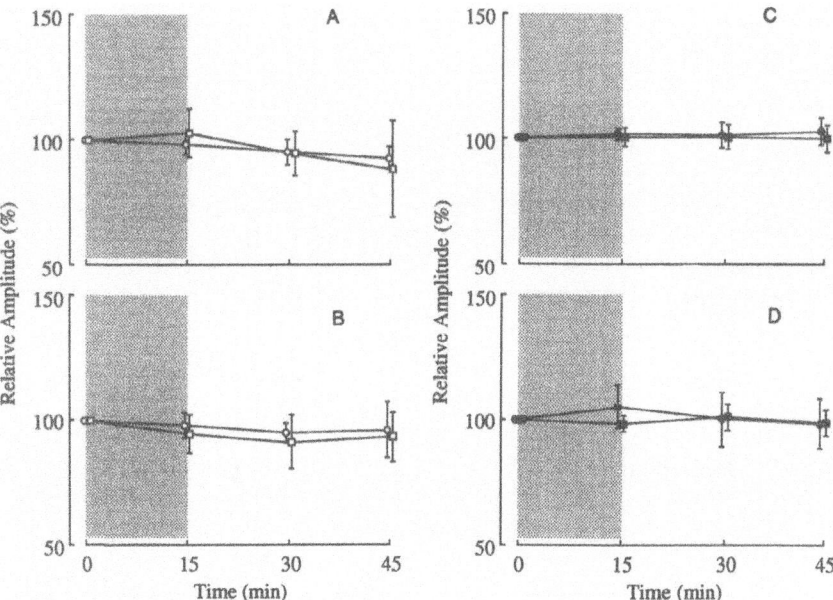

Figure 2. Changes in amplitude of the b-wave (A) and the second peak (O₂) of the OPs (B) by perfusing the eye-cups of albino rabbits with solutions containing low-molecular-weight heparin. ○, 5 IU/ml; ☐, 20 IU/ml. The amplitude values obtained during perfusion with solutions containing low-molecular-weight heparin are expressed as percentages of those obtained at the end of the initial perfusion of the control solution (time 0), (tested solution/control solution) x 100 (%), and plotted against time after onset of perfusion with the solution containing low-molecular-weight heparin. The shaded areas indicate the period of perfusion of the solutions containing low-molecular-weight heparin. Each point and vertical bar represent the mean ± SD.

Figure 3. Changes in amplitude of the a- (C) and b-waves (D) by perfusing the eye-cups of albino rabbits with a colchicine-containing solution. ●, 25 μg/ml; ■, 50 μg/ml. Other conditions were the same as in Fig. 2.

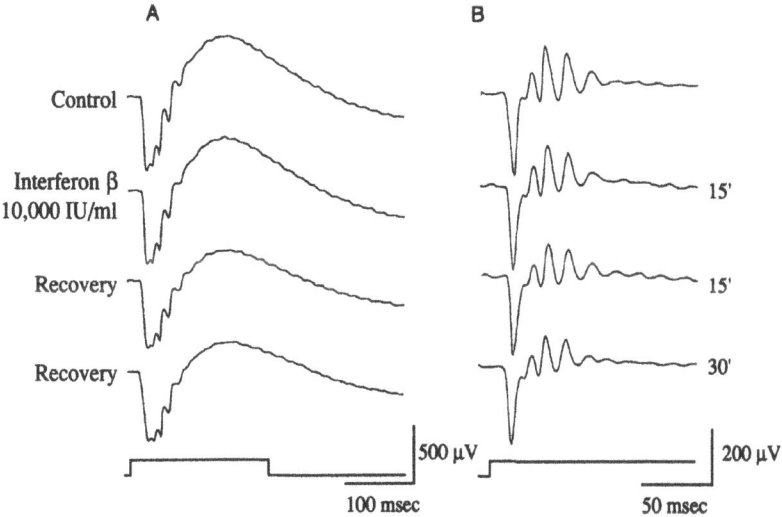

Figure 4. Effects of 10,000 IU/ml interferon β on the eye-cup ERG of the albino rabbit. The second tracing from the top shows responses during perfusion for 15 minutes with a solution containing interferon β. Other conditions were the same as in Fig. 1.

DISCUSSION

Native heparin is a long-chain glycosaminoglycan consisting of alternating *N*-acetylglucosamine and glucuronic acid residues. The average molecular weight of native heparin is 12,000 to 15,000 daltons (range, 6,000 to 25,000 daltons). Low-molecular-weight heparin, a derivative of native heparin, has an average molecular weight of 5,000 daltons. The heparin derivatives with a molecular weight of less than 5,000 daltons retain the ability to catalyze factor Xa degradation but do not affect thrombin activity or prolong the activated partial thromboplastin time of plasma, a test for the survival time of thrombin in plasma[6]. Therefore, low-molecular-weight heparins are thought to cause fewer hemorrhages than native preparations when used in equal antithrombotic concentrations[6].

Heparin and low-molecular-weight heparin may be used during intraocular surgery to inhibit fibrin formation or for prophylaxis of PVR by stopping DNA and RNA synthesis[7]. Systemic administration of heparin during vitrectomy may reduce postoperative fibrin formation, but increase intraoperative bleeding[8]. Intraocular use of low-molecular-weight heparin for prophylaxis of fibrin formation has been evaluated. Iverson et al[9] reported that intraocular infusion of 5 IU/ml low-molecular-weight heparin during lensectomy, vitrectomy, and retinotomy inhibited intraocular fibrin formation in the rabbit model. Kondo et al[10] showed that intraocular fibrin formation was significantly reduced in rabbit eyes infused with a solution containing 5 IU/ml of low-molecular-weight heparin during extracapsular cataract extraction. In our study, the eye-cup ERG remained unchanged during perfusion with 5 IU/ml and 20 IU/ml low-molecular-weight heparin. Although further investigation is required in primates and humans to determine the safe and effective concentration, low-molecular-weight heparin may be useful as a pharmacologic agent to prevent and treat fibrin formation after intraocular surgery.

Interferon has been used to treat intraocular viral infection and intraocular malignant neoplasms. Interferon has recently been used to treat choroidal neovascular membranes in age-related macular degeneration[11] Antiviral effects of interferon alone are not sufficiently potent. Interferon, however, can be effective when used in combination with antiviral drugs such as acyclovir or ganciclovir[3]. The antitumor properties of interferon through natural killer cells in retinoblastoma[4] or intraocular melanoma[5] were reported. An effective therapeutic intraocular concentration is difficult to attain in most of systemically-applied drugs. Further, systemic use of interferon may cause adverse effects such as high fever or general malaise. Therefore, an intravitreal injection and intravitreal irrigation during vitrectomy may be possible routes to treat intraocular viral infection. Peyman and associates [12-15] investigated the electrophysiologic and histologic effects of intraocular interferon on the retina. They reported that no retinal toxicity was observed with a single intravitreal injection of 42,000 IU/0.1 ml interferon α[13], 640,000 IU/0.1 ml interferon α-2a[14], or 166,600 IU/0.1 ml interferon β[12] in albino rabbits. In the present study, the perfusion of 10,000 IU/ml interferon β in the eye-cups of the albino rabbits did not change the ERG. If 166,600 IU interferon β, a nontoxic intravitreal dose[12], evenly diffuses in the rabbit vitreous cavity, the concentration in the vitreous would be approximately 98,000 IU/ml. Although further *in vivo* studies have to be conducted, intravitreal irrigation with 5,000 to 10,000 IU/ml interferon β may be acceptable to treat intraocular viral infections.

Colchicine is neurotoxic and causes depolymerization of microtubules by binding to tubulin, the protein subunit of microtubules. Lemor et al[1] reported that 10^{-7} mol/l colchicine inhibited cell migration in 44% of RPE cells, 46% of astrocytes and 93% of fibroblasts. Colchicine administered at very low concentrations may inhibit the proliferation and migration of cells involved in PVR, and may be useful in the management of PVR. Oral administration of colchicine reduced the incidence and severity of traction retinal detachment in an animal model[2], but not in the human[16]. Because oral administration of colchicine often causes adverse effects in hematogenous organs, genitalia, liver or kidney, topical use including intravitreal injection and intravitreal irrigation during vitrectomy would be preferable. Karlsson et al[17] reported that an intravitreal injection of 2.5 μg colchicine induced profound effects on the axonal transport of protein and morphologic changes in the retinal ganglion cells in albino rabbits. Vaccarezza et al[18] observed marked alterations in several feline retinal structures caused by an intravitreal injection of 20 μg colchicine. Davidson et al[19] observed abnormal structures in the retinal ganglion cells and photoreceptors after an intravitreal injection of as little as 1 μg of colchicine in the monkey. The retina appears to be more vulnerable to intravitreal colchicine in the monkey than in some lower animals[19]. According to these reports, an intravitreal injection of colchicine may be toxic to ocular tissues even at low doses. Although 25 and 50 μg/ml colchicine perfusion did not change the eye-cup ERG of the albino rabbits in the present study, further *in vivo* trials must be performed to determine the safe and effective intravitreal concentrations of colchicine for clinical use.

Acknowledgments

We thank Prof. K. Kawasaki for his encouragement and advice with the manuscript. We also thank Kissei Pharmaceutical Co., Ltd. for supplying low-molecular-weight heparin and Daiichi Pharmaceutical Co., Ltd. for supplying interferon β.

REFERENCES

1. M. Lemor, S. de Bustros, and B. M. Glaser, Low-dose colchicine inhibits astrocyte, fibroblast, and retinal pigment epithelial cell migration and proliferation, *Arch. Ophthalmol.* 104: 1223 (1986).
2. M. Lemor, J. H. Jeo, and B. M. Glaser, Oral colchicine for the treatment of experimental traction retinal detachment, *Arch. Ophthalmol.* 104: 1226 (1986).
3. N. Ishida, Strategies for antiviral chemotherapy, *Atarashii Ganka* 9: 173 (1992).
4. Y. Ohashi, T. Sasabe, T. Nishida, and R. Manabe, Natural killer cells kill human retinoblastma cells, *Jpn. J. Ophthalmol.* 28: 370 (1984).
5. T. Yokoyama, O. Yoshie, H. Aso, T. Ebina, N. Ishida, and K. Mizuno, Role of natural killer cells in intraocular melanoma metastasis, *Invest. Ophthalmol. Vis. Sci.* 27: 516 (1986).
6. S. Hamano, M. Kinukawa, H. Komatsu, S. Ikeda, and N. Sakuragawa, Effects of low molecular weight heparin (FR-860) on coagulative and fibrinolytic activities, *Folia Pharmacol. Japon* 94: 243 (1989).
7. M. S. Blumenkranz, M. K. Hartzer, and D. Iverson, An overview of potential applications of heparin in vitreoretinal surgery, *Retina* 12: S71 (1992).
8. R. N. Johnson, and G. Blankenship, A prospective, randomized, clinical trial of heparin therapy for postoperative intraocular fibrin, *Ophthalmology* 95: 312 (1988).
9. D. A. Iverson, H. Katsura, M. K. Hartzer, and M. S. Blumenkranz, Inhibition of intraocular fibrin formation following infusion of low-molecular-weight heparin during vitrectomy, *Arch. Ophthalmol.* 109: 405 (1991).
10. H. Kondo, H. Hayashi, and K. Oshima, Fibrin prophylaxis with low molecular weight heparin during intraocular surgery, *Jpn. J. Ophthalmic Surg.* 6: 597 (1993).
11. J. N. P. Kirkpatrick, A. D. Dick, and J. V. Forrester, Clinical experience with interferon alfa-2a for exudative age-related macular degeneration, *Br. J. Ophthalmol.* 77: 766 (1993).
12. S. Vegh, J. Vernot, G. A. Peyman, and R. Fiscella, Toxicity of intravitreal interferon, *Ophthalmic Surg.* 17: 103 (1986).
13. S. K. Dharma, G. A. Peyman, J. Vernot, and R. Fiscella, Toxicity of intravitreally administered alpha-interferon, *Ophthalmic Surg.* 18: 51 (1987).
14. M. A. Karaçorlu, G. A. Peyman, S. Cruz, K. F. Soike, Lack of toxicity of intravitreally administered interferon alpha-2a, *Ophthalmic Surg.* 23: 833 (1992).
15. K. Ohki, G. A. Peyman, A. Candel, and R. Fiscella, Toxicity of intravitreal interferon in combination with acyclovir after lensectomy and vitrectomy, *Folia Ophthalmol. Jpn.* 38: 158 (1987).
16. D. H. Berman and G. M. Gombos, Proliferative vitreoretinopathy: Does oral low-dose colchicine have an inhibitory effect? A controlled study in humans, *Ophthalmic Surg.* 20: 268 (1989).
17. J. O. Karlsson, H. A. Hansson, and J. Sjöstrand, Effect of colchicine on axonal transport and morphology of retinal ganglion cells, *Z. Zellforsch.* 115: 265 (1971).
18. O. L. Vaccarezza, E. Pasqualini, and J. P. Saavedra, Retinal alterations induced by intravitreous colchicine, *Virchows Arch. Abt. B Zellpath.* 12: 159 (1973).
19. C. Davidson, W. R. Green, and V. G. Wong, Retinal atrophy induced by intravitreous colchicine, *Invest. Ophthalmol. Vis. Sci.* 24: 301 (1983).

NORMAL ERG ON RHESUS MONKEYS (Macaca mulatta) :
PRELIMINARY RESULTS OF A TECHNIC
USING SUBCUTANEOUS ELECTRODES

Serge G. Rosolen,[1] Hugues Malecki,[2] and Catherine Vandermercken [3]

[1] Clinique Vétérinaire, 119 Boulevard Voltaire, 92600 Asnières, France
[2] Centre d'Etudes et de Recherches de Médecine Aérospatiale, BP 73
    91220 Brétigny-sur-Orge, France
[3] Institut Technique d'Etude du Médicament, 93 avenue de Fontainebleau
    94276 Le Kremlin-Bicêtre Cedex, France

INTRODUCTION

The electroretinogram (ERG) is composed of responses of many different retinal cell types. Many studies have been made to separate the ERG into components and to link different components to different retinal structures. In theese studies, authors used microelectrodes and intact eyes of laboratory animals (Heynen and van Norren, 1985). However, in most clinical situations or during the course of toxicity studies, this technic is not suitable because it does not allow long-term studies on the same animal. Our first goal was to find a technic that permit to record global ERGs from the same animal at different times.

Meanwhile, it is well recognized that it is difficult to obtain electroretinographic samples in awake primates using a classical type of recording electrodes, because of difficulties in keeping a contact lens electrode in constant contact with the cornea (Satoh et al., 1980). However, various types of contact lens electrodes have been evaluated and improved for ERGs examination in tranquilized primates (Buist and Heywood, 1982) or in conscious dogs (Sato et al., 1982). Further, a comparison of electroretonograms recorded with contact lens versus needle electrode has been made in anesthetized dogs (Steiss et al., 1992). Our second goal was to obtain ERGs from tranquilized macaques using subcutaneous electrodes, because these electrodes seemed to us better adapted for use in conscious primates.

In this paper we report an experiment from the CERMA on a technic using subcutaneous electrodes that permit ERG recording without contact with the eyeballs. Our aims were to assess a sampling and recording technic of a global electroretinogram by flash, in rhesus monkeys, and to get basic data for this population of macaques. In order to validate the technic, basic requirements were the inocuousness of the technic, its reliability and reproducibility, the ease of use and to put the capturing device into position, the time taken to test one animal, and the absence of measuring artefact.

MATERIALS AND METHODS

Electroretinography was carried out on 48, clinicaly normal captive-breed rhesus monkeys (*Macaca mulatta*), of both sexes (15 females and 33 males). The age of animals ranged from 2 months to 18 years and their weights were between 0.9 and 16.7 kg. The animals were housed singly and light/dark cycles for males were established on a 16/8 ratio. The light/dark cycles for females were based on a 12/12 ratio. The protocol of this experiment has been reviewed by the veterinary unit of the CERMA.

Monkeys were tranquilized with ketamine hydrochloride (Imalgène 1000, Rhône Mérieux, Lyon, France), 10 mg/kg of body weight, IM. Pupils were dilated with tropicamide (Mydriaticum, MSD-Chibret, Paris, France) and phenylephrine (Néosynéphrine 10% Chibret, MSD-Chibret, Paris, France), 20 minutes before recording. The electrodes were put into position after a minimum of 15 minutes of dark adaptation. The animals were then placed in a dark room.

The recordinf electrodes consisted of needle electrodes placed subcutaneously (0.2 mm cross section). A neutral electrode was placed in the occipital area, then two reference electrodes were inserted at the ear-temple junction. The two active electrodes were inserted in the lower eyelids.

The monitoring and recording system (SPECTRAL, SEREME Corp. Nimes, France), included an analysis time of 250 ms. The photostimulator was used to present 30 light flash stimuli of 10 msec duration, with a 1 flash per second frequency.

Three series of flashes were carried out with blue light (blue filter Wratten 440 nm) white light (250 cd/m^2) and red light (red interferential 635 nm). The stimulator was placed about 20 cm in the front of the animal's face (stimulation field $> 30°$). A and B wave latency and amplitude were measured by adding steady state phase ERGs.

Statistical analysis: differences among group means (age, sex, laterality) are currently analysed using t test and analysis of variance (ANOVA), with a significance level of $p < 0.05$.

RESULTS

Practical assessment

Ten minutes were necessary to carry out the positioning of the electrodes and the trhee series of flashing stimulations.Additional sedation was not required. One case of a lower eyelid haematoma was observed 12 hours later, which was reduced in 24 hours using classical medicines.

Global description of ERGs

The flash ERFG steady state was early observed after 2 or 3 flashes. A and B waves were distinct in the 3 light stimulations. B1 and B2 waves were somtimes visible with the white light stimuli. Proximity-induced artefacts, as interference, were reduced although electrodes leads were 30 cm long. The artefacts due to the animals movements were rare and never superimposed within an A-B complex. We never observed artefact linked to eyelid fluttering. High voltage B-waves were somtimes out of range of the monitoring system.

Morphological and arthmetical analysis

A-waves were observed as sharp-peaked and were split into two parts 15% of the time. B-waves had domed peaks during blue-light stimulations, showing a predominance of B2-wave. They had a sharp-peaks followed by a rounded peak with red-light stimulations (B1-B2 complex). B-complex was similar with white-light flashes, with a round-peaked B2 wave. The polarity values ratio of the A-B complex distinguished a positive ERG with blue-light flashes, a negative or equalized ERG with white-light flashes and a positive or overpositive ERG with red-light flashes.

Variation factors

Studies of the effects of sex and age on ERGs are in progress. Results are presented in the following table.

Table 1. Description of measured parameters of ERGs (n=48)

Stimulation colour	Measured parameter	Means (standard dev.) msec. or µV	Min.	Max.
white	A-wave latency	14.12 (2.34)	11	21
	A-wave amplitude	-27.74 (5.99)	-36	-11
	B-wave latency	34.17 (1.62)	30	37
	B-wave amplitude	23.12 (10.06)	-2	40
blue	A-wave latency	16.50 (1.50)	13	19
	A-wave amplitude	-19.91 (7.56)	-34	-6
	B-wave latency	37.17 (2.65)	33	46
	B-wave amplitude	33.99 (5.86)	15	40
red	A-wave latency	16.58 (2.58)	10	24
	A-wave amplitude	-10.72 (4.80)	-21	-3
	B-wave latency	39.67 (3.43)	32	52
	B-wave amplitude	30.29 (6.41)	16	39

DISCUSSION-CONCLUSION

In this study, a simple and brief technique provided results comparable to published data dependent upon to dark-adapted state. Morphological aspects of ERGs using subcutaneous electrodes are similar to ERGs using corneal lens electrodes. It seems that the effects of mechanical and environmental variables are minimized in this procedure. Artefacts seems to have a negligible occurrence.

The procedure is adapted from the recommendations for standardization issued by the ISCEV (Marmor et al., 1989). ERGs obtained with blue-light flashes (scotopic ERG) showed a predominance of B2-wave and a shark-peak A wave. ERGs with red-light flashes are photo-scotopic mixed flash ERGs. On dark-adapted eyes, ERG with white flashes is a mixed response. Procedural alterations are required to obtain a photopic flash ERG.

Results of this study show the potential of the technic as an easy tool in clinical diagnosis. It seems further possible to use this technic in pharmacological an toxicological studies. However additional study may be required to define optimal electrodes placement.

Acknowledgments

This study was supported by the Société Française d'Etudes et de Recherches en Ophtalmologie Vétérinaire (SFEROV), Fondation Ophtalmologique A.de Rothschild, 25-29 rue Manin, 75940 Paris Cedex 19, France.

REFERENCES

Buist, D.P., and Heywood, R., 1982, A standardized procedure for electroretinographic examination of rhesus monkeys (*Macaca mulatta*), *Lab. Anim. Sci.*, 32(1):91-93.

Heynen, H., and van Norren, D., 1985, Origin of electroretinogram in the intact macaque eye- 1. Principal component analysis, *Vision Res.*, 25(5):697-707.

Marmor, M.F., Arden, G.B., Nisson, S., Zrenner, E., 1989, Clinical standard for ERG, *Arch. Ophthalmol.*, 107:816-819.

Sato, S., Sugimoto, S., and Chiba, S., 1982, A procedure for recording electroretinogram and visual evoked potential in conscious dogs. *J. Pharmacol. Methods*, 8:173-181.

Satoh, H., Fukuda, N., Kuriki, H., Maki, Y., Nomura, M., Saji, Y., and Nagawa, Y., 1980, A procedure for recording electroretinogram (ERG) in conscious monkeys, and effect of some drugs (author's transl.), *Nippon Yakurigaku Zasshi*, 76(7): 581-594.

Steiss, J.E., Storrs, D.P., and Wright, J.C., 1992, Comparisons of electroretinograms recorded with a contact lens versus needle electrode in clinicaly normal dogs, *Prog. Vet. & Compar. Ophthalmol.*, 2(4):143-146.

EFFECTS OF QUININE
ON THE ELECTRORETINOGRAM OF THE BEAGLE DOG

Olivier Loget[1] and Gérard Saint-Macary[2]

[1]Pharmakon Europe
Domaine des Oncins - BP 0118
69593 L'Arbresle Cédex
France

[2]Synthélabo Recherche
Département d'Etude sur la Sécurité du Médicament
2-8 Route de Rouen
78840 Gargenville
France

SUMMARY

Ocular electrophysiologic examinations are occasionnally required to evaluate the functional capability of the retina of laboratory animals treated with a test article which may have a detrimental effect on retinal function. In order to test the sensitivity of the SYNTHELABO RECHERCHE electroretinograph and to quantify potential functional changes, an ocular electrophysiologic study was performed in beagle dogs which received quinine hydrochloride by intravenous infusion at different dose levels. Quinine is known to affect the visual capability[2, 8, 15, 25, 27, 28, 29] to decrease the amplitude and to increase the latencies of the eletroretinogram[2, 5, 7, 14, 27] and therefore permits definition of degrees of change.

MATERIALS AND METHODS

The study was carried out using six beagle dogs which were allocated to three groups, each consisting of one male and one female. The dogs were housed singly in pens (85 cm x 190 cm) in an air-conditionned, protected building with a 12 hours light (artificial) / 12 hours dark lighting cycle. The animals were fed with pelleted commercial diet and received water ad libitum via an automatic watering system. Before treatment, all the dogs underwent clinical ophthalmoscopic, slit-lamp and electroretinographic examinations to ensure that they were free from pathological disorders. The ocular reflexes were also evaluated. The ERG's were recorded after a period of dark adaptation lasting 30 minutes. At the beginning of this

LATENCY

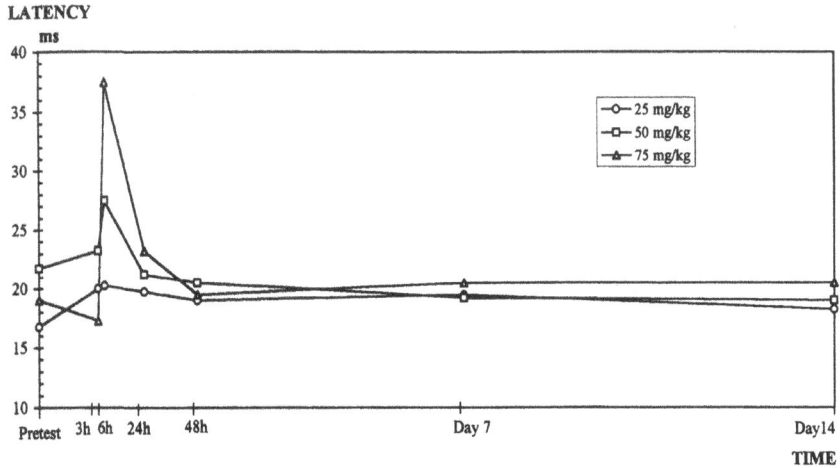

Figure 1. Changes in the "a" wave latency following quinine injection at 3 dose levels.

LATENCY

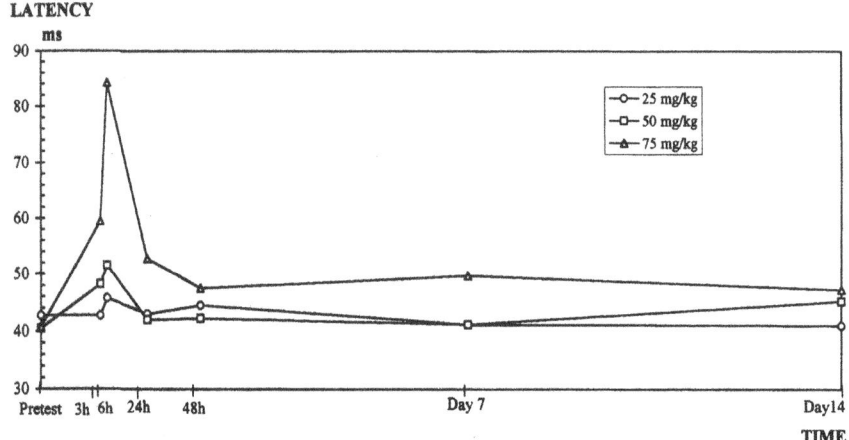

Figure 2. Changes in the "b" wave latency following quinine injection at 3 dose levels.

period and again 15 minutes later a mydriatic agent (Tropicamide, Mydriaticum, M.S.D. Chibret, Paris, France) was instilled into the eyes. At the end of the dark adaptation period, 32 consecutive white stimulations were performed (3 stimulations of 10 ms per second, at an intensity of 2 lux, at 20 cm from the eyes). Each final plot was obtained after averaging the results of the 32 plots obtained over the 250 ms following the light flashes. The latencies of the "a" and "b" waves were recorded. Electroretinograms were recorded once the day before quinine treatment and then 3, 6, 24, 48 hours after treatment as well as 7 and 14 days after treatment. Quinine hydrochloride was administered by the intravenous route, at the dose volume of 3.5 ml/kg, using a 50 ml syringe (Braun), a filter (minisart NML-SM 16534 Sartorius) an external catheter (Braun length 150 cm, diameter 2.7 mm), a trocar for intravenous injection made of Teflon (Intraflon 2 - vygon ref.: 121-10, length: 30 mm, diameter 1.0 mm G: 20) and a perfusor (Secura Braun).

The first treated animal was a female which received 75 mg/kg of quinine hydrochloride by slow manual intravenous injection over 2 minutes. Although this injection was performed slowly, no perfusor was used and it lasted only two minutes. This injection period was too short. Consequently, after injection, the dog was agitated. Thereafter, it had convulsions and died 22 minutes after the injection. Due to these marked clinical signs followed by death, no ophthalmological examinations were performed after injection and it was decided to increase the injection period and to choose dose levels up to 75 mg/kg.

Consequently, the subsequent dose levels and injection period length were defined as follows :
- 25 mg/kg, 30 minutes in one 11.5 kg female and one 14.2 kg male;
- 50 mg/kg, 45 minutes in one 9.7 kg female and one 11.9 kg male;
- 75 mg/kg, 75 minutes in one 11.0 kg female and 160 minutes in one 11.8 kg male.

The injection rate used for the second female which received 75 mg/kg of quinine was 30 ml/hour. This injection also produced marked clinical signs. Thus, the injection rate was decreased to 15 ml/hour for the male.

After treatment, the dogs were observed for at least 2 hours and thereafter examined clinically twice daily for fourteen days. The ocular reflexes (corneal palpebral, pupillary direct and consensual) were evaluated and ophthalmoscopic and biomicroscopic examinations were performed pretest and one and fourteen days after treatment.

RESULTS

Clinical signs

During injection, and for a few hours thereafter, animals showed different degrees of mucous membrane congestion, loss of balance, hypersalivation, episodic vomiting (except in low dose animals), decubitus (except in low dose animals). Agitation, convulsions, spasmodic maxillary movements, pedalling, polypnea and tachycardia were also noted in high dose animals.

Conventional ophthalmologic examinations

Conventional ophthalmologic examinations did not show abnormalities except in high dose animals where the menace response completely disappeared, due to a permanent loss of vision, about 2 hours after the end of infusion.

Electroretinographic changes

The latency of the "a" and "b" waves generally showed a dose-related increase. All times post treatment were measured from the mid point of the injection period.

Table 1. Quinine– Waves "a" and "b" mean latency increases.
(ms and %)

OCCASIONS		WAVE "a"			WAVE "b"		
		Dose level mg/kg			Dose level mg/kg		
		25	50	75	25	50	75
+ 3 hours	ms	3.25	1.50	-1.75	0.00	7.75	18.75
	%	19.40	3.70	-9.20	0.00	18.70	46.01
+ 6 hours	ms	3.50	5.75	18.50	3.00	11.00	45.50
	%	21.00	7.00	97.40	7.00	26.50	106.75
+ 24 hours	ms	3.00	-0.50	4.25	0.25	1.50	12.00
	%	17.90	-2.30	22.40	0.60	3.60	29.45
+ 48 hours	ms	2.25	-1.25	0.50	1.75	1.75	6.75
	%	13.40	-5.75	2.60	4.10	4.20	6.55
+ 7 days	ms	2.75	-2.50	1.50	-1.50	0.75	9.00
	%	16.00	-11.49	7.90	-3.50	1.80	22.10
+ 14 days	ms	1.50	-2.75	1.50	-1.75	3.75	6.50
	%	9.00	-12.60	7.90	-4.10	9.30	15.95

Table 2. Quinine– Changes in the "a" and "b" wave latencies.
(ms)
Dose Level: 25mg/kg

OCCASIONS		WAVES "a" and "b"					
		WAVE "a"			WAVE "b"		
		M	F	m	M	F	m
- 24 hours = pretest	LE	17.00	15.00	16.00	46.00	40.00	43.00
	RE	17.00	18.00	17.50	45.00	40.00	42.50
	m	17.00	16.50	16.75	45.50	40.00	42.75
+ 3 hours	LE	21.00	19.00	20.00	45.00	43.00	44.00
	RE	19.00	21.00	20.00	40.00	43.00	41.50
	m	20.00	20.00	20.00	42.50	43.00	42.75
+ 6 hours	LE	19.00	20.00	19.50	47.00	46.00	46.50
	RE	24.00	20.00	22.00	46.00	44.00	45.00
	m	21.50	20.00	20.25	46.50	46.00	45.75
+ 24 hours	LE	22.00	20.00	21.00	43.00	45.00	44.00
	RE	20.00	17.00	18.50	38.00	46.00	42.00
	m	21.00	18.50	19.75	40.50	45.50	43.00
+ 48 hours	LE	20.00	16.00	18.00	44.00	47.00	45.50
	RE	18.00	22.00	20.00	40.00	47.00	43.50
	m	19.00	19.00	19.00	42.00	47.00	44.50
+ 7 days	LE	19.00	21.00	20.00	42.00	43.00	42.50
	RE	20.00	18.00	19.00	40.00	40.00	40.00
	m	19.50	19.50	19.50	41.00	41.50	41.25
+ 14 days	LE	20.00	18.00	19.00	43.00	41.00	42.00
	RE	16.00	19.00	17.50	41.00	39.00	40.00
	m	18.00	18.50	18.25	42.00	40.00	41.00

M = Male   F = Female   m = mean

LE = Left Eye   RE = Right Eye

Table 3. Quinine– Changes in the "a" and "b" wave latencies.
(ms)
Dose Level: 50mg/kg

OCCASIONS		WAVES "a" and "b"					
		WAVE "a"			WAVE "b"		
		M	F	m	M	F	m
- 24 hours	LE	21.00	23.00	22.00	41.00	39.00	40.00
= pretest	RE	21.00	22.00	21.50	41.00	41.00	41.00
	m	21.00	22.50	21.75	41.00	40.00	40.50
+ 3 hours	LE	21.00	24.00	22.50	48.00	52.00	50.00
	RE	25.00	23.00	24.00	43.00	50.00	46.50
	m	23.00	23.50	23.25	45.50	51.00	48.25
+ 6 hours	LE	31.00	29.00	30.00	52.00	50.00	51.00
	RE	25.00	25.00	25.00	50.00	54.00	52.00
	m	18.00	27.00	27.50	51.00	52.00	51.50
+ 24 hours	LE	22.00	20.00	21.00	41.00	42.00	41.50
	RE	22.00	21.00	21.50	43.00	42.00	42.50
	m	22.00	20.50	21.25	42.00	42.00	42.00
+ 48 hours	LE	19.00	19.00	19.00	42.00	42.00	42.00
	RE	23.00	21.00	22.00	42.00	43.00	42.50
	m	21.00	20.00	20.50	42.00	42.50	42.25
+ 7 days	LE	18.00	18.00	18.00	42.00	42.00	42.00
	RE	19.00	22.00	20.50	41.00	40.00	40.50
	m	18.50	22.00	19.25	41.50	41.00	41.25
+ 14 days	LE	17.00	21.00	19.00	44.00	50.00	47.00
	RE	18.00	20.00	19.00	43.00	40.00	41.50
	m	17.50	20.50	19.00	43.50	45.00	45.25

M = Male   F = Female   m = mean

LE = Left Eye   RE = Right Eye

Table 4. Quinine– Changes in the "a" and "b" wave latencies.
(ms)
Dose Level: 75mg/kg

OCCASIONS		WAVES "a" and "b"					
		WAVE "a"			WAVE "b"		
		M	F	m	M	F	m
- 24 hours	LE	22.00	22.00	22.00	38.00	43.00	40.50
	RE	16.00	16.00	16.00	43.00	39.00	41.00
= pretest	m	19.00	19.00	19.00	40.50	41.00	40.75
	LE	17.00	19.00	18.00	64.00	57.00	60.50
+ 3 hours	RE	17.00	16.00	16.50	60.00	57.00	58.50
	m	17.00	17.50	17.25	62.00	57.00	59.50
	LE	33.00	39.00	36.00	96.00	76.00	86.00
+ 6 hours	RE	44.00	34.00	39.00	86.00	79.00	82.50
	m	38.50	36.50	37.50	91.00	77.50	84.25
	LE	23.00	23.00	23.00	61.00	46.00	53.50
+ 24 hours	RE	25.00	22.00	23.50	61.00	43.00	52.00
	m	24.00	22.50	23.25	61.00	44.50	52.75
	LE	18.00	23.00	20.50	50.00	45.00	47.50
+ 48 hours	RE	18.00	19.00	18.50	49.00	46.00	47.50
	m	18.00	21.00	19.50	49.50	45.50	47.50
	LE	20.00	23.00	21.50	57.00	46.00	51.50
+ 7 days	RE	21.00	18.00	19.50	50.00	46.00	46.00
	m	20.50	20.50	20.50	53.50	46.00	49.75
	LE	20.00	23.00	21.50	55.50	47.00	51.25
+ 14 days	RE	21.00	18.00	19.50	45.50	41.00	43.25
	m	20.50	20.50	20.50	50.50	44.00	47.25

M = Male   F = Female   m = mean

LE = Left Eye   RE = Right Eye

"a" wave (Tables 1 - 4). In animals treated at the dose level of 25 mg/kg, at three hours, the mean "a" wave latency has increased by 3.25 ms when compared with the pretest value. Three hours later, the mean increase reached 3.5 ms. Twenty-four hours after injection, the mean increase was less marked (3 ms), therafter the "a" wave latency tended to return to the pretest value and fourteen days later, it was only 1.5 ms higher than pretest. In animals treated at the dose level of 50 mg/kg, the increase was less marked at 3 hours, but reached + 5.75 ms after a further 3 hours. However, no further increase was observed: all values were below those observed pretest (+ 24 h: - 0.50 ms, + 48 h : - 1.25ms, + 7 days: - 2.5 ms and + 14 days: - 2.75 ms). In animals treated at the dose level of 75 mg/kg, at three hours, the mean "a" wave latency was below the pretest value. Three hours later it was markedly increased (+ 6 h : + 18.5 ms). Thereafter mean latency tended to return to the pretest value (+ 24 h: + 4.25 ms) and was very close to this value at + 48 h (+ 0.5 ms) and thereafter (+ 7 days and + 14 days: + 1.5 ms).

"b" wave (Tables 1 - 4). In animals treated at the dose level of 25 mg/kg the "b" wave latency was not affected three hours after injection. Three hours later, the mean latency had a 3 ms increase. Twenty-four hours after the injection the "b" wave latency was only 0.25 ms longer than pretest. However, the mean "b" wave latency was slightly increased (+ 1.75 ms) fourty-eight hours after injection. Seven and 14 days after injection, all values were below pretest. In animals treated at the dose level of 50 mg/kg, marked mean "b" wave latency increases were observed early (+ 3 h: + 7.75 ms, + 6 h: + 11 ms). Thereafter the increases were less marked and the latencies tended to return to the pretest values (+ 24 h: + 1.5 ms, + 48 h: + 1.75 ms, 7 days: + 0.75 ms, 14 days: + 3.75 ms). In animals treated at the dose level of 75 mg/kg, "b" wave latency increases occurred very early and were very marked (+ 3 h: + 18.75 ms, + 6 h: + 45.50 ms). Thereafter the latencies tended to decrease but never reached pretest value (+ 24 h: + 12 ms, + 48 h: + 6.75 ms, + 7 days: + 9 ms, + 14 days: + 6.5 ms).

DISCUSSION

In beagle dogs, quinine induces marked but, to some extent, reversible alterations in the ERG's. Early marked increases in a and b waves latencies were observed in this study and confirmed findings of Zahn et al[29]. These changes occurred earlier and lasted longer in animals treated at the dose level of 25 mg/kg. In these animals, the latency increase occurred earlier for the "a" wave than for the "b" wave (Figures 1,2). An explanation could be a primary, direct neurological effect on photoreceptors followed by an effect on Müller cells[4, 6, 8, 9, 13, 15], although it was not confirmed histopathologically. Moreover, it is difficult to verify this hypothesis, as other dose levels induced earlier changes in the "b" wave[3, 16, 21, 22, 25]. Changes in the "b" wave were dose-related and occurred very early (at + 3 hours with high dose levels and at + 6 hours with the low dose level) and were negligible from + 24 hours, except at the dose level of 75 mg/kg, where changes were probably not reversible. These early and, to some extent, permanent changes in "b" wave latency were consistent with the neurotoxic effect of quinine on glial cells[4, 6, 8, 9, 13, 15]. This study was also usefull to estimate significant percentage increases in ERG latencies in order to easily interpret ERG's from studies to test new drugs.

REFERENCES

1. H. Almeida, Quinine amblyopia. Quartely Bulletin of the Northwest University, *Medical school*. 35:217 (1961).

2. P. Bacon, D.J. Spalton, S.E. Smith, Blindness from quinine toxicity. *Br. J. Ophthalmol.* 72 (3):219(1988).

3. B.L. Braverman, D.S. Koransky, M.M. Kubvin, Quinine amaurosis. *Am. J. Ophthalmol.* 31:331 (1948).

4. G.S. Brinton, E.W. Norton, J.R. Zahn, Ocular quinine toxicity. *Invest. Ophthalmol. Visual Sci.* suppl. 276 (1979).

5. G.S. Brinton, E.W. Norton, J.R. Zahn, R.W. Knighton, Ocular quinine toxicity. *Am. J. Ophthalmol.* 90 (3):403 (1980).

6. T.A.S. Buchanan, R.W. Lyness, A.D. Collins, T.A. Gardiner, D.B. Archer, An experimental study of quinine blindness. *Eye.* 1:522 (1987).

7. B. Calissendorf, Melanotropic drugs and retinal functions. Acta Ophthalmol. 54 (1):109 (1976).

8. C.R. Canning, S. Hague, Ocular quinine toxicity. *Br. J. Ophthalmol.* 72 (1):23 (1988).

9. M.T. Carapancea, Synchronic quinine toxicity in visual retina and superior nervous centres. *Photochem. Photobiol.* 45 (suppl.):36S (1987).

10. M.T. Carapancea, Déséquilibres oculaires expérimentaux, correspondant aux troubles oculaires cliniques, dans l'intoxication quininique. *Rev. Roum. Physiol.* 10 (4):299 (1973).

11. M.T. Carapancea, Caractères du seuil toxique oculaire de la quinine. *Rev. Roum. Morphol. Embryol. Physiol.* 14 (1):27 (1977).

12. J. Chabot, P. Verin, J. Bouchard, L'électrorétinogramme dans l'intoxication par la quinine. *Bull. Soc. Ophtal. Fr.* 63:531 (1963).

13. G.W. Cibis, H.M. Burian., F.C. Blodi, Electroretinogram changes in acute quinine poisoning. *Arch. Ophthalmol.* 90:307 (1973).

14. P. Dickinson, J. Sabto J., R.H. West, Management of quinine toxicity. *Aust. J. Ophthalmol.* 11 (4):265 (1983).

15. L.P. Fong, D.V. Kaufman, J.E.K. Galbraith, Ocular toxicity of quinine. *Med. J. Aust.* 141 (8):528 (1984).

16. J. Francois, A. De Rouck, E. Gambie, Retinal and optic evaluation in quinine poisoning. *Ann. Ophthalmol.* 4:177 (1972).

17. E.A. Gall, Report of the pathology panel : National halothane study. *Anesthesology.* 29:233 (1968).

18. D. Giannini, Dell'inffluenza dei disturbi di circola sulla patogenesi della alterazioni funzionali el anatomiche del nervo otticoe della retina negli avvelamenti da chinino. *Ann. Ottalmol. Clin. Oculist.* 62:1069 (1934).

19. L.S. Goodman, A. Gillman, "The pharmacological basis of therapeutics. 7th Ed.". Mac Millan, New York. 1041:1044 (1985).

20. K. Hommer, R.G. Frey, Einzelreiz - und Flimmer-ERG im akuten Stadium der Chininvergiftung. *Doc. Ophthal.* 18:392 (1964).

21. K. Hommer, Die Wirkung des Chinins, Chlorochins, Jodoacetats und Chlordiazepoxids auf das ERG des isolierten Kaninchennetzhaut. *Graefes Arch. Ophthal.* 175:111 (1968).

22. K. Hommer, Über die Chininvergiftung der Netzhaut mit einer Bemerkung zur experimentellen Chlorochinvergiftung. *Klin. Monatsbl., Augenheilkd.* 152, 6:785 (1968).

23. G. Le Breton Oliveau, E. Audoueineix, E.R.G. clinique et intoxication par la quinine. *Bull. Soc. Opht. France.* 4/5:431 (1980).

24. O. Loget, L'électrophysiologie sensorielle oculaire chez les animaux de laboratoire. Vet. Med. Thesis, Nantes (1990).

25. J. Moloney, M. Hillery,M. Fenton, Two year electrophysiology follow-up in quinine amblyopia. *Acta Ophthalm.* 65 (6):731 (1987).

26. C. J. Pycock, Retinal neurotransmission. *Surv Ophthalmol.* 29:355 (1985).

27. S. Sato, Toxic effects on the visual system of diaminophenoxybutane, quinine and ethambutol in conscious dogs. *Fund. Appl. Tox.* 5:777 (1985).

28. Y. Yospaiboon, T. Lawtiantong, S. Chotibutr, Clinical observations of ocular quinine intoxication. *Jpn. J. Ophthalmol.* 28 (4):409(1984).

29. J.R. Zahn, G.F. Brinton, E. Norton, Ocular quinine toxicity followed by electroretinogram, electro-oculogram, and pattern visually evoked potential. *Am. J. Optom. Physiol. Opt.* 58 (6):492 (1981).

EFFECT OF DIFFERENT VEHICLES ON OCULAR KINETICS/DISTRIBUTION

Marco Fabrizio Saettone

Department of Pharmaceutical Sciences
University of Pisa, 56100 Pisa (Italy)

INTRODUCTION

Purpose of the present review is to present some essential facts and figures concerning drug delivery to the eye from topical preparations.

Drugs are always delivered to the organism in an appropriate vehicle, or dosage form, i.e. in a medium allowing administration by the desired route (oral, rectal, s.c., iv., ocular, etc.) and in the desired amount (dosage). As illustrated in Fig. 1, an ophthalmic dosage form results from the combination of drug(s) with a series of pharmacologically "inert" components, which should ensure an optimal performance of the preparation in terms of localization to the absorption site, delivery, physiological compatibility, patient acceptance, etc.

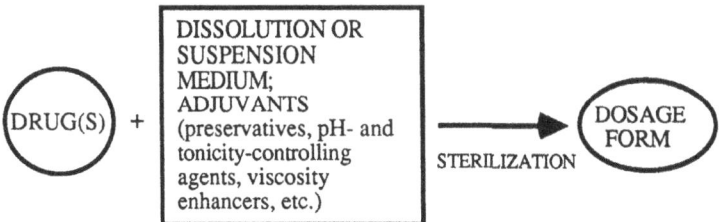

Figure 1. Essential components of an ophthalmic dosage form.

Much time and effort has been devoted in recent years to the improvement and optimization of traditional ocular vehicles, which have been not inappropriately defined by Lee and Robinson[1] as "fairly primitive and inefficient". In the words of Hughes and Mitra[2] "ophthalmic drug delivery is one of the most interesting and challenging endeavors facing the pharmaceutical scientist....The anatomy, physiology and biochemistry of the eye render this organ exquisitely impervious to foreign substances....The challenge to the formulator is to circumvent the protective barriers of the eye without causing permanent tissue damage....The primitive ophthalmic solutions, suspensions and ointment dosage forms are clearly no longer sufficient to combat some present virulent diseases...".

The pharmacokinetics and constraints of ocular drug absorption have been thoroughly reviewed in a number of excellent papers [3-12]. They will be briefly discussed in the folowing paragraphs, before examining some recent approaches to deliver drugs more efficiently to the eye.

DRUG ABSORPTION AND DISPOSITION IN THE EYE

The time pattern of drug absorption and disposition in the eye following topical administration is a complex phenomenon, influenced by the drug, the vehicle, and by anatomical/physiological factors. In order to understand the pharmacokinetics of ocular drugs it is necessary to consider the absorption, distribution and disposition of drugs in three areas of the eye: (a) the preocular (precorneal) area, (b) the cornea, and (c) the interior of the eye. A picture of the pathways for absorption, and of their complex interrelations is given in Fig. 2.

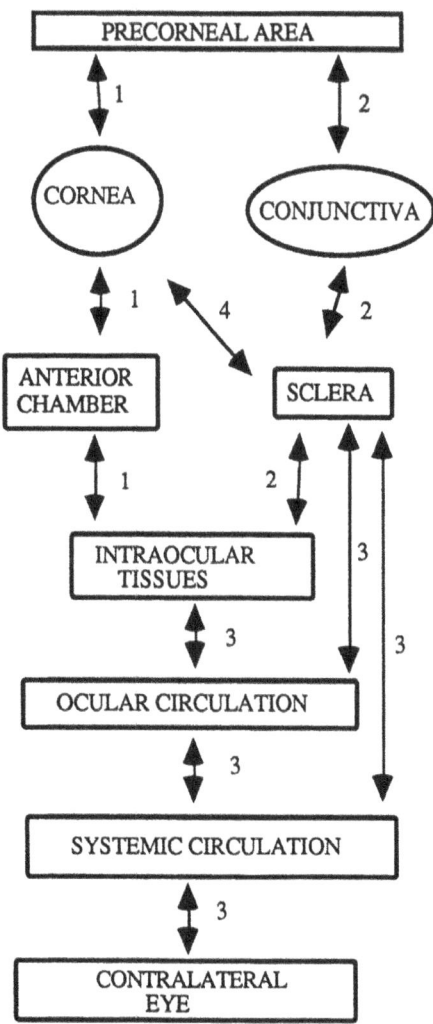

Figure 2. Ocular penetration pathways for topically applied drugs. Key: 1 = transcorneal pathway; 2 = noncorneal pathway; 3 = systemic return pathway; 4 = lateral diffusion (From Ref. 13).

It is a common knowledge that the ocular bioavailability of drugs is very poor. The absorption of drugs in the eye is severely limited by some protective mechanisms that insure the proper functioning of the eye, and by other concomitant factors. These mechanisms and factors include:

      1) the drainage of instilled solutions;
      2) lacrimation and tear turnover;
      3) metabolism;
      4) tear evaporation;
      5) non-productive absorption/adsorption;
      4) poor corneal and scleral permeability to foreign substances;
      5) possible binding by the lacrimal proteins.

The drainage of the administered dose *via* the nasolacrimal system into the nasopharynx and the gastrointestinal tract takes place when the volume of fluid in the eye exceeds the normal lacrimal volume of 7-10 microliters. Thus, the portion of the instilled dose (1-2 drops, corresponding to 50-100 microliters) that is not eliminated by spillage from the palpebral fissure is quickly drained, and the contact time of the dose with the absorbing surfaces (cornea and sclera) is reduced to a maximum of 2 minutes. A pharmacokinetic scheme illustrating the precorneal fluid dynamics and the distribution/disposition of pilocarpine in rabbits is shown in Fig. 3.

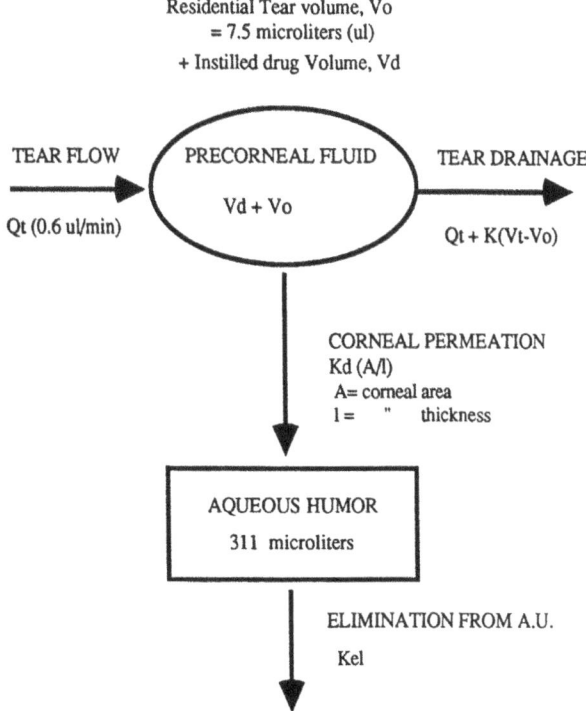

Figure 3. Pharmacokinetic scheme illustrating the distribution of pilocarpine from the tear fluid into the aqueous humor (modified, from Ref. 14).

The lacrimation and the physiological tear turnover (16% per minute in humans in normal conditions) can be stimulated and increased by the instillation even of mildly irritating solutions. The net result is a dilution of the applied medication, and an acceleration of drug loss. It is now definitively established that the rate at which instilled solutions are removed from the eye varies linearly with instilled volume. In other words, the larger the instilled volume, the more rapidly the instilled solution is drained from the precorneal area. This is illustrated in Fig. 4.

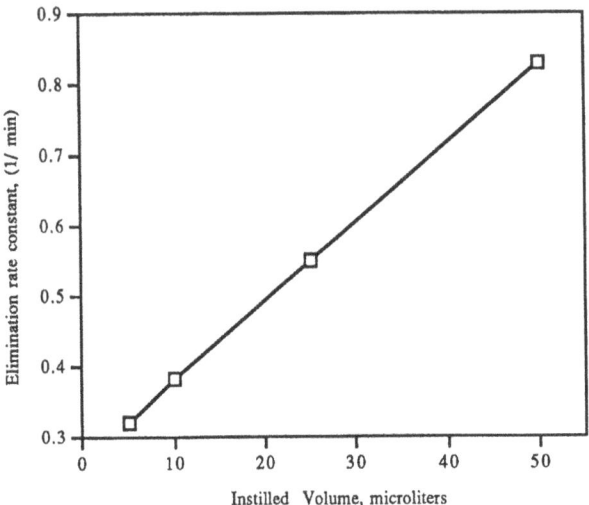

Figure 4. Relationship between the rate constant for decline in volume and volume instilled (from Ref. 15).

Ideally, a high concentration of drug in a minimum drop volume would be desirable. It has been shown[16] that approximately equal tear film concentrations result from the instillation of 5 microliters of 1.61×10^{-2} M pilocarpine nitrate or from 25 microliters of 1.0×10^{-2} M solution. The 5 microliter dose contain only 38% as much pilocarpine, yet its bioavailability is greater due to decreased drainage loss. Thus, smaller instilled voumes might: a) reduce drainage loss and increase contact time, leading to improved drug activity, and b) reduce systemic side-effects through reduction in drainage loss. However, there is a practical limit to the concept of minimum dosage volume. Droppers delivering small volumes are difficult to design and to produce. Furthermore, their practical usefulness could be reduced by the fact that most patients cannot detect the administration of small volumes.

The conjunctival absorption, which occurs *via* the vessels of the palpebral and scleral conjunctiva, concurs in reducing the drug available for absorption into the eye. The mentioned factors, associated with possible drug binding by the lacrimal proteins, may result in transcorneal absorption of 1% or less of the drug applied topically as a solution. Typical transcorneal absorption rate constants range from $1 \cdot 10^{-3}$ to $5 \cdot 10^{-3}$ min^{-1}, while the overall rate constant for loss from the eye ranges from 0.5 to 0.7 min^{-1} (i.e., the rate of loss can be 500 to 700 times greater than the rate of absorption).

As the preceding discussion has made clear, solutions instilled onto the eye have, due to drainage, only a very limited time period during which they can be absorbed transcorneally. Protein binding in the tear fluids can further reduce the amount of free drug available for absorption, and hence can affect ocular bioavailability. The average total protein content (albumin, globulins, lysozyme) of human tears is about 0.7%, and the albumin content is about 0.4%. Many factors, including certain pathological conditions, may result in increased tear protein content. Furthermore, if it is considered that the appreciable turnover of tears is a continuous source of fresh protein, it will be realized that drug-protein binding in the precorneal fluids can result in reduced bioavailability. Another pictorial representation of the drug and fluid movements in the eye, where the proteins contents have been evidenced, is given in Fig. 5.

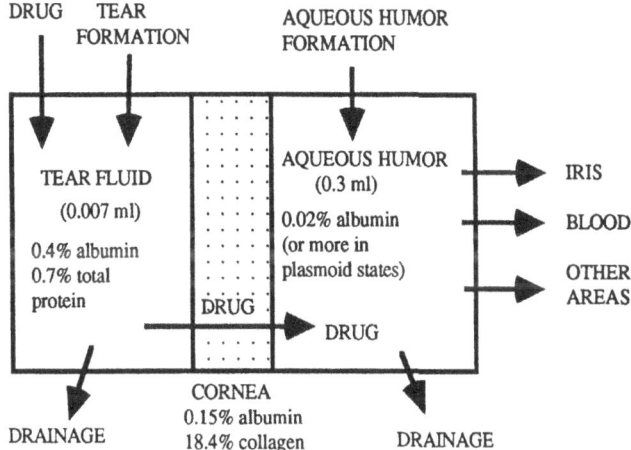

Figure 5. Pictorial representation of the drug and fluid movements in a portion of the human eye, and of the protein contents of the different eye compartments. (Modified, from Ref. 17).

Any instilled drug which has not been swept away from the precorneal area by the drainage apparatus, and has further escaped the effects of protein binding, is subject to metabolic degradation in the tear film (Cf. Fig. 6). Drug metabolism in the precorneal area (which, clearly, will be a function of the susceptibility of individual drugs), is a potential mechanism which can contribute to the loss of biological activity of topically applied medications.

Evaporation of the tear film from the precorneal area can cause changes in the concentration of instilled drug solutions, and therefore can affect the rate of drug transport across the ocular membranes.

Topically applied drugs are potentially available for absorption by the scleral and palpebral conjunctiva (Cf. pathway 2, Fig. 2). Such routes of loss are referred to as "non productive" absorption, since it is well documented that drugs which penetrate the conjunctiva are rapidly removed for the eye by local circulation, and undergo systemic absorption. A direct transscleral access to some intraocular tissues, however, cannot be excluded.

Subject to experimental conditions, the relative effectiveness of the factors involved in precorneal drug removal are, in the case e.g. of pilocarpine, the following: drainage≈vaso-dilation>nonconjunctival loss>induced lacrimation≈conjunctival absorption>normal tear turnover.

In conclusion, the fluid dynamics in the precorneal area of the eye have a huge effect on ocular drug absorption and disposition. When the normal fluid dynamics are altered by e.g., tonicity, pH, or irritant drugs or vehicles, the situation becomes even more complex. The formulation of ophthalmic drug products must take into account not only the stability and compatibility of a drug in a given formulation, but also the influence of that formulation on precorneal fluid dynamics.

The concepts exposed in the preceding paragraphs are summarized in Fig. 6, which illustrates the various factors and pathways involved in the ocular disposition of formulations applied topically to the eye.

As said, ophthalmic drugs topically applied are intended to exert a local effect on the eye or to penetrate the cornea. However, after being placed in the conjunctival sac, a significant amount of the drug is available for systemic absorption, and may produce systemic side-effects. These effects are frequently not anticipated, recognized, or treated appropriately. The main pathways for systemic absorption of ocular medications are illustrated in Table 1.

The issue of the occurrence of systemic absorption of ophthalmic medications is probably very old, even if it has been apparently neglected until recent times. This is testified by the advice given almost 2000 years ago by the famed Latin scientist Pliny the Elder (23-

79 A.D.): "Diagora's collyrium should be compounded without opium, otherwise severe toxic effects might result".

A few figures on systemic absorption of ocularly applied drugs are given in Table 2.

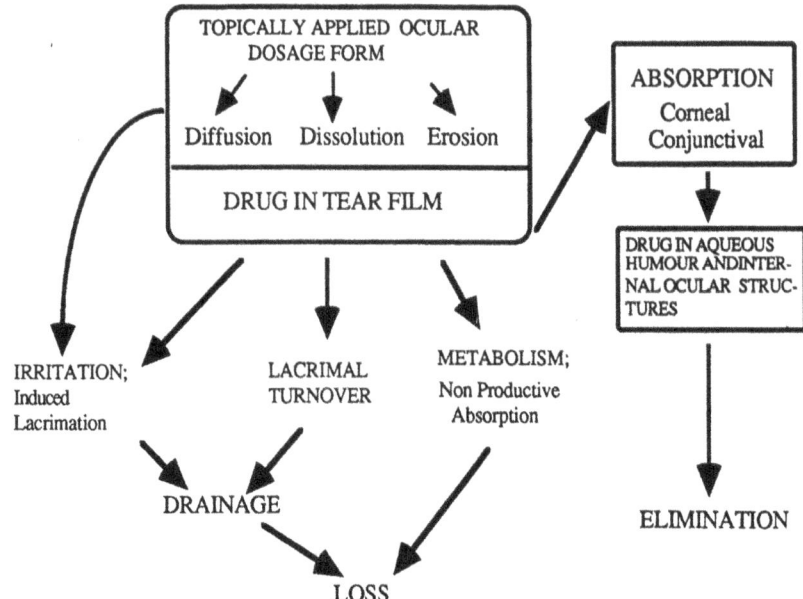

Figure 6. Schematic illustration of the ocular disposition of topically applied formulations (From Ref. 18).

Table 1. Routes for systemic absorption of topical ocular medications.

1) Conjunctival, episcleral and intraocular vessels;
2) Nasal mucosa (The rate and extent of absorption are comparable to intravenous administration);
3) G.I. Tract (Access occurs by swallowing the drug after it has traversed the naso-lacrimal duct and the nasopharynx).

TRADITIONAL OPHTHALMIC VEHICLES

The traditional ophthalmic dosage forms (solutions, suspensions and ointments) have been described and discussed in detail.[18-20] As indicated in the introduction, the characteristic parts of an ophthalmic dosage form, i.e., the drug and the other ingredients of the vehicle, occupy the same general relationship to each other as they do in other drug solutions, suspensions and ointment products. However, as discussed in the preceding paragraphs, the eye itself has several specific characteristics (physical and physiological) that affect the expected performance of each of these components.

Solutions are undoubtedly the most commonly used and accepted forms. They are relatively simple to make, filter and sterilize. Suspensions, while not as common as solutions, are widely used for formulations involving anti-inflammatory steroids (e.g., prednisolone alcohol and acetate). Early resistance to these forms, based on the emotional fear that "particles in the eye are bad", has largely been overcome as particle sizes have been reduced, and as the benefits of these dosage forms have been demonstrated.

Table 2. Percent of Topically Applied Dose Absorbed Into the Systemic Circulation.

Drug	% systemically absorbed
Cortisol	30-35
Dipivalylepinephrine	65
Epinephrine	55
Flurbiprofen	74
Imirestat	50-75
Inulin	3
Insulin, with 1% Na glycocholate	5
Timolol	80
Levobunolol	46
[D-Ala^2]Metenkephalinamide	36
Tetrahydrocannabinol	23

(From Ref. 21)

Ointments have for years presented some problems, since they could not be filtered to eliminate particulate matter; they could not be made truly sterile; and no adequate tests had been devised to indicate the suitability of added preservatives. In time most of these problems have been solved and sterile, filtered ophthalmic ointments have appeared on the market. These preparation, however, still occupy a position of minor importance.

Two particular physical factors in ocular formulations which, among others, have been attentively investigated are the drug solubility and form, and the vehicle viscosity.

As already said, some drugs do not penetrate easily the corneal epithelium because of their unfavorable physo-chemical characteristics, and are eliminated by tear dilution and subsequent washout much faster than commonly supposed. This produces an undesired drug load for the systemic circulation when adequate concentrations are used to provide the desired ophthalmic effect.

The prodrug approach[22] has been resorted to in some instances to improve the ocular/systemic absorption ratio, as in the case of dipivalylepinephrine (Dipivefrin, DPE), a lipophilic prodrug of epinephrine (EP), an antiglaucoma topical drug. The majority of topical EP, administered as a 2% solution, enters the systemic circulation, as a result of systemic absorption through the nasal mucosa, and has been reported many times to produce systemic α- and β-adrenergic symptoms. DPE has no apparent systemic effect, because the enzymatic release of EP occurs most efficiently in the cornea, which is better penetrated by the more lipophilic DPE. The rationale for the realization of prodrugs is illustrated in Fig. 8.

In the case of poorly soluble drugs, as the steroids, two aspects of the "solubility" parameter are relevant to ocular absorption: the presence in the cul-de-sac of the eye of a reservoir of insoluble particles could lead to a sustaining effect, and different esters of the drug could show different transcorneal permeation characteristics.

While normal saline is an acceptable vehicle for ophthalmic drugs, slightly viscous solutions are generally recognized as more satisfying to use for the patients. Increasing the viscosity has also been proposed as a means to increase the bioavailability of drugs, since to an increased viscosity should correspond an increased time of residence of the medication in the eye. However, there appears to be only a narrow band of acceptable viscosity, since the products must have negligible visual effects, should not obstruct the puncti and canaliculi, and should be filterable and sterilizable.

In summary, if maximal ocular penetration of a drug is desired, the physical and physiological parameters of the eye suggest viscosities of 1 to 15 Cps for comfort and minimal visual effects, and drug forms with a sufficient lipophilic character (log PC $\geq$ 2).

ADVANCED DELIVERY SYSTEMS

In recent years, the prolongation of the retention time of delivery systems on the eye surface has been the object of extensive investigation. Parallel investigations have been

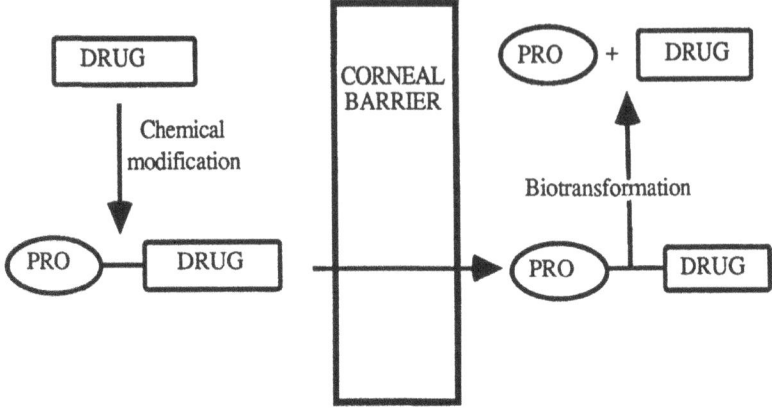

Figure 8. Rationale for the improvement of corneal drug penetration by the use of a prodrug (From Ref. 22).

dedicated to methods for improving transcorneal penetration of traditional and of innovative therapeutic agents, such as protein and peptide drugs, and for reducing systemic absorption of topically applied drugs. Exhaustive reviews on different advanced delivery systems can be found in two recently published books.[23,24]

Some recently developed systems aim at enhancing the magnitude of the pulse entry of the drug. These systems offer the advantage of prolonging the effect and increasing the time before another pulse is needed. However, in some cases pulse increases are accompanied by corresponding increases in side-effects. Other delivery systems are designed to provide controlled, continuous drug delivery, with the dual goal of avoiding or minimizing the initial pulse (with its associated side-effects), and of avoiding the prolonged period of underdosing which often occurs between drug administrations. This approach allows using drugs with shorter half-lives, and safer using of drugs which do have serious side-effects.

The following approaches will be briefly described:

1) In-situ activated gel-forming systems;
2) mucoadhesives;
3) inserts;
4) penetration enhancers.

In-Situ Activated Gel-Forming Systems

These (liquid) vehicles undergo a viscosity increase upon instillation in the eye, thus promoting precorneal retention.[25] Such a change in viscosity can be triggered by a change in temperature, pH or electrolyte composition. Poloxamer 407 (a polyoxyethylene-polyoxypropylene block copolymer) is a polymer whose solution viscosity increases when its temperature is raised to the eye temperature, Cellulose acetophthalate (CAP) is a polymer whose solution undergoes coagulation when its original pH of 4.5 is raised by the tear fluid to pH 7.4. Both systems, however, are characterized by a high polymer concentration (25% for Poloxamer 407, and 30% for CAP). By contrast, Gelrite®, is a polysaccharide (low-acetyl gellan gum) which forms clear gels at a much lower concentration, in the presence of mono or divalent cations typically found in tear fluids.[26] In fact, the concentration of Na^+ in tears, 2.6 g/l, is sufficient to cause gelation of the solution upon topical instillation in the conjunctival sac. Compared to an equiviscous solution of hydroxyethylcellulose, a moderate improvement in ocular absorption was observed when timolol maleate (0.25%) was instilled in 0.6% Gelrite® in albino rabbits. Similar favorable results were obtained in terms of peak and duration of activity in 45 patients with intraocular pressure greater than 23 mm Hg, following the topical instillation of 0.008% timolol maleate in Gelrite®, when compared with 0.008% timolol maleate in buffer solution.

Mucoadhesive Formulations

This approach relies on vehicles containing polymers which will attach, via non-covalent bonds, to conjunctival mucin (a glycoprotein), thus remaining in contact with precorneal tissues until mucin turnover causes elimination of the polymer.[27]

Mucoadhesive polymers are usually hydrocolloids with numerous hydrophilic functional groups, such as carboxyl, hydroxyl, amide and sulfate. These groups can establish electrostatic interactions, hydrophobic interactions, van der Waals intermolecular interactions, and hydrogen bonding with underlying substrates. For many polymers, hydrogen bonding appears to play a significant role in mucoadhesion, and thus the presence of water seems to be a prerequisite for a majority of the mucoadhesive phenomena.

When macromolecular hydrocolloids with hydrophilic functional groups are placed in aqueous media, they swell and expand into a gel or network. Interpenetration and entanglement of this network with the mucin substrate can be partly responsible for the mucoadhesive properties. Therefore, mobility and flexibility of the polymer chains is a prerequisite for strong mucoadhesion.

Mucoadhesive polymers have been divided into synthetic and naturally occurring. The following synthetic polymers have been evaluated for mucoadhesion, with variable results: hydroxypropylcellulose, polyacrylic acid, high molecular weight (>200,000) polyethylene glycols, dextrans, hyaluronic acid, polygalacturonic acid, etc.

Active investigations on potentially mucoadhesive polymers as ingredients for ophthalmic vehicles are underway in many laboratories, and hopefully they will eventually lead to the development of more efficient ocular delivery systems.

Inserts

Ophthalmic inserts are solid devices, intended to be placed in the conjunctival sac and to deliver the drug at a comparatively slow rate.[28] These devices might present valuable assets, such as:

1) increased ocular permanence with respect to standard vehicles, hence a prolonged drug activity and a higher drug bioavailability;
2) accurate dosing (all of the drug is theoretically retained at the absorption site);
3) possible reduction of systemic absorption, which occurs freely with standard eyedrops *via* the nasal mucosa;
4) better patient compliance, resulting from a reduced frequency of medication and a lower incidence of visual and systemic side-effects;
5) possibility of targeting internal ocular tissues through non-corneal conjunctival-scleral) penetration routes;
6) increased shelf life with respect to eyedrops, due to the absence of water;
7) last but not least, possibility of providing a constant rate of drug release.

The different types of inserts have been classified on the basis of their physical characteristics, as follows:

a) soluble inserts (undergoing gradual dissolution and/or surface erosion once placed in the conjunctival cul-de-sac: eg. Collagen Shields);
b) insoluble inserts (including medicated contact lenses, constant-rate release devices such as the Ocusert®, etc.).

The latter device, developed by Alza Corp., Palo Alto, California, is a diffusion unit consisting of a drug reservoir (e.g., pilocarpine HCl in an alginate gel) enclosed by two release-controlling membranes made of ethylene-vinyl acetate copolymer, and enclosed by a white ring which allows positioning of the system in the eye. The Pilo-20 Ocular Therapeutic System has a release rate of 20 mg/hr for 7 days, and the Pilo-40 system a release rate of 40 mg/hr for 7 days. The former releases a total of 3.4 mg in 7 days, the latter 6.7 mg. In order to maintain constant release of drug, and in accordance with the principles of diffusion, there must be an excess of drug maintained in the reservoir. Therefore, the Pilo-20 system contains a total of 5.0 mg pilocarpine, and the Pilo-40 system, 11.0 mg. The latter also contains di(2-ethylhexyl)-phthalate, about 90 mg of which is released during the life of the system to facilitate a more rapid release of drug through the membrane. Clinical studies with the pilocarpine Ocusert® have demonstrated that slow release of the drug can effectively control the increased intraocular pressure in glaucoma, with a minor incidence of side-effects, such as miosis, myopia, browache.

Furthermore, these and other inserts, both erodible and nonerodible (as e.g. medicated contact lenses, collagen shields, the Minidisc) have been shown capable to diminish the systemic absorption of ocularly applied drugs, as a results of a decreased drainage into the nasal cavity, which is one of the major systemic absorption sites of topical ocular medications. This is particularly important, if one considers the potential systemic toxicity of some recently introduced drugs, such as the beta-blockers. Another potential advantage of insert therapy is the possibility of promoting non-corneal drug penetration, thus increasing the efficacy of some hydrophilic drugs which are poorly absorbed through the cornea.

Ocular Penetration Enhancers

The use of appropriate corneal penetration promotors is a potentially interesting, still little-explored approach to improving the bioavailability of topical ocular drugs.[29] Depending on their structure, penetration enhancers may improve corneal drug transport by two methods: by influencing the paracellular or the transcellular pathway. Unfortunately, some agents, while effective, cause transient irritation or produce irreversible damages to the corneal tissues.

In a recent study carried out in the laboratory of the present author,[30] the effect of different agents, known for their capacity of altering the permeability of biological membranes, was tested on "in vitro" permeation through rabbit corneas of three ophthalmic drugs possessing different lipophilic character: timolol maleate (TM), levobunolol hydrochloride (LB) and cyclopentolate hydrochloride (CY). (Octanol/water distribution coefficients = 0.051, 0.197 and 0.247, respectively).

Table 3. Effect of various enhancers on transcorneal permeation of timolol maleate (TM), Levobunolol HCl (LB) and Cyclopentolate HCl (CY).

ENHANCERS		HL[a], %	DRUGS		
			TM	LB	CY
			Permeation	Coefficient,	cm/s $.10^6$
GBR[b]		80.4	3.6	23.0	18.0
BZ	(0.02%)	86.4	9.6	22.8	21.7
Brij® 35	(0.05%)	81.4	5.5	16.4	30.8
Brij®78	(0.05%)	81.6	14.0	27.5	29.2
Brij®98	(0.05%)	82.9	3.2	12.8	24.0
DIG[c]		87.4	14.0	26.9	15.3
EDTA	(0.5%)	78.4	0.17	0.13	10.0
TC	(0.025%)	81.7	5.3	0.94	10.0
SAP	(0.05%)	88.4	40.3	30.3	25.8

[a]Corneal hydration level; [b]Glutatione Bicarbonate Ringer (no enhancer); [c]Corneas pretreated with 100 mM DIG for 10 min. (From Ref. 30).

The tested enhancers were benzalkonium chloride (BZ), polyoxyethylene glycol lauryl ether (Brij® 35), Polyoxyethylene glycol stearyl ether (Brij® 78), Polyoxyethylene glycol oleyl ether (Brij® 98), ethylenediaminetetraacetic acid, Na salt (EDTA), digitonin (DIG), sodium taurocholate (TC) and saponine (SAP). The results of the study are summarized in Table 3. In the absence of enhancers, the corneal permeability of the less lipophilic TM was lower than those of LB and CY, in agreement with literature data. In general, the enhancers increased the rate of permeation of TM more than those of the other two, more lipophilic drugs. Three enhancers, however (BZ, DIG and SAP), altered substantially the normal hydration state of the cornea, expressed by the hydration level, HL, thus indicating the possible occurrence of corneal damage. Brij® 78, which produced a 3.9-fold increase of the permeability coefficient (PC) in the case of TM, and 1.2-1.6-fold increases in the case of LB and CY, respectively, appeared as the most promising agent. Of particular interest was the significant PC reduction of TM and LB caused by EDTA, known to produce ultrastructural changes in the corneal epithelium, resulting in increased paracellular permeability. The results obtained with SAP may warrant further investigations: lower concentrations of this enhancer might be active without producing corneal damage.

CONCLUSIONS

In spite of continuous progress in the understanding of principles and processes governing ocular drug absorption and disposition, and of indisputable advances in the efficacy of delivery systems, several challenges, enunciated by Lee and Robinson a few years ago,[1] still confront the field of ophthalmic drug delivery. These are: a) the extent to which the protective mechanisms of the eye can be safely altered to facilitate drug absorption; b) delivery of drugs to the posterior portion of the eye from topical dosing; c) topical delivery of macromolecular drugs; d) improved technology, allowing non-invasive monitoring of drug transport in the eye, and e) predictive animal models for all phases of ocular drug evaluation.

It is hoped that the present review, notwithstanding its incompleteness, will provide some useful information to readers (such as clinicians, toxicologists, etc.) not directly involved in the formulation, development and testing of ophthalmic dosage forms.

REFERENCES

1. V.H.L. Lee and J.R. Robinson, Review: Topical ocular drug delivery: recent development and future challenges, *J. Ocul. Pharmacol.*, 2:67 (1986).
2. P.M. Hughes and A.K. Mitra, Overview of ocular drug delivery and iatrogenic ocular cytopathologies, *in* "Ophthalmic Drug Delivery Systems", A.K. Mitra, ed., M. Dekker, Inc., New York (1993).
3. Patton, T.F., Ocular drug disposition characteristics, *in* "Ophthalmic Drug Delivery Systems", J.R. Robinson, ed., American Pharmaceutical Association, Washington, 1980.
4. S.P. Eriksen, Physiological and formulation constraints on ocular drug bioavailability, *in* "Ophthalmic Drug Delivery Systems", J.R. Robinson, ed., American Pharmaceutical Association, Washington, 1980.
5. S. Mishima, Clinical pharmacokinetics of the eye, *Invest. Ophthalmol. Vis. Sci.*, 21:504 (1981).
6. J.W. Shell, Pharmacokinetics of topically applied ophthalmic drugs, *Surv. Ophthalmol.*, 26:207 (1982).
7 D.M. Maurice and S. Mishima, Ocular pharmacokinetics, *in* "Pharmacology of the Eye", M. Sears, ed., Spinger Verlag, Berlin (1984).
8. J.W. Shell, Ophthalmic drug delivery systems, *Surv. Ophthalmol.*, 29:117 (1984).
9. N.L. Burstein and J.A. Anderson, Corneal penetration and ocular bioavailability of drugs, *J. Ocular Pharmacol.*, 1:309 (1985).
10. D.M. Maurice, Kinetics of topically applied ophthalmic drugs, *in* " Ophthalmic Drug Delivery, Biopharmaceutical, Technological and Clinical Aspects", M.F. Saettone, M. Bucci and P. Speiser, eds., Springer Verlag, Berlin, 1987.
11. R.D. Schoenwald, Ocular Pharmacokinetic studies, *in* "Ophthalmic Drug Delivery Systems", A.K. Mitra, ed., M. Dekker, Inc., New York (1993).
12. V.H.L. Lee, Precorneal Corneal and postcorneal factors, *in* "Ophthalmic Drug Delivery systems", A.K. Mitra, ed., M. Dekker, Inc., New York (1993).
13. I. Ahmed and T.F. Patton, Disposition of timolol and inulin in the rabbit eye following corneal versus non-corneal absorption, *Int. J. Pharm.*, 38:9 (1987).
14. K.J. Himmelstein, I. Guvenir and T.F. Patton, Preliminary pharmacokinetic model of pilocarpine uptake and distribution in the eye, *J. Pharm. Sci.*, 67:603 (1978).
15. S.S.Chrai, T.F. Patton, A. Mehta and J.R. Robinson , Lacrimal and instilled fluid dynamics in rabbit eyes, *J. Pharm. Sci.*, 62:1112 (1972).
16. T.F. Patton, Pharmacokinetic evidence for improved ophthalmic drug delivery by reduction of instilled volume, *J. Pharm. Sci.*, 66:1058 (1977).
17. T.J. Mikkelson , S.S. Chrai and J.R. Robinson, Altered bioavailability of drugs in the eye due to drug-protein interaction, *J. Pharm. Sci.* 62:1648 (1973).

18. G. Hecht, R.E. Roehrs and C.D. Shively, Design and evaluation of ophthalmic pharmaceutical products, *in* "Modern pharmaceutics", G.S. Banker and C.T. Rhodes, eds., M. Dekker, Inc., New York, 1979.

19. J.D. Mullins and G. Hecht, Ophthalmic preparations, *in* "Remington's pharmaceutical sciences", A.R. Gennaro, ed., Mack Publishing Co., Easton, 1990.

20. O. Olejnik, Conventional systems in ophthalmic drug delivery, *in* "Ophthalmic Drug Delivery systems", A.K. Mitra, ed., M. Dekker, Inc., New York (1993).

21. V.H.L. Lee, Precorneal corneal and postcorneal factors, *in* "Ophthalmic Drug Delivery systems", A.K. Mitra, ed., M. Dekker, Inc., New York (1993).

22. V.H.L. Lee, Improved ocular delivery by use of chemical modification (prodrugs), *in* "Biopharmaceutics of Ocular Drug Delivery", P. Edman, ed., CRC Press, Boca Raton (1993).

23. Various authors, "Ophthalmic Drug Delivery systems", A.K. Mitra, ed., M. Dekker, Inc., New York (1993).

24. Various authors, "Biopharmaceutics of Ocular Drug Delivery", P. Edman, ed., CRC Press, Boca Raton (1993).

25. R. Gurny, H. Ibrahim and P. Buri, The development and use of in situ formed gels, triggered by pH, *in* "Biopharmaceutics of Ocular Drug Delivery", P. Edman, ed., CRC Press, Boca Raton (1993).

26. A. Rozier, C. Mazuel, J. Grove and B. Plazonnet, Gelrite®, a novel, ion-activated, in-situ gelling polymer for ophthalmic vehicles. Effect on bioavailability of timolol, *Int. J. Pharm.*, 57:163 (1989).

27. R. Krishnamoorthy and A.K. Mitra, Mucoadhesive polymers in ocular drug delivery, *in* "Ophthalmic Drug Delivery systems", A.K. Mitra, ed., M. Dekker, Inc., New York (1993).

28. M.F. Saettone, Solid polymeric inserts/disks as drug delivery devices, *in* "Biopharmaceutics of Ocular Drug Delivery", P. Edman, ed., CRC Press, Boca Raton (1993).

29. J. Liaw and J.R. Robinson, Ocular penetration enhancers, *in* "Ophthalmic Drug Delivery systems", A.K. Mitra, ed., M. Dekker, Inc., New York (1993).

30. M.F. Saettone, P. Chetoni, R. Cerbai and G. Mazzanti, Effect of different enhancers on "in vitro" transcorneal penetration of drugs, Proceedings, 21st International Symposium on Controlled Release of Bioactive Materials, Nice (France), June 27-30, 1994, Vol 21:591 (1994).

DRUG DISTRIBUTION STUDIES IN SINGLE LENS LAYERS THROUGH THE APPLICATION OF A SECTIONING TECHNIQUE

Masami Kojima

Department of Ophthalmology, Kanazawa Medical University, Uchinada, Japan

INTRODUCTION

The pharmacodynamics of a drug need to be clarified before it can enter the market. The intraocular penetration of drugs which are expected to be used for a long term such as anti-cataract or anti-glaucoma drugs is a significant problem that we have to fully resolve before commencing their use in clinical trials. The previous studies concerning intralenticular drug penetration have been performed on entire lens samples, because of technical problems with analysis. In those investigations, the drug concentration obtained was an average value of the whole lens. In cases where small doses of the drug penetrated into only a limited area, the drug concentration in the entire lens might have been shown as below a detected level. In 1987, a new technique that overcame this disadvantage was introduced into the lens research field as a microsectioning analysis of the lens [1]. Utilizing this technology, regional lens layer analysis became possible and much new information was obtained which was not possible from the previous methodology [1,2]. Recently, the author applied this regional lens layer analysis to a drug penetration study in the lens and we found that highly localized low drug concentrations which were not detected in the entire lens samples could be detected with regional lens analysis [3]. This demonstrates that entire lens analysis is an inadequate method of detecting such low concentrations in the lens. In this study, the author again attempted to investigate intralenticular drug dynamics utilizing a lens sectioning technique.

MATERIALS AND METHODS

In this experiment, an aldose reductase inhibitor and a steroid were nominated as the sample drugs.

Topographic Distribution of Aldose Reductase in the Lens

The activity of the target enzyme of aldose reductase inhibitor (ARI), aldose reductase (AR), was measured in diabetic and normal rats before and after ARI treatment. 29 female 7 week old Brown Norway rats were divided into 4 groups: Group 1 (normal control, n=5), Group 2 (normal +ARI, n=6), Group 3 (diabetes control, n=8), Group 4 (diabetes+ARI, n=10). Diabetic rats were induced by injecting 70 mg/kg Streptozotocin into the tail vain. 10 days after diabetes induction, the rats which showed a higher than 300 mg/dl blood glucose level were selected as diabetic rat models. An ARI, 5 μl of 0.4% AD-5467 ophthalmic solution (Senju/Japan) or vehicle solution (without AD-5467) was instilled into the cul de sac 4 times daily. 9 days after the start of ARI or vehicle treatment, the lens changes were documented by a Scheimpflug camera (EAS-1000, Nidek). Thereafter, the rats were sacrificed according to the guidelines for animal experiments at Kanazawa Medical University, and the lenses were enucleated for AR activity measurement. The enucleated lenses were frozen and mechanically divided into an equatorial ring which corresponded to 20% of the lens diameter and an inner central cylinder portion corresponding to 80% of the lens diameter, with a 3 mm trephine. The central cylinder was sectioned into 5 single lens layers: the anterior shallow cortex, deeper cortex, nucleus, posterior deeper cortex, and posterior shallow cortex. The details of the sectioning technique were reported previously [3]. AR activity was measured according to Hayman & Kinoshita [4].

ARI Penetration into the Lens

5 μl of 0.4% AD-5467 were administered 5 times at 5 minute intervals in both eyes of 7 week old Brown Norway rats. AD-5467 concentrations in the eye tissues were measured 0.5, 1, 2, 4, 6, 12, 24, 36, and 48 hours after the final instillation. After rinsing the enucleated eyeballs with isotonic sodium chloride solution and blotting dry, the anterior chamber of the examined eye was punctured with a 26 gauge needle and the aqueous humor was corrected by capillary attraction. Lenses were removed from the enucleated eye balls by the posterior approach, rinsed with an isotonic sodium chloride solution, blotted dry and immediately frozen on a special plate for lens microsectioning and kept below -20°C. The enucleated lenses were divided into 6 lens layers including the equatorial ring through the procedure described above. To provide enough sample materials for drug concentration determination, the corresponding lens layers of the right and left lenses were combined as one analytical sample. 3 ml of methanol including 10 ng/ml of internal standard (AD-5491) were added to each lens section and then homogenized. AD-5467 was extracted from a homogenate solution and protein denaturation by means of 30 minute shaking at 37°C. After centrifugation at 10,000 G for 20 minutes, the supernatant was concentrated by evaporation. 300 μl of the mobile phase was added and injected into the high performance liquid chromatography (HPLC) system. The HPLC conditions were as follows: Drug detection wave length was UV 310 nm. The column was an Inertsil ODS-2, and the column temperature was 35°C. The composition of the mobile phase was 50 mM $N_aH_2PO_4$ (pH 6.5) : CH_3CN = 6 : 4.

Prednisolone Penetration into the Eye

Thirty-one adult pigmented rabbits (Japanese Mongrel) weighing from 1.5 to 3.0 kg were used in this study. The rabbits were randomly divided into short term and long term study groups. Rabbits in the short term study were divided into three groups and those in the long term were divided into two subgroups according to the drug administration methods.

Short Term Study Group

Eye Drop Instillation group (15 rabbits): 40 microliters of 0.1 % prednisolone acetate suspension (Nitten, Japan) were instilled five times into the cul de sacs of both rabbit eyes at five minute intervals. 15, 30, 60 and 120 minutes after the final instillation, the rabbits were sacrificed according to the guidelines for animal experiments in Kanazawa Medical University. Both eyeballs were enucleated to measure the drug penetration.

Retrobulbar Injection Group (4 rabbits): 1 mg/kg of 1 % prednisolone acetate suspension (Shionogi, Japan) was injected into the retrobulbar tissues of both eyes, separately. Sampling times were after 60 and 120 minutes after the injection.

Muscle Injection Group (4 rabbits): 1 mg/Kg of 1 % prednisolone acetate suspension was injected into the buttock muscles. Sampling times were 60 and 120 minutes.

Long Term Study Group

Eye Drop Instillation Group (4 rabbits): 40 microliter of 0.1 % prednisolone acetate suspension were instilled five times each at five minute intervals three times daily into the cul de sacs of both rabbits eyes. The total dosage of applied prednisolone acetate was about 1 mg/day. The drug instillation was continued for twenty-nine days. 60 minutes after the final instillation, samples were collected following the same procedures as those performed in the short term study.

Retrobulbar Injection Group (4 rabbits): 1 mg/Kg of 1 % prednisolone acetate suspension was injected into the retrobulbar tissues of both rabbit eyes for 29 days. The sampling time was 60 minutes after the final injection.

Sample Preparations

Aqueous Humor: After the enucleated eyeballs had been rinsed with isotonic sodium chloride solution and blotted dry, the anterior chamber of the examined eye was punctured with a 26 gauge needle and 200 microliters of the aqueous humor were taken as the materials.

Cornea: Following the removal of the eyes, the cornea was dissected from the limbus and then the central part of the cornea was punched out with a 9 mm trephine and washed with an isotonic sodium chloride solution and blotted dry. After measuring the wet weight of the removed corneal flap, it was transferred to homogenizing vessels, and then briefly minced with scissors. The tissues were homogenized in an ice bath with an appropriate-fold volume of 10% ethanol using a homogenizer (Poly Tron®). This homogenate was adjusted to the final concentration of 10% (w/v wet weight) homogenate and prednisolone was extracted by shaking for 3 hours at room temperature. 200 microliters of the supernatant were taken as a sample extract after centrifugation at 10,000 G for 30 minutes.

Lens: Lenses removed from the enucleated eyeballs through the anterior approach were rinsed with an isotonic sodium chloride solution, blotted dry and immediately frozen on a special plate for lens microsectioning technique and kept under -20°C for the following procedures. A frozen lens was divided into an equatorial ring portion which corresponded to 20% of the lens diameter and an inner cylinder portion corresponding with 80% of the lens diameter, with 7.0 - 8.0 mm trephine. The inner cylinder portion was separated into three layers: the anterior cortex, nucleus and posterior cortex. Sliced lens sections were weighed and homogenized with 10% ethanol 1 : 5 dilution weight per volume. The homogenized solution was centrifuged at 10,000 G for 30 minutes. 200 μl of supernatant were prepared. Dexamethasone was used as an internal standard for HPLC analysis. The drug was extracted by dichlormethane [5,6].

Vitreous: After removing the corneal flap and the lens, the remaining eyeball was frozen immediately in liquid nitrogen, afterwhich the central part of the frozen vitreous was withdrawn and centrifuged at 800 G for 30 minutes. 200 μl of the vitreous were used for HPLC analysis.

Serum: 1 ml of blood was taken from a marginal ear vein. The blood was allowed to stand for one hour at room temperature to obtain serum in the usual manner. 200 μl of the serum obtained by centrifugation were prepared for HPLC analysis.

Determination of HPLC conditions: A Shimadzu C-R7A Liquid Chromatograph System was utilized. A column was revered-face SHIN-PACK CLC-SIL. The mobile phase was composed by $CH_2CL_2:C_2H_5OH:H_2O = 95.5 : 4 : 0.5$.

The flow rate was 1 ml per minute and UV absorbance was set at 243.5 nm.

Further details of HPLC methods will be published in another article.

In Vitro Prednisolone Penetration Study

Freshly enucleated pig lenses were divided into 8 groups. The complete vitreous was removed in the lens groups A-1 to A-4, and the adherent parts of the vitreous were left in groups B-1 to B-4. The grouping scheme is shown in Figure 1.

These lenses were incubated with or without a divided chamber according to the method of Iwata and Horiuchi [17]. 2 μg/ml prednisolone acetate concentration were used. The lenses of groups A-1, A-2, B-1, and B-2 were incubated in a closed chamber system, groups A-3, A-4, B-3, and B-4 were incubated in a divided chamber system for 4 hours. Prednisolone acetate was applied from the lower vessel. Lenses in groups A-1 and A-2 without vitreous were incubated in a closed chamber system with the anterior part of the lens standing up or down in the incubation chamber, respectively. Groups B-1 and B-2 had the same conditions as groups A-1 and A-2, but the adherent parts of the vitreous were left in these lenses. Group A-3 lenses were placed in the divided chamber with the posterior side up, so that the lens anterior side was always attached to the prednisolone containing medium. The posterior side of the lenses in group A-4 always faced the drug containing medium. Group B-3 had the same condition as group A-3, but the lenses were with vitreous. Group B-4 lenses had the same condition as group A-4, but again with vitreous.

The upper chamber was filled with TCM-199 without prednisolone. After incubation, the lenses were rinsed with a TCM-199 without prednisolone acetate, blotted dried and

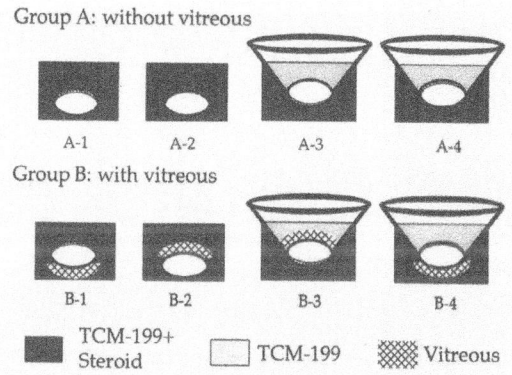

Figure 1. Grouping scheme.

immediately frozen for lens sectioning. The lens sectioning procedure was almost all the same as described above, but in this study, the lens was divided into 4 parts: the equatorial ring, the anterior cortex, nucleus, and posterior cortex.

The drug concentration in each lens section was measured by the HPLC system described above.

RESULTS

Early diabetic cataractous changes were observed in the diabetic control group by slit lamp examination 9 days after ARI treatment. In contrast, the AD-5467 treatment diabetes group (DM+ARI) showed a very slight lens change at the anterior subcapsular region (Figure 2).

Topographic Distribution of Aldose Reductase in the Lens

The aldose reductase activity corresponded highly with region; it was distributed in a U-shaped pattern almost symmetrical to the center of the normal lenses. The highest AR activity was found in the equatorial region part, followed by the anterior and posterior cortex layers, and the lowest was in the nucleus (Figure 3).

19 days after diabetic induction, AR activity of the diabetic control group was significantly higher ($p<0.05$) than normal in all the lens layers, except the equator.

On the other hand, the AR activity of the ARI treated group was significantly lower than that of the diabetes control group at the equator, anterior and posterior cortices. AR activity of the ARI treated normal group (normal+ARI) showed no big difference compared to the normal control group, however, higher AR activity was observed in the anterior and posterior deeper cortices and nucleus (Figure 3).

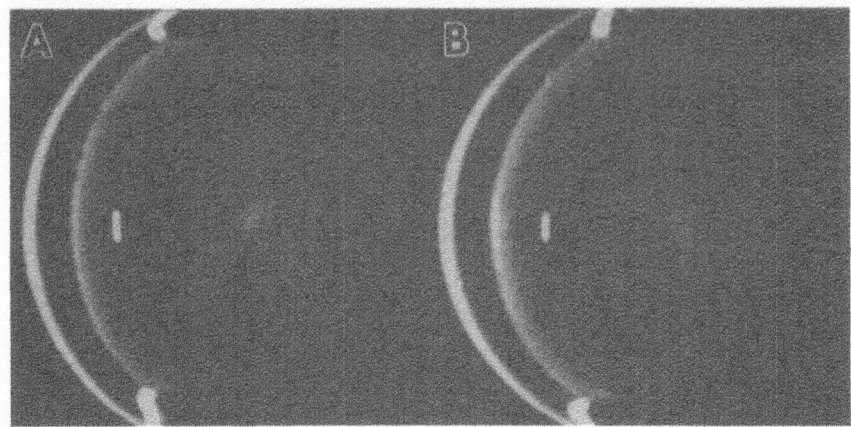

Figure 2. The representative lens condition 9 days after the start of ARI treatment. A: DM+ARI group. B: DM control group.

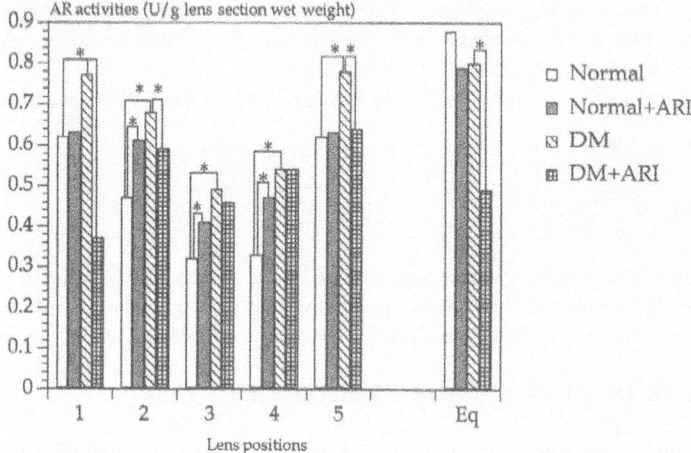

Figure 3. Aldose reductase activity in all groups. The asterisk indicates statistical difference ($p < 0.05$, t-test). The figure on the horizontal axis (1-5) indicates the position of the lens sections. 1 is the anterior side and 5 is the posterior side. Eq. means the equatorial part.

ARI Penetration into the Lens

Figure 4 shows the time course of ARI penetration into the eye. The pattern of ARI penetration into the eye had a two-phase peak. The highest concentration of AD-5467 was observed in the aqueous humor 30 minutes after the final instillation, afterwhich AD-5467 concentration in the aqueous humor gradually decreased. The ARI penetration in the lens detected from the early phase until 6 hours after the final instillation was highest in the equator followed by the anterior cortex, and the posterior cortex. No drug penetration was detected in the nucleus. During the late phase, however, after 12 hours, a low drug concentration was detected in the nucleus (Figure 4).

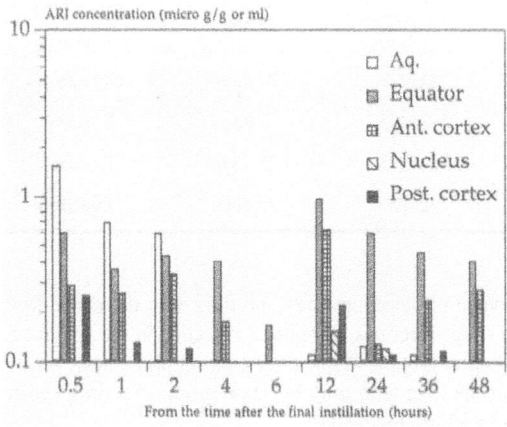

Figure 4. The time course of AD-5467 penetration into the eye. Aq. means aqueous humor.

Prednisolone Penetration into the Eye

A prednisolone acetate suspension eye drop showed good penetration into the ocular tissues (Table 1). In the eye drop instillation group, the highest concentration in the cornea was seen 15 minutes after the final instillation, thereafter it reducing gradually. The drug concentrations in the aqueous humor and the vitreous showed their highest peaks after 29 continuous drug instillation. The highest drug concentration in the serum was observed in the long term retrobulbar injection group. All of the highest drug concentrations detected from the lens samples were obtained from the long term eye drop application group (Table 1).

An accumulation of prednisolone acetate was not observed in the cornea after 29 days of repeated administration, however, varying grades were seen in the vitreous and the serum after the same term of administration (Figure 5).

The drug penetration mode into the lens was detected in the anterior cortex layer and the equatorial ring from 15 to 120 minutes and 30 and 60 minutes after the final instillation, respectively, in the short term drug administration group.

No detectable drug concentrations were found in the nucleus or the posterior layer.

However, after 29 days of continuous drug administration, it was detectable in the equatorial ring, the anterior cortical layer, and the posterior cortex, but not in the nuclear layer (Figure 6).

Table 1. The highest concentrations of prednisolone acetate in different tissues.

	Concentration (ng/ml or g)	Time	Group	n=
Cornea	4777±969	15 minutes	Eye drop	6
Aqueous humor	260±49	29 days	Eye drop	6
Serum	160±27	29 days	Retrobulbar injection	4
Vitreous	41±22	29 days	Eye drop	6
Lens (equator)	199±123	29 days	Eye drop	6
Lens (anterior)	126±105	29 days	Eye drop	6
Lens (posterior)	42±27	29 days	Eye drop	6

In the retrobulbar drug injection study, no drug was detectable from any ocular tissues receiving one shot drug injections, in spite of detection in the serum of both short and long term drug administration groups. A low drug concentration, however, was detected from the vitreous samples of the long term drug injection group. No drug penetration was found the lens after one shot injection (Figure 7).

After 29 days of continuous injection, a trace level of the drug was detected from the equatorial ring and the posterior cortex. It was <50 ng/g of the lens section's wet weight (data not shown).

In the rabbits receiving one shot injections into the muscle, no drug penetration into the ocular tissues was found. The drug concentration in the serum 60 and 120 minutes after the injection was 96.8 ng/ml and 127.6 ng/ml, respectively.

One rabbit died during the long term eye drop administration and two rabbits died during the long term retrobulbar injection (data not shown).

In Vitro Prednisolone Penetration Study

The prednisolone distribution was not homogeneous in the lenses of the groups either with or without vitreous. The highest drug penetration was observed in the equatorial ring followed by the anterior and posterior cortices. A slight prednisolone concentration could be detected in the nucleus when the lens was incubated without vitreous (Figure 8). In the closed chamber incubation system, prednisolone concentration was not effected by the position of the lens placement or the absence or presence of vitreous.

Figure 9 demonstrates the prednisolone distribution in the lens with a divided chamber incubation system. When prednisolone was applied from the anterior side (A-3, B-3), the highest drug penetration in the lens layer was observed in the anterior cortex followed by the equator. No drug concentration was detected in the nucleus or the posterior cortex. There was a tendency of higher drug concentrations in the anterior cortex and equator of the groups

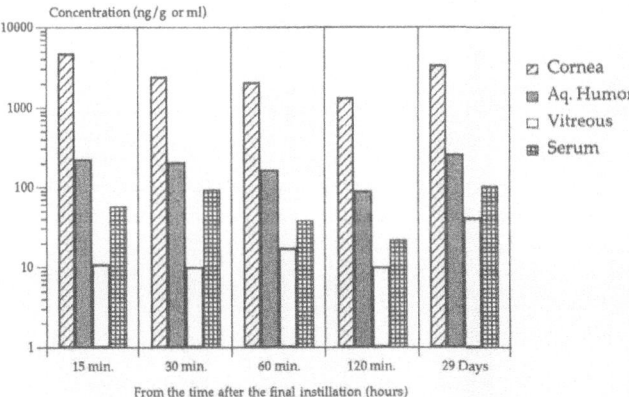

Figure 5. The prednisolone concentrations in different tissues and the time courses of the eye drop groups.

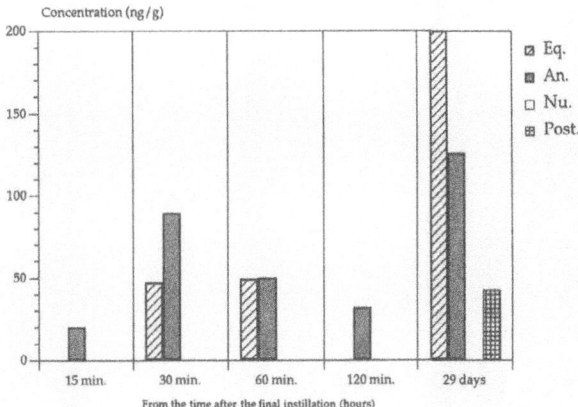

Figure 6. The prednisolone concentrations in the lenses of the eye drop groups. (Eq : Equator, An.: the anterior cortex, Nu.: nucleus, Post.: the posterior cortex)

with no vitreous. When the drug was applied from the posterior side (A-4, B-4), drug penetration was found only in the posterior cortex, followed by the equator. No drug penetration was detected in the nucleus or the anterior cortex. A comparison of drug concentrations in the posterior cortex between the groups with and without vitreous showed significantly higher levels without vitreous than with vitreous (Figure 9). In the case of lens incubation without vitreous, the posterior side drug application group showed much higher drug penetration in the lens layer of the drug applied side than that of the anterior drug application group.

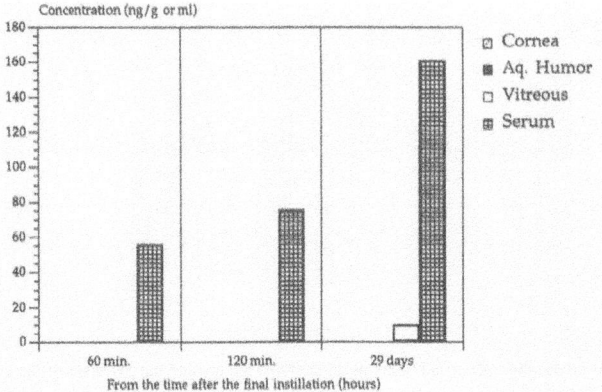

Figure 7. The prednisolone concentrations in different tissues and the time courses of the retrobulbar injection groups.

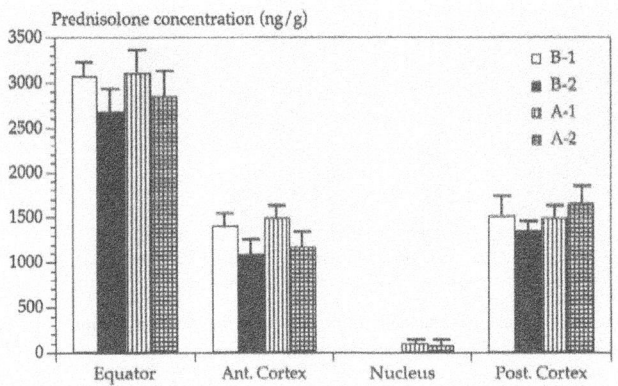

Figure 8. The prednisolone distribution in the lens. The data demonstrated the mean±SE of drug concentration in each lens layer after incubation the lens for 4 hours in a closed chamber system. A-1: Lens position being the anterior pole up (without vitreous), A-2: the anterior pole down (without vitreous), B-1: the anterior pole up (with vitreous), B-2: the posterior pole down (with vitreous).

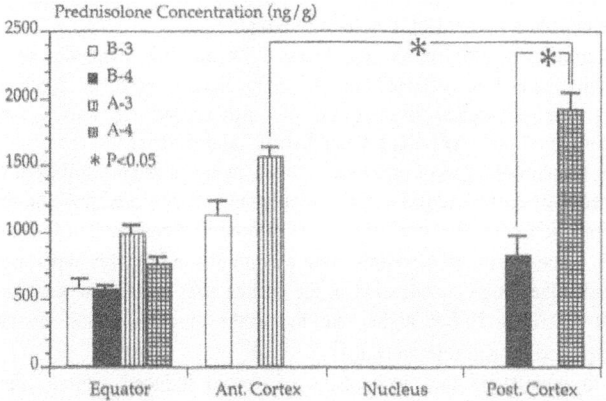

Figure 9. The prednisolone distribution in the lens after incubating for 4 hours in a divided chamber system. The data indicated the mean±SE in each lens layers. A-3: Lens position being the anterior pole down (without vitreous), A-4: the anterior pole up (without vitreous), B-3: the anterior pole down (with vitreous), B-4: the anterior pole up (with vitreous)

DISCUSSION

How the drug reaches the target organ or tissues when applied locally is a very important factor in the study of lens pharmacokinetics yet this aspect has not been fully investigated in all kinds of drugs. In the case of a pharmacological target organ or tissue, the drug therapy must reach the intraocular components. The efficacy of the drug depends on its corneal permeability. Many features influence this factor, such as instilled volume, osmolality, pH, viscosity, drugs and adjuvant, and lipophilic/hydrophilic characteristics etc., which make it difficult to determine the corneal permeability of drugs in general. However, it seems that we have to fully resolve these problems for newly developing drugs before we can commence using them in clinical trials. The main problem for drug therapy is to allow a sufficient amount of drug to reach the pharmacological targets. In this study, the author nominated an aldose reductase inhibitor to test for drug therapeutic problems and a corticosteroid for drug toxicity.

It is well known that the target enzyme, aldose reductase (EC 1.1.1.21) for aldose reductase inhibitor, is not homogeneously distributed in the lens [8]. In this study AR distribution in the lens was also shown to be highly related to lens layer. The highest AR activity was seen at the equator, followed by the anterior and posterior cortices, and the lowest amount of activity was found at the nucleus. After the induction of diabetes, the AR activity in diabetic rat lenses was significantly higher than normal in all the lens layers, except the equator. Conversely, the AR activity of an ARI treated rat lens 9 days after the start of ARI administration was significantly lower than that of the ARI non-treated diabetes control group. The drug penetration results showed that the main ARI drug penetration lens parts were in the equator, the anterior and posterior cortices. The ARI penetration into the nucleus part might be expected in cases of long term treatment.

The ARI penetration detected in the lens layers from the drug dynamics study and the AR enzyme activity reduction detected in the lens layers were in complete agreement. Furthermore, morphological observation of ARI treated rat lenses remained almost transparent compared with ARI non-treated diabetic control lenses.

In spite of the contribution of previous authors, many problems still exist concerning the pharmacokinetics of corticosteroid in the ocular tissues. Since prednisolone acetate uptake is high in the lipid rich corneal epithelium, it has commonly been used in the ophthalmological field [6,9]. This is the reason why prednisolone was nominated for this experiment.

In this study, the drug concentration in the cornea after instillation was the highest of all the tissues. It was 10 to 20 fold higher than that in the aqueous, which was almost the same data as that reported by Kupferman et al.[10].

In order to understand the mechanisms of steroid induced cataract, the route of the administered steroid into the crystalline lens should be clarified. Although intralenticular corticosteroid penetration studies have been performed [8], the methodologies applied were different from those of the authors'. This study aimed to investigate topographic lenticular drug distribution together with the route of drug penetration into the ocular tissues by using a convenient HPLC technique combined with a newly applied microsectioning method.

Regarding intralenticular drug concentration after topical instillation, the highest concentrations of prednisolone acetate were observed in the cornea, the aqueous and the serum 15 and 30 minutes after topical drug administration. That in the vitreous was at a trace level during almost the entire observation period (Figure 5). A low level concentration of prednisolone acetate was detectable only in the anterior part 15 minutes after. The highest drug concentration in the lens was noticed in the anterior cortex 30 minutes after. The drug penetration into the equatorial ring was detectable after 30 minutes and continued to be noticed after 60 minutes. From the above penetration pattern of instilled prednisolone acetate into the eye, the main route of the drug penetration was considered to be via the cornea to the aqueous and into the lens (Figures 5,6). By another administration method of retrobulbar injection, the drug was detectable in the serum during the short term observation period after 60 and 120 minutes and on the 29th day of the long term continuous administration study, while only traces of the drug were found in the vitreous 29 days after drug injection (Figure 7). Traces of the drug were noticed in the equatorial ring and the posterior cortex on the 29 days, however, no drug was detectable in other parts of the lens. These results suggest that prednisolone acetate administered retrobulbar injection may enter the lens from the posterior side. The results principally supported the concept of the steroid delivery route into ocular tissues from the periocular tissues [10, 11, 18].

The other purpose of this study was to investigate the possibility of making an in vitro model of drug distribution into the lens, in order to avoid sacrificing many animals for this kind of experiment.

With the whole lens incubation methods, using a closed chamber in which the condition of the outer lens circumstances was a homogeneous steroid concentration, no significant differences in drug concentration due to the position of the lens placement or the absence or presence of vitreous were seen. This means that a whole lens incubation with a closed chamber system is an inadequate method of detecting the route of drug penetration into the eye. The prednisolone concentration was 2 times higher in the equator than in the other lens layers. This might be due to the differences in the sample area which faces the drug. The estimated area of the equator is 2 times larger than that of the other lens layers.

A divided chamber was reported by Iwata[7] for the purpose of artificially creating the conditions of the anterior chamber and the vitreous cavity. In the divided lens chamber incubation without vitreous, the drug penetration in the lens layer was detected in the anterior cortex and the equator, but not in the nucleus or the posterior cortex. In contrast, when the drug was applied from the posterior side, drug penetration was detected in the posterior cortex and the equator, but not in the anterior cortex or the nucleus. In the case of lens incubation without vitreous, the posterior side drug application group showed a much higher drug penetration in the lens layer of the drug applied side than that of the anterior drug application group. The author would like to think that this difference is due to the absence or presence of the epithelial cell layer.

When a lens was incubated in the presence of a vitreous in a divided chamber which is much more similar to the physiological condition, the prednisolone penetration pattern in the lens was almost the same as that of the lens incubated without vitreous. However, when a drug was applied from the posterior lens side, the presence of the vitreous made a big difference to the amount of drug penetration into the lens. This phenomenon may be explained by a certain amount of drug being trapped by the vitreous.

The data from lens incubation in the presence of a vitreous in a divided chamber are similar to the results from in vivo drug penetration studies on rabbits. Since the data from drug distribution in the lens by eye drop application is very similar to the data from the anterior side drug application with a divided chamber, the main route of drug penetration into the lens must be diffusion from the anterior side. The drug distribution pattern from the posterior drug application by retrobulbar injection was found to be almost the same as that from the posterior drug application with a divided chamber indicating that the route of drug penetration into the eye might be via the sclera, the choroid, the vitreous, and the lens.

In conclusion, the application of a regional lens sectioning technique to the study of drug penetration yields more precise data. When used in combination with Scheimpflug photography, regional enzymatic analysis and regional drug penetration study provide a better understanding of the mechanisms of lens changes that occur in distinct regions of the lens due to cataractogenesis or drug side-effects. Furthermore, the combination of the regional lens sectioning technique and the divided chamber lens incubation system was able to reduce the number of experimental animals sacrificed.

Acknowledgments

The author thanks Professor Sasaki for his kind revision of the manuscript. The excellent technical assistance of Dr. Ying Bo Shui and Mr. Yoshimasa Abe is gratefully acknowledged.

REFERENCES

1. A. Müller, B. Möller, V. Dragomirescu, O. Hockwin, Profiles of enzyme activities in bovine lenses, in: "Drug-induced ocular side effects and ocular toxicology," O.Hockwin, ed., Karger, Basel (1987).
2. M. Kojima, Enzyme distribution pattern of rats lenses and changes during naphthalene cataract development, Ophthalmic Res 24:73 (1987).
3. M. Kojima, O. Hockwin, and K. Sasaki: A new approach to drug penetration study, Lens and Eye Toxicity Res 9(3&4):547 (1992).
4. S. Hayman and H.J. Kinoshita, Isolation and properties of lens aldose reductase, J Biol Chem 240: 877 (1965).
5. J.Q. Rose, and W.J. Jusko, Corticosteroid analysis in biological fluids by high-performance liquid chromatography. J Chromatogr, 163:273 (1979).
6. F. Tsuji, H. Hikishima, K. Sasaki, and A. Tsuji A, Intraocular penetration of steroid high performance liquid chromatographic determination. Journal of the Eye, 3:396 (1985).
7. S. Iwata and M. Horiuchi, Structural characteristics of lens and its drug-response. J Pharm Soc J, 102: 935 (1982).
8. Y. Akagi, H. Tasaka, H. Terubayashi, P.F. Kador, and J.H. Kinoshita, Aldose reductase localization in rat sugar cataract, in: "Polyol pathway and its role in diabetic complications," N. Sakamoto, J.H. Kinoshita, P.F. Kador, N. Hotta, eds., Excerpta Medica, Amsterdam, New York, Oxford (1988).
9. H.M Leibowitz, and A. Kupferman, Kinetics to topically administered prednisolone acetate, Arch Ophthalmol, 94: 1387 (1976).
10. A. Kupferman, and H.M. Leibowitz, Biological equivalence of ophthalmic prednisolone acetate suspensions. Am J Ophthalmol 82:109 (1976).

OCULAR PHARMACOKINETICS OF SOME PROTEOLYTIC DRUGS IN THE COURSE OF TOPICAL APPLICATION: LONG TERM OBSERVATION

G.S. Polunin, M.N. Ivanov, A.A. Fedorov, A.N. Ovchinnikov

Research Institute of Eye Diseases, Russian Academy of Medical Science, Moscow, Russia

ABSTRACT

We have made a comparative study of the effects which occurred when some proteolytic enzymes of animal, vegetable and microbial origin and kallikrein-trypsin inhibitors were applied to either unchanged or impaired ocular tissues and fluids. The analysis was based on the experimental data and on clinical research.

This comparative study was instrumental in defining the following main lines of approach to enzymotherapy:

- selection of an enzyme in line with its specific form of action and the specific features of a pathological formation;
- definition of optimum therapeutic dosage forms;
- selection of a method of attack on pathological formation;
- creation of favorable condition for prolonging the duration of action of an enzyme drug in an impaired tissue.

We have worked out some new ways of employing known enzymes and indications for using these enzymes in the complex treatment of a variety of diseases and disorders, including vitreous hemorrhages and uveitis of various etiology, microsurgical and laser treatment of glaucoma, cataract extraction and non-surgical treatment of chalazion, scar of eyelids and obstruction of nasolacrimal ducts.

INTRODUCTION

At present, ophthalmological clinics use some proteolytic drugs (chymotrypsin, fibrinolysin, streptase, urokinase, lekosim). Attention is drawn to these products mostly because they display fibrinolytic activity or because the use of some of them leads to lysis of hemorrhages and exudates.[1-4]

Some researchers point out that, after a thorough study of specific properties of certain proteolytic enzymes has been made, one can expect to increase their potential therapeutic activity. In 1971 Prof. M.M. Krasnov[5] reported that a specific protease which normally destroys kallikrein and trypsin was instrumental in reconstructing the anterior eye segment. In 1979 G.A. Kisiliov and L.V. Kovaliova discovered that papain increases trabecular permeability. It was also reported that immobilization of streptase prolonged its fibrinolytic effect[7] and that lekosim prevented growth of connective tissue.[8]

A clinician has a task in each case of enzyme use, i.e. inducing lysis of fibrin or clot of blood, of destroying certain pathological formations of ocular tissues, preventing scar growth, etc. One can find the solution of such problems through a purposeful search for specific proteolytic drugs and careful selection of their dosages, as well as by defining the optimum performance criteria for such drugs and an appropriate course of treatment.

MATERIALS AND METHODS

The material and methods have previously been published. References to this information can be found in the relevant sections below.

We made experimental and clinical investigations. The enzymes of animal origin such as fibrinolysin (St. Petersburg Co. of Medical Drugs, Russia), chymotrypsin (Moscow Co. of Medical Drugs), and urokinase-ukidan (Serono Pharm. Praparate GmbH Freiburg i Br.), vegetable origin such as lekosim (Lek. Co., Slovenia), and microbial origin such as kollalysin (Inst. for vaccine and serum, St. Petersburg, Russia), protelin (Inst. of Organic Chemistry, Moscow, Russia), and streptase (Germany) were employed. Enzyme solutions were prepared immediately before their administration. The drugs were administered by instillations, subconjunctival injections, or electrophoresis. Chinchilla rabbits were used in our experiments. Our purpose was to study the penetration of enzymes through the cornea and the action of proteases on normal and pathological tissues. Indications of enzyme application in therapy and microsurgery of some eye diseases were defined.

We followed patients with different eye pathology: intraocular hemorrhages of various etiology, glaucoma, cataract, keratoiridociclytes, chalazion, dacryocystitis and scar deformations of eyelids. All patients were divided into groups and subgroups. This will be discussed below.

RESULTS

Penetration of Proteolytic Drugs, Administered by Different Methods, into Anterior Chamber Fluid

The animals were divided in 15 groups, with 6 animals in each group. The enzyme products of animal origin (fibrinolysin, chymotrypsin, urokinase), vegetable origin (lekosim) and microbial origin (streptase, kollalysin, protelin) were employed.[9]

Drugs were administered by means of topical instillation, subconjunctival injection or electrophoresis (current 0.5 mA, exposure 10 min). A combination of the above mechanisms was employed as well. Anterior chamber fluids were extracted by way of syringe with puncturing of the anterior chamber at hourly intervals following the administration of the drugs. Anson's biochemical method was used for assessing the proteolytic activity of anterior chamber fluid.

As a result of our experiments, we established[10] (Tab. 1) that the peak activity of anterior chamber fluid was attained following administration of direct action enzyme drugs of vegetable (lekosim) and microbial (protelin) origin.

Table 1. Proteolytic activity of aqueous humor after parabulbaric injection of some drugs.

Drugs	Dosage (1st injection)	Activity	Time after injection (hours)					
			1	2	3	4	5	6
Control	–	–	3.1±1.5	2.6±1.8	2.9±2.0			
Lekosim	1.0 Fip	–	9.7±2.8	9.2±3.4	4.5±3.2	4.2±2.1	3.6±2.4	3.2±1.6
Protelin	0.1%	8 PU/g	11.2±2.8	9.2±1.8	4.0±2.4	3.8±2.0	4.0±1.8	2.8±2.0
Protolysin	0.2%	2000 PA U/g	8.2±3.0	8.0±3.2	3.6±1.8	3.6±2.2	3.4±1.6	
Collalysin	10.0 KU	–	6.6±3.1	5.7±2.8	3.8±2.2	4.0±2.2	3.8±1.6	
Terralysin	0.3%	2.5 PU/g	4.8±1.5	3.6±1.5	3.0±2.4			
Streptase	5000 IU	–	4.2±1.7	4.7±1.8	2.8±1.6	3.2±1.6		
Urokinase	5000 IU		3.9±1.4	3.2±1.8	3.0±1.8			
Fibrinolysin	16 U		4.1±1.6	3.8±1.6	2.6±1.8			
Chymotrypsin	1 mg	–	3.2±1.8	3.6±1.2	3.1±1.6			
Collitin	1 mg	–	3.5±2.2	3.2±1.6	2.8±1.2			

Direct action enzyme drugs of animal origin (chymotrypsin) and plasmin activator (streptase) produced a moderate increase of activity of anterior chamber fluid. Peak proteolytic activity was recorded one hour following administration of drugs; irrespective of the mechanisms by which enzymes were introduced, high proteolytic concentrations occurred for an average of 3 hours and then started to decrease drastically.

Subconjunctival injection of 1.0 Fip lekosim with subsequent electrophoresis proved to be the means of attaining maximum proteolytic activity of anterior chamber fluids.

Effect of Proteases and Kallikrein-trypsin Inhibitor on Reparative Processes in Cornea

We have performed some experiments on rabbits (36 animals) in order to evaluate the action of proteases and kallikrein-trypsin inhibitors - gordox (Gedeon Richter, Hungarn).[11] Thermal burns of the cornea were made at 20 points parallel to the limbus by means of a globe-shaped electrode (0.5 mm diameter) at 100°C.

As the result of these experiments,[11] we found that instillation of the kallikrein-trypsin inhibitors 5 times daily accelerated the reparative processes in the cornea. Complete epithelialization was recorded at an average at 7.2±0.4 days following administration of drugs, whereas in a control group of rabbits respective values averaged at 8.5±0.3 days. In animals receiving treatment with proteases, complete epithelialization was observed at 10.4±0.5 days after initiation of treatment. It is significant that the scar characteristics were not the same. After medication with proteases the cornea was essentially transparent at the burn sites in 87% of the animals and the impaired section was reduced in thickness to 0.5 mm. In other rabbits solid fibrous scars (wall-eye) developed and the cornea was thickened to 1.1±0.1 mm. We thus arrived at the conclusion that proteases prevented fibrosis and were instrumental in conserving injury surface shape.

Performance of Proteolytic Drugs in Laser Goniopuncture

Our histological studies (light microscopy) of the anterior chamber angle of the eye which we made on rabbits before and after argon application[12] revealed some common types of inflammation around the laser application focus. The burn surface was then covered with fibrin and fibroblasts started to migrate there to form a fibrous structure, i.e. a fibrous scar developed.

The anterior chamber angle in the eyes treated with proteolytic drugs differed from the one in the control group. It, unlike the latter one, was not completely filled with cells similar to fibroblasts. It was observed that fibrinous conglomerations dissipated and a delicate scar developed.

Specific Effects of Lekosim Application in Crystalline Lens

The aim of our first series of experiments (21 rabbits were divided in groups, with 3 animals in each group) was to find out how enzymes administered in various dosages affected the linkage between lens fibres in cortical masses.[16]

0.15-0.2 ml dosages of lekosim solution (0.1 Fip in 1.0 ml) of different concentrations were administered into cortical masses following the extraction of the lens nucleus. Enzyme exposure was for 5 minutes. Isotonic solution was administered to animals in a control group.

It was discovered that the lens fibres were tightly linked with each other and with the lens capsule following an injection of isotonic solution, and the space between the fibres was intensively colored by toluidin-blue (dye for proteoglycans). Administration of lekosim destroyed the linkage between fibres, inducing their disintegration down to small groups and their separation from the capsule. The action of kollalysin was less pronounced since the linage between separate fibres and between the fibres and the capsule only partially disintegrated.

Our experiments have shown that the administration of enzymes in the manner to the lens did not induce any significant changes in the corneal endothelium. Examination of zonulaciliaris, retina, and vitreous body revealed no tissue changes.

Application of Proteolytic Drugs in Treatment of Vitreous Hemorrhages

Patients with intraocular hemorrhages of various etiology (267 patients)[13] but in cases with compensation of the main pathological process and in the absence of hemorrhages relapses were treated. Proteolytic drugs, when administered in therapeutic dosages (0.7 Fip in 0.2 ml of isotonic solution) by subconjunctival injection (made every other day, 5 injections per one course, treatment courses were repeated every 6 months), favored prevention of blood clots and accelerated blood resorption.

The peak therapeutic effectiveness was recorded when a direct action multicomponent enzyme drug (lekosim) was used in combination with plasmin activators (urokinase, streptokinase).

Application of Some Enzymes in Microsurgery and Laser Treatment of Glaucoma

We have worked out methods of proteolytic drug use for limiting the scarring of new ways of outflow, which were brought into being by microsurgical and laser treatment of glaucoma[14,15]:

(1) Administration of lekosim in combination with subsequent electrophoresis, following microsurgical operations of glaucoma reduced intraocular pressure to the norm in half of patients who had a tendency to have an increase in intraocular pressure. Lekosim in 1.0 Fip dosages was administered repeatedly up to 10 times by injection into the zone of filtration.

(2) Subconjunctival injections of lekosim in patients (143 patients) with initial stage open angle glaucoma, brought intraocular pressure to normal levels in 70% of patients (3 years observation). Lekosim in 1.0 Fip dosages was administered repeatedly up to 5 times by subconjunctival injections into the zone of argon laser application (Tab. 2, tab. 3).

(3) Medication with gordox before and after laser iridectomy of uveal glaucoma (87 patients) was inducive to saving coloboma in the iris of 18 patients, and the rest needed further laser treatment. A single 100000 KU dosage of gordox was administered by intravenous injection before iridectomy and the same dosages were given repeatedly for five days following iridectomy.

Lekosim Application in Microsurgery of Cataract

In patients with extracapsular cataract extraction (58 patients), the local

Table 2. Intraocular pressure (mm Hg) in patients treated by laser trabeculopuncture (LTP) combined with lekosim.

Procedure	Number of patients	Pressure (average)						P
		Start	1 day	1 week	1 month	3 months	6 months	
LTP	20	27.4	22.0	26.9	22.5	24.7	27.6	<0.05
Lekosim	20	28.0	27.3	27.5	28.4	27.6	27.9	<0.05
LTP+lekosim	20	29.1	22.1	22.5	23.1	22.2	22.3	<0.001

Table 3. Treatment results of glaucoma patients at 3 years after laser trabeculopuncture combined with subconjunctival injections of lekosim.

	Improvement	No change	Worsening
1. Hydrodynamic parameters	72.0%	26.0%	2.0%
2. Field of vision	13.5%	82.0%	4.5%
3. Acuity of vision	-	86.5%	13.5%

Table 4. Volume of washing fluid needed for removing lens mass during extracapsular cataract extraction.

Washing fluids	Volume of washing fluid
Saline solution + lekosim	69.6%
Saline solution + kollalysin	82.4%
Saline solution	100%

administration of lekosim under the lens capsule (1.0 Fip of lekosim in 0.2 ml of saline/isotonic solution, 4 minutes exposure) decreased the volume of irrigation fluid (Tab. 4), needed for the removal of lens mass by 34% and made unnecessary further mechanical cleaning of the posterior capsule[16].

Topical Improvement of Lekosim in Keratoplasty

Early administration of lekosim following penetrating keratoplastic treatment of ulcers in viral keratoiridociclytes (22 patients) favored exudate resorption and prevented the development of anterior synechiae which was one of the most frequent postoperative complications following such operations. A 1.0 Fip dosage of lekosim was administered in this case by subconjunctival injection.[10]

Intravitreal Application of Lekosim in Treatment of Hemorrhages

The study of intravitreal application of lekosim (0.05 Fip in 1.0 of saline solution) in treatment patients with traumatic hemophthalmia was carried out on 22 persons (17-54 years). The data of ophthalmological and electrophysiological examination of the retina were classified as positive. Lekosim was administered by injection into the central vitreous body. Prior to injection incisions of sclera were made at 5-6 mm from limbus. The incisions were 2/3 of the sclera thickness. The treatment course comprised 1-3 injections given repeatedly every two weeks. The transparency of the vitreous body and increase of visual acuity (0.2-1.0) were recorded 3 month following the treatment. No complications were observed in patients who received this treatment.

Enzymotherapy of Nasolacrimal Duct Obstructions

The medical liquid cleansing of the nasolacrimal canal was made in three groups of patients. Dosages of 10-12 Fip of lekosim in 2 ml of saline/isotonic solution were used for cleansing in the first group of patients (47 patients), chymotrypsin solution was used in the second group (44 patients), and a saline/isotonic solution was used in the third group (42 patients). The degree of obstruction of the nasolacrimal canal was checked by an x-ray contrast method. The duration of the obstruction ranged from 1 month to 2.5 years. Liquid cleansing of lacrimal ducts was given twice a week.

It was recorded that the permeability of the nasolacrimal canal was restored in 22 patients (45%) who received treatment with lekosim. The duration of obstruction in the majority of these patients ranged between 1 and 4 months. The permeability was restored in 19 patients (41%) who received treatment with chymotrypsin. In a control group of patients, restoration of permeability was recorded for 2 patients only (Tab. 5).

Table 5. Restoration of nasal-lacrimal duct permeability depending upon therapy employed.

Washing solution	Number of patients	Permeability restoration
Lekosim solution	47	44.5%
Chymotrypsin solution	44	41.2%
Saline solution	42	4.8%

Enzymotherapy of Scar Deformations of Eyelids

We followed 43 patients aged 14-65. The time of observation ranged between 6 and 24 months. The scar life ranged from one month to 25 years. Doses of 1.5-2.0 Fip of lekosim in 0.2 ml of saline/isotonic solution were administered once a week repeatedly 5-10 times. Good cosmetic results were observed in 15 (34%) patients who did not need further surgery.

Lekosim Treatment of Chalazion

We have worked out a new method of treating chalazion by injecting lekosim into a pathological formation [17]. The doses of 1-5 Fip of lekosim in 0.1-0.5 ml of saline/isotonic solution were dependent on a size of the pathological formation (smaller injection volumes in smaller lesions). Complete resorption of chalazion following 1-3 injections was recorded for 17 patients out of the total number of 28 persons who received this treatment, and in 9 patients complete resorption was recorded after 4-6 injections (8 months observation).

Enzyme Therapy of Cataract

We have proved that lekosim administered by parabulbar injections was inducive in decreasing optical density of the posterior capsule and cortical layers of lens. The data of microdensitometry and photos of optical cuts of lens bore ample evidence of it. [18]

It has been revealed that in treatment of cortical cataract in patients with diabetes mellitus, administration of lekosim by parabulbar injection in combination with Sencatalin instillations was more effective for reducing optical density than Sencatalin as monotherapy. [19]

It is evident that a further study of enzyme drugs looks very promising and that new possibilities will be opened in therapy and microsurgery of eye diseases thanks to new enzyme drugs.

DISCUSSION

We have worked out new methods of enzyme therapy based on the results of our study and managed to show the performance of enzyme drugs was dependent both on the pathogenesis of an eye disease and on changes at the ultrastructural, cellular, and molecular levels of ocular tissues.

Small concentrations of enzymes can be used for the diffusive penetration of ocular tissues by electrophoresis and parabulbar injections. In such cases one can induce lysis of hemorrhages and exudates and restores the transparency of eye optical media. At the same time, small concentrations of enzymes can have an effect on metabolism in tissues and, in particular, on accelerating fluid metabolism and increasing the diffusion of drugs into ocular tissues. The latter point needs some further investigation.

Large concentrations of enzymes can be used as a peculiar biological instrument for removing such pathological changes in ocular tissues which are inoperable. To widen the range of indications for the use of large concentrations of enzymes in ophthalmotherapy, one has to design special instruments for local administration of enzyme drugs.

Enzyme drugs thus can be used as a difference from the usual biological instrument which makes possible to prevent unwanted development of fibrosis, restore transparency of eye optical media, and improve metabolic processes an deliver of necessary drugs to a site of impairment.

REFERENCES

1. G.S. Polunin, O.V. Zobnin, Proteolytic enzymes and kallikrein-trypsin inhibitors in ophthalmology, Vestnik Ophthalmol. (Russia) 2:9 (1977).
2. G.L. Starkov, V.I. Savinich, Enzymotherapy in Ophthalmology, Kemerovo, Russia (1977).
3. V.F. Danilichev, Therapeutic Effectiveness of Some Proteolytic Enzymes in Treatment of Eye Diseases, M.D. thesis, Leningrad, Russia (1983).
4. M. Wolf, K. Ransberger, Enzymotherapy, Vantage Press, NY (1972).
5. M.M. Krasnov, Surgical Reconstruction of the anterior eye segment. Vestnik Ophthalmol. (Russia) 5:66 (1971).
6. G.A. Kiselev, T.B. Kovaleva, Papain in microsurgery, Kasan Medical J. (Russia) 1:32 (1978).
7. R.A. Gundorova, V.P. Makarova, A.D. Romatshenko, E.D. Gamm, Study of the therapeutic and toxicity effects of the streptodecase, Vestnik Ophthalmol. (Russia) 4:37 (1985).
8. M.N. Pavlova, T.I. Podosheva, O.N. Polakov, Effect of papain on the normal and pathological changes in connective tissue, in: Proteolytic Enzymes of the Carica Papaya (Lekosim) in Medical Practice, Moscow, Russia (1978).
9. G.S. Polunin, M.N. Ivanov, N.A. Zvereva, Ocular pharmacokinetics of some proteases, J. of Medical Abstracts (Russia) VIII:11:6 (1990).
10. G.S. Polunin, Indication and Methods of Enzymotherapy in Ophthalmology, M.D. thesis, Moscow, Russia (1990).
11. G.S. Polunin, Proteolytic enzymes and inhibitors of proteases in

treatment of thermal burns of cornea (in experimental study). 3rd
Russian Ophthalmology meeting, Rostov-Don, Russia 2:192
(1975).

12. G.S. Polunin, Protelin drug in lasertrabeculopuncture and
laseriridectomy (experimental study), Vestnik Ophthalmol.
(Russia) 2:9 (1977).

13. G.S. Polunin, Clinical topography of hemophthalmia, Vestnik Ophthalmol.
(Russia) 1:38 (1982).

14. G.S. Polunin, V.S. Akopyan, Increase of therapeutic effectiveness of
lasertrabeculopuncture by administration proteolytic enzymes, in:
Lasermethods of Treatment in Ophthalmology, Moscow, Russia
(1983).

15. G.S. Polunin, V.S. Akopyan, N.M. Drozdova, Kallikrein-trypsin
inhibitor in laseriridectomy of uveaglaucoma, in: Lasermethods of
Treatment in Ophthalmology, Moscow, Russia (1983).

16. M.N. Ivanov, Proteolytic enzymes in extracapsular cataract extraction,
M.D. thesis, Moscow, Russia (1990).

17. G.S. Polunin, M.N. Ivanov, Lekosim therapy of chalazion, Vestnik
Ophthalmol. (Russia) 3:44 (1985).

18. M.M. Krasnov, G.S. Polunin, Impact of certain proteolytic agents on the
developments of different types of cataract, in: Risk Factor of
Cataract Development, Dev. ophthalmol. Basel, Karger, 17:199
(1988).

19. G.S. Polunin, Influence of certain drugs on the densitometry results of
optic lens sections, Ophthalmic Res., 22 (suppl 1):85 (1990).

NEW METHOD OF REVERSE INTRAATERIAL DRUG INFUSION INTO FINAL PERIORBITAL CHANNELS OF OPHTHALMIC ARTERY IN URGENT TREATMENT OF TOXIC OPTICNEUROPATHY

D.L. Bayandin, O.K. Vorobyeva, and Y.G. Klimchenko

Research Institute of Eye Diseases
Russian Academy of Medical Science
Electromechanical Research Institute, Moscow, Russia

ABSTRACT

Advantages of intraarterial drug infusion method into the eye blood supply region with the help of automatic thermoinfusion device were shown in comparison with the traditional methods. They were the following: absence of side influence on intraocular and regional hemodynamics, the direct drug infusion into the eye blood supply region, simplicity and convenience of the device use for medical staff and patients. The drug infusion method was used in clinic in 21 patients with retrobulbar toxic neuritis, 23 procedures of infusion system implantation were performed. It patients were in the control group. In the result of infusion therapy by TRENTAL and ACTOVEGIN medications in turn during 120 hours acuity vision increase was achieved practically in all patients. Acuity vision increased from 0.03-0.06 to 0.3-0.0. A central scotoma disappeared. Conductivity of axial bundle of the optic nerve restored from 28-32 Hz to 38-40 Hz. Improvements of vision functions were not marked in the control group of patients.

INTRODUCTION

It is known, that ingestion of various highly concentrated chemical neurotoxic agents such as alcohol and its substitutes, nicotine, industrial poisons, vapors of ethylated petrol and so on into a human body, results usually in injuries of axons and ganglions cells of retina. This leads to an atrophy of the optic nerve and, as a result, to the loss of vision. The basic principles in treatment of toxic opticneuropathy involve both an effective evacuation of the toxic agent and maintenance and intensification of retinochoroidal blood circulation. Artificial increase of number of active capillaries and optimization of blood circulation are ensured by intraarterial drug infusions through the ophthalmic region. This method was proposed by academician M.M. Krasnow in 1976.

In the last few years the method of intraarterial drug infusion through the region of the ophthalmic artery has been used for treatment of vascular diseases of the retina and optic nerve, especially in acute cases of the disease, for example alcoholic intoxications.

However there are no based data about the choice of one or another arterial channel of the ophthalmic region for the implantation of the infusion catheter because the existing anatomic variety of face vessel architectonics makes difficult this stage of infusion therapy.

The method of drug infusion via catheter introduced into artery is an important stage of intraarterial infusion therapy (IAIT). In traditional devices for drug infusion such as syringe or systems on the supports the level of infusion pressure can exceed the pressure not only in the area of the nearest vessel branch but in more large arterial trunks. The use of devices of common type does not always afford to provide for direct drug infusion in eye blood supply region. The use of infusion medium for IAIT may cause hyperhydratation of regional reveal tract and the great vessels when infusion pressure is move higher that leads to the risk of intraocular or intracranial pressure increase.

New drug superchargers working without the use of infusion medium appeared last years. They are perspective for the use in ophthalmology.[1]

The aim of the present investigation was anatomo-topographic and experimental clinic basis of the arterial collector choice for fixing of the infusion system. This tactics afforded to determine the surgical criteria fop fixing of the infusion catheter into one of the face or orbit arteries. A method for direct drug infusion in the eye blood supply region was developed.

MATERIALS AND METHODS

Anatomo-topographic value of the versions and diameter ranges of periorbital extraocular branches of the orbital artery was studied on the sectional material (17 cadavers of the both sex at the age from 34 to 75 years). Experimental studies of drug pharmacokinetics via the arteries of the periorbital area were performed on the days (4 animals, 8 eyes). Roentgenocontrast examination of the head arteries was experimentally performed on the roentgen apparatus of the ARMAN firm (Germany). The infusion catheter was fixed by Arnautov's method (certificate for the invention of the USSR N1997402/28-13 of 15.10.1973). The influence of TRENTAL and AGAPOURIN medications dissoluble in the infusion medium and medications improving oxygen penetration 'into the retina tissue such as ACTOVEGIN and SOLCOSERYL were studied experimentally.

The ultrasonic apparatus invented in the Scientific Surgical Center of the Russian Medical Academy was used for the determination of the versions of extraocular periorbital bloodstream and the choice of the artery. The apparatus affords to value the direction and the average linear blood flow velocity in the vessels and perform topical auscultating localization of the arteries for successful catheter implantation. The versions of periorbital blood circulation were studied in the nonchosen group of 60 patients. Those patients had vascular pathology of the optic nerve of ischemic type (toxic retrobulbar neuritis, partial atrophy of the optic nerve - 21 patient, 23 operations on the implantation of the arterial infusion system and 11 patients from the control group). The fluorescent angiography of the fundus was performed all the patients before the operation on the OPTON's funduscamera for the value of perfusion and vascular wall of the microcirculation channel.

The following methods as visometry, quantitative perimetry, campimetry with the use of photostress, the tests of entoptic phenomena (autoopthalmoscopy, the determination of mecharophosphen, quantitative frequency of flickers confluence) and methods of electrophysiologic diagnostics? The determination of threshold of retina electrical sensitivity and conductivity of the optic nerve, the registration of electroretinogram) were used for the estimation of the eye function.

Prothrombin index and blood clotting time were studied in all patients before operation. The neurologic state was examined in some patients. All these investigations were performed before the operation, when discharging from the clinic and every 6 month after the procedure.

The fixation of infusion catheter was performed on the microsurgical method with the use of vascular micro-instrumentation (microhemoclips, infusion Polymeric catheter with inner diameter of 0.4 mm and external diameter of 0.6 mm with canula of LUER type and also PORTEX catheter (USA) with inner diameter of 0.5 mm and external diameter of 0.8 mm with canula of RECORD type. The operations were performed under OPTON operation microscope (Germany).

The drug infusion into arterial channel was performed by own method with the help of automatic thermoinfusion device with drug dosatory (DLTH) invented in the Electromechanical Research Institute (Russia) the volume of which was 10.0 and 30.0 ml.

RESULTS AND DISCUSSION

Anatomo-morpholoyic investigations showed that in more than 3/4 of cases linear diameter of supraorbital artery of the section was from 0.6 to 1.5 mm. The inner lumen of the arteries were preserved in spite of the signs of arteriosclerotic process in intima. These cases are convenient for the successful catheter implantation of drug infusion.

It was noted that in 1/4 of cases the diameter of the supraorbital artery was less than 0.5 mm or 0.1 mm and represented a bundle of small vessels instead of one trunk. These vessels were disposed in synovial case and passed separately ("scattered" version of arterial component of supraorbital vascular-neural bundle).[2]

The state of periorbital circulation was studied in 60 patients at the age from 24 to 55 years old because in 25% of cases there was no real possibility of fixing infusion catheter into a. supraorbitalis.

Three main versions of circulation in periorbital area were established (Table 1). These versions were indications for choice of the vessel for intraarterial infusion and basis for more oriented drug pharmakinetics to the eye blood supply region.

The first version of periorbital circulation state was observed more often. It is characterized for physiologic state of blood circulation of this region.

The second version included analogic asculatatory signs, however a weakened influence of outer carotid artery compression on periorbital circulation was marked. As supposed, it is a symptom for initial changes in vascular wall (rigidity, lumen vessel stenosis). Difficulties may appear when the catheter is fixing due to insufficient elasticity of artery walls.

The third version evidenced about reduced character of circulation through these branches. Compression tests may show a prevailed influence of circulation from the pool system of the outer carotid artery. Periferic extracranial segments of outer carotid artery is advisable to use as arterial collector for intraarterial infusion therapy in this case.

As shown, our experimental angiographic investigations use the traditional streaming method of drug infusion into the face artery only partially provides its infusion into a.ophthalmica. It is explained by the fact that an infusion fluid pressure reated in catheters exit multiply exceeds systolic pressure level in the ophthalmic artery. That is why a considerable part of the infused drug (more than 99% is spread outside of eye blood supply pool). Thus, this method may be considered as "relative" regional intraarterial infusion therapy (Fig. 1-a).

Table 1. Ultrasonic versions of periorbital blood circulation in nonchosen group of patients for choice of arterial collector.

Versions of blood circulation and % cases	Direction of blood circulation and auscultatory tone characteristics	Linear speed of circulation cm/sec (LSC)	Influence of artery compression	Choice of artery
I (70%)	anterograde Clear arterial tone	8-9	Increase of 8-9 to 14-16 cm/sec 3-5 sec. later	a. Supraorbitalis
II (10%)	anterograde clear arterial tone	8-9	Does not influence or LSC is increased to 12-14 cm/sec 15 sec. later	a Supraorbitalis
III (20%)	weakening or absence of arterial tone, sometimes amplification of retrograde tone	4-12	weakening of auscultatory tone	brch of a. tempor. superficial.

A principally other system of drug infusion into arteries was used (Fig. 2). The main difference is the absence of hydrodynamic wave when an infused drug is introduced. The action of systems of such type is based on the effect of continuous "fluent" drug push out from the compact sealed frame connected with the infusion catheter. The patient's blood becomes the basic infusion medium into which drug enters by microdrops. The functioning of the device is based on the utilization of the human body temperature.

The device is fixed on the patient's skin 20 - 30 min later drug column gradually fills in the catheters lumen, a fragment of supraorbital artery with tied up distal segment thus reaching the lumen of the ophthalmic artery. The part of drug which may be lost (through collaterals or vaso-vasorum of supraorbital artery itself) is insignificant. Thermocoagulation of small additional branches is performed in case of their revealing during fixing of the catheter. In this case this procedure provides for full drug infusion in the eye blood supply region. It may be called a "direct" regional infusion therapy of the eye (Fig. 1-b).

The other advantage of this method is autonomy of the device action. The device is fixed on the patient,s neck and does not limit his movements. The patient who receives the infusion therapy does not require stay in the bed and constant observation by medical staff (Fig. 3). There are practically no mechanical reasons which can prevent to infuse drug into the catheter. "Push out" pressure is 400-500 mm of Mercury and resting of catheters exit port against any obstacle excludes possibility of its thrombosing and stopping of the system.

The method of intraarterial drug infusion was used in clinic in patients with vascular ischemic alcoholic intoxications of the retina and the optic nerve.

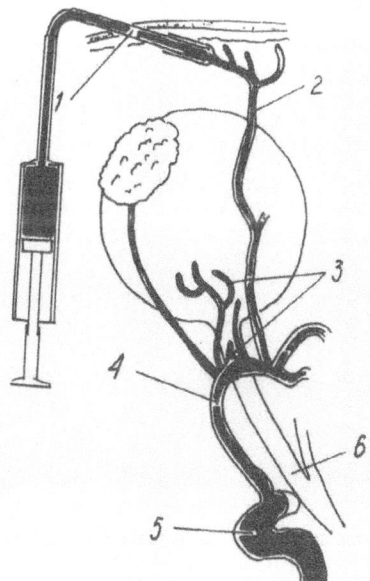

Figure 1-a. Picture for principles "relative" intraarterial infusion therapy of the eye (scheme). 1) syringe infusion; 2) a. supraorbitalis; 3) a.a. ciliaris posterioris brevis et a. centralis retinae; 4) a. ophthalmica; 5) a. carotis interna; 6) n. opticus.

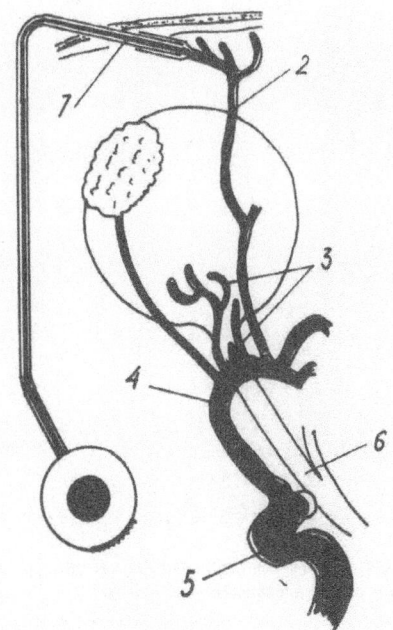

Figure 1-b. Picture for principles "direct" intraarterial infusion therapy of the eye (scheme). 2) a. supraorbitalis; 3) a.a. ciliaris posterioris brevis et a. centralis retinae; 4) a. ophthalmica; 5) a. carotis interna; 6) n. opticus; 7) DLTN pump infusion.

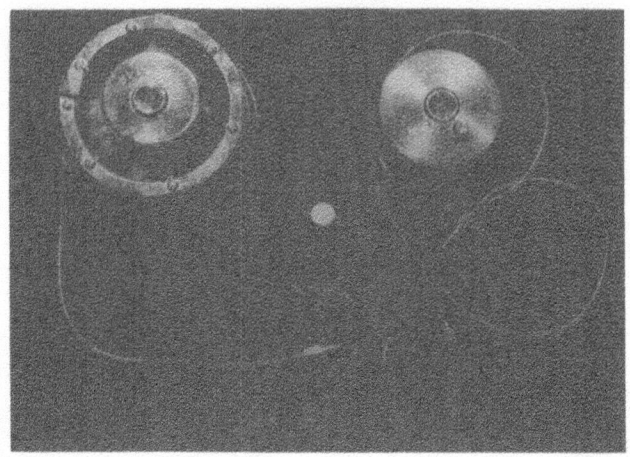

Figure 2. Portable thermoinfusion pumps DLTN, drug chamber volume 30.0 and 10.0 ml.

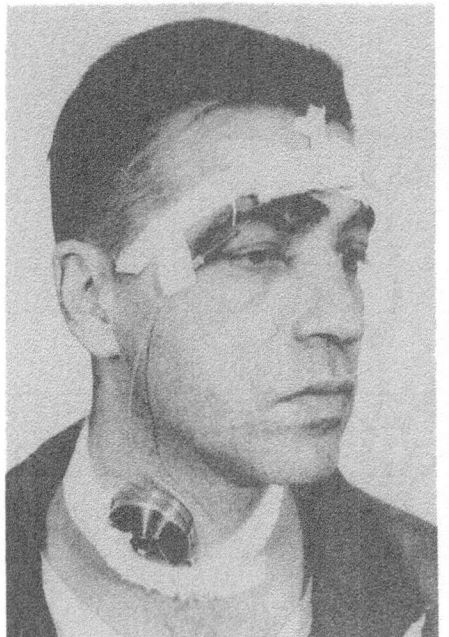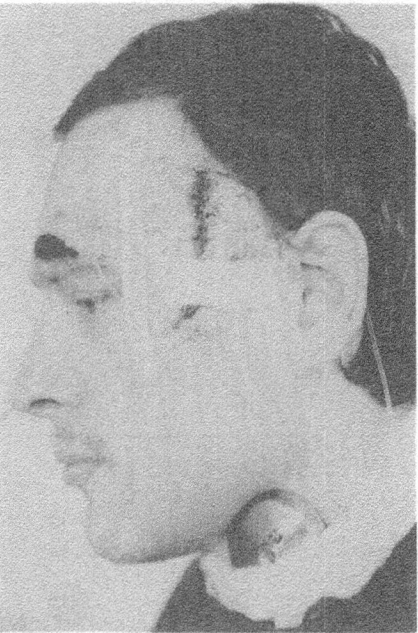

Figure 3. Patients during IAIT of the eyes through ophthalmic blood supply region, infusion systems were implanted into a.supraorbitalis or into a.temperalis superficialis.

The chosen patients had toxic retrobulbar neuritis and their mean age was 32 years old. The systemic diseases were absent.

When studying the vessels of periorbital region the first version of blood circulation was revealed in 12 patients. To these patients the implantation of infusion catheter was performed in the supraorbital artery. Three patients had the second version of periorbital blood circulation. The wall of supraorbital artery of one patient was rigid that caused technical difficulties for
catheterization. In further thrombosing of the artery occurred on the second day after procedure and the catheter was removed. Other complications were not observed in process of intraarterial infusion therapy. The duration of this therapy was 5 days (100-120 hours of infusion by Trental and Actovegin medications in turn). The functional results of the treatment are presented in Table 2.

Table 2. Acuity vision and electrophysiological data in patients with toxic neuritis before and after intraarterial infusion therapy via supraorbital arteries (direct regional intraarterial infusion therapy).

Data	Number of patients		
Acuity Vision	Before procedure	5 days after infusion	6 months after infusion
0.01 - 0.03	4	1	1
0.04 - 0.06	3	-	-
0.07 - 0.09	5	3	3
0.10 - 0.30	-	4	4
0.60 - 0.90	-	4	4
	Mean Data		
Threshold of electric sensitivity (mkA)	90-120	40-85	40-85
Lability of the optic nerve (Hz)	28-34	32-38	36-38
Quantitative frequency of flickers confluence (bright2,Hz)	28-34	32-38	36-38

Note: As shown in the table, acuity vision increase is achieved practically in all patients. Improvements of vision functions were not marked in the control group.

CONCLUSION

On the basis of anatomic investigations of the vessels of ophthalmic region, periorbital blood circulation and ultrasonic examinations a surgical tactics of artery choice was developed for infusion eye therapy.

Own method of drug infusion into arteries of ophthalmic region with the help of infusion pump does not affect the vessel wall and offers to perform "direct" infusion eye therapy. The infusion of intraarterial therapy in the eye blood supply region in patients with opticneuropathy showed vision function improvement in the majority of patients. Acuity vision from 0.03 to 0.08 increased from 0.3 to 0.8, a central scatoma disappeared. Lability of the optic nerve restored from 28 to 32 Hz to 38-40 Hz. When fixing infusion catheter in the branch of superficial temporal artery, acuity vision did not exceed 0,1. Lability of the optic nerve remained 30-32 Hz. Vision functions did not change in the control group.

REFERENCES

1.   A.I. Abrosimovt Y.G. Klimchenko, S.A. Tyulyandin, Infusion therapy of diseases with the use of portable thermoinfusion devices with dosimetry of drugs (Review of literature), *Bull. of Inst-of Scientific Inform.* [Russia] 8:8(1988).

2.   D.L. Bayandin, I.V. Kaltashyov, A.A. Fyodorow, Anatomic and topographic variants of supraorbital artery, *Veitnit Ophthalmol.* [Russia] 4:54(1991).

3.   D.L. Bayandin, D.A. Yeryomin, O.K. Pereverzina, A.A. Fyodorov, Experimental study of Trental and Actovegin effects on the organ of vision in injection of these drugs into the end of periorbital branches of the apthilmic artery, *Vestnik Ophthalmol.* [Russia] 4-6:23(1992).

4.   D.L. Bayandin, A.A. Tsagikyan, Yu.G, Klimchenko, Method of retrograde intraarterial drug infusion into final periorbital channels of the opthalmic artery, *Thesis of Yll All-Russian opthalmol-congress.* Moscow,Russia:126)(1994).

5.   A.I. Yeremenko, Long-term intracarotid drug infusion in the treatment of urgent vascular opticneurapathy, *Thesis of YII All-Union opthalmol-congress*, [Moscow,Russia] 3:78(1985).

6.   Y.F. Kovalenko, O.A. Osipov at al., Efficacy of regional intraarterial infusion in treatment of the optic nerve atrophy, *Thesis of the reports of the Second symp. on Refractive surgery*, IOL implantation and complex treatment of the optic nerve atrophy, [Moscow,Russia]. 192(1991).

7.   M.M. Krasnow, L.G. Arnautova, A new method of retrograde intraarterial administration of medical agents in a. opthalmica in the treatment of eye diseases, *Vestnit Opthalmol.* [Russia] 6:46 (1976).

8.   M.M. Krasnow, Analysis of intraocular hemodynamics peculiarities and possibilities of therapeutic action on it in the treatment of glaucoma and blood supply deficit, *Vestnit Opthalmol.* [Russia] 6:36 (1989).

9.   L.V. Kucherenko, Efficacy of infusion therapy via superficial temporal artery in eye diseases, *Synopsis of the scientific work for the degree of the degree of medical doctor* [Odessa, Ukraine],(1991).

10.   P.L. Dedrick, Arterial drug infusions, pharmacokinetic problems and pitfalls, *Journal Natl. Cancer Inst.* 2:84(1989).

EVALUATION OF THE EFFECT OF THE VEHICLE ON OCULAR DISTRIBUTION AND BIOAVAILABILITY OF BETAXOLOL

Jeffrey Grove, Gilles Chastaing, Marie-Paule Quint, Annouk Rozier, and Bernard Plazonnet

Centre de Recherche
Laboratoires Merck, Sharp & Dohme-Chibret
63203 Riom Cedex, France

INTRODUCTION

Ocular bioavailability is generally accepted to be extremely low compared to bioavailability obtained from conventional oral doses. Indeed, whereas ocular bioavailability is of the order of 1-3% (Lee and Robinson, 1986) a similar oral bioavailability would probably not be commercially acceptable. There is, therefore, a great potential need for improvement of the ocular bioavailability of almost all ophthalmic agents that penetrate the eye for their pharmacological effect.

Numerous approaches that have been tried to increase bioavailability include modification of the compound by formation of prodrugs (Bundgaard et al, 1988; Sugrue et al, 1988), modification of the vehicle (viscosifying agents, Green and Downs, 1975; Gelrite®, Rozier et al, 1989) control release devices, eg inserts, (Maichuk, 1975) nanoparticles (Li et al, 1986), liposomes (Niesman, 1992) pharmacosomes, (Orhan Vaizoglu & Speiser, 1986), resins (Jani et al, 1994) and bioadhesive polymers (Park & Robinson, 1987; Thermes et al, 1992). The list is by no means exhaustive, but with the exception of the prodrugs the aim has been usually to increase the pre-corneal residence time of the compound in order to prolong the period available for trans-corneal penetration.

We have reported on the effect of increasing vehicle viscosity on the ocular bioavailability of the beta-adrenergic agent L-653,328 (Grove et al, 1990). It has been suggested that since L-653,328 is a prodrug the vehicle could exert an influence on the corneal esterases. We have therefore examined the effects of vehicle on another ß1-antagonist, betaxolol, that is not metabolised in the cornea and have also compared the bioavailability with commercially available formulations.

MATERIALS AND METHODS

Betaxolol hydrochoride was obtained from Alcon Laboratories, Kayersberg, France and Betoptic®, 0.5% and Betoptic 'S'®, 0.25% were purchased from commercial pharmacies. Carbopol 934P was supplied by B.F. Goodrich Chemicals, Europe. Albino rabbits were supplied by Charles River, France.

Instillation

Rabbits were placed in wooden restraining boxes and bilateral instillations of one drop of 30 μL of the test material were made into the conjunctival sac and the lower lid was brought gently up to meet the upper.

The following formulations were evaluated:-
(A) 0.25% betaxolol solution.
(B) 0.5% Betoptic®
(C) 0.25% Betoptic 'S'®
(D) 0.25% betaxolol solution in Carbopol 934P

Ingredients of the solutions A and D, other than betaxolol or betaxolol-resin, were the same as those of as 0.5% Betoptic® and 0.25% Betoptic 'S'®, respectively. In other words, benzalkonium chloride 0.01%, EDTA 0.01% and sodium chloride 0.85% were added and the pH adjusted to 6.5. The viscosity of the 0.25% betaxolol in Carbopol was 97 cps and that of Betoptic 'S'®, was 80 cps.

The animals were euthanized at 10, 20, 30, 60, 90, 120 and 180 minutes by rapid injection of a lethal dose of sodium pentobarbital into the marginal ear vein. Ocular tissues were subsequently sampled for measurement of their drug content by an HPLC-fluorescence assay.

Preparation of Extracts for HPLC

Corneas, aqueous humor and iris + ciliary body extracts were prepared in a similar manner to that previously described (Grove et al, 1990).

Chromatography

A Hewlett Packard Model 1090 fitted with an automatic injector and an HP 3385A integrator were used with a Shimadzu RF-530 fluorimeter as detector. The excitation and emission wavelengths were 274 and 300 nm, respectively. Separation was effected by reverse-phase chromatography, on a Brownlee 5 μ Cyano column (100 x 4.6 mm) fitted with the appropriate guard column (30 x 4.6 mm) using isocratic elution with acetonitrile/0.6% phosphoric acid (40:60) at a flow rate of 1.5 mL/min and a temperature of 40 °C. Under these conditions the retention time for betaxolol and metoprolol, the internal standard, were 6.3 and 7.1 minutes, respectively.

RESULTS

The ocular concentrations in cornea, aqueous humor and iris + ciliary body following instillation of (A) 0.25 betaxolol, (B) 0.5% Betoptic®, (C) 0.25% Betoptic 'S'® and (D) 0.25% betaxolol in Carbopol 934P are presented in Tables 1, 2, 3 and 4, respectively.

Ocular bioavailability was assessed by calculation of the $AUC_{(0-3h)}$ of the concentration time profiles for each of the ocular sites. Maximum concentrations of betaxolol were observed in the cornea at the first sampling (10 minutes) followed by peak concentrations in the aqueous humor and iris + ciliary body at 20 or 30 minutes post-instillation (Figure 1). The vehicles did not appear to modify the time to C_{max}. Ocular bioavailability increased in the order A < C < B < D, with solution D having about twice the ocular bioavailability as solution A (See Figure 1).

Discussion

For years, addition of a viscous polymer to achieve an increase in the penetration of an ophthalmic drug has been claimed to be maximum at about 15-20 cps (Blaug and Canada, 1965; Alder et al., 1971; Patton and Robinson, 1975; Eriksen, 1980). A recent review concluded that "increasing solution viscosity had a limited utility in causing a marked improvement in the amount of drug absorbed" into the eye (Lee and Robinson, 1986).

Table 1. Concentrations of betaxolol following instillation of 30 µL of Formulation A

Minutes	Cornea (µg/g)	Aqueous Humor (µg/mL)	Iris + Ciliary Body (µg/g)
10	27.73 ± 3.38	0.60 ± 0.13	2.24 ± 0.27
20	15.34 ± 1.30	0.53 ± 0.05	1.81 ± 0.19
30	14.69 ± 1.66	0.72 ± 0.10	2.13 ± 0.23
60	12.83 ± 1.18	0.71 ± 0.10	1.20 ± 0.12
90	6.63 ± 0.63	0.28 ± 0.03	0.66 ± 0.08
120	5.30 ± 0.61	0.23 ± 0.06	0.87 ± 0.18
180	2.46 ± 0.35	0.09 ± 0.02	0.26 ± 0.04
AUC(µg/g or mL)	27.0	1.14	3.10

Table 2. Concentrations of betaxolol following instillation of 30 µL of Formulation B

Minutes	Cornea (µg/g)	Aqueous Humor (µg/mL)	Iris + Ciliary Body (µg/g)
10	33.39 ± 3.28	0.66 ± 0.06	2.83 ± 0.21
20	30.73 ± 4.05	1.23 ± 0.16	3.62 ± 0.53
30	21.78 ± 2.90	1.02 ± 0.08	2.45 ± 0.27
60	12.15 ± 1.56	0.79 ± 0.10	1.49 ± 0.15
90	11.54 ± 2.41	0.57 ± 0.08	1.78 ± 0.35
120	5.19 ± 0.54	0.24 ± 0.02	0.98 ± 0.18
180	4.99 ± 1.14	0.18 ± 0.03	0.88 ± 0.14
AUC (µg.h/g or mL)	36.2	1.61	4.70

Concentrations are Mean ± SEM (n=12)

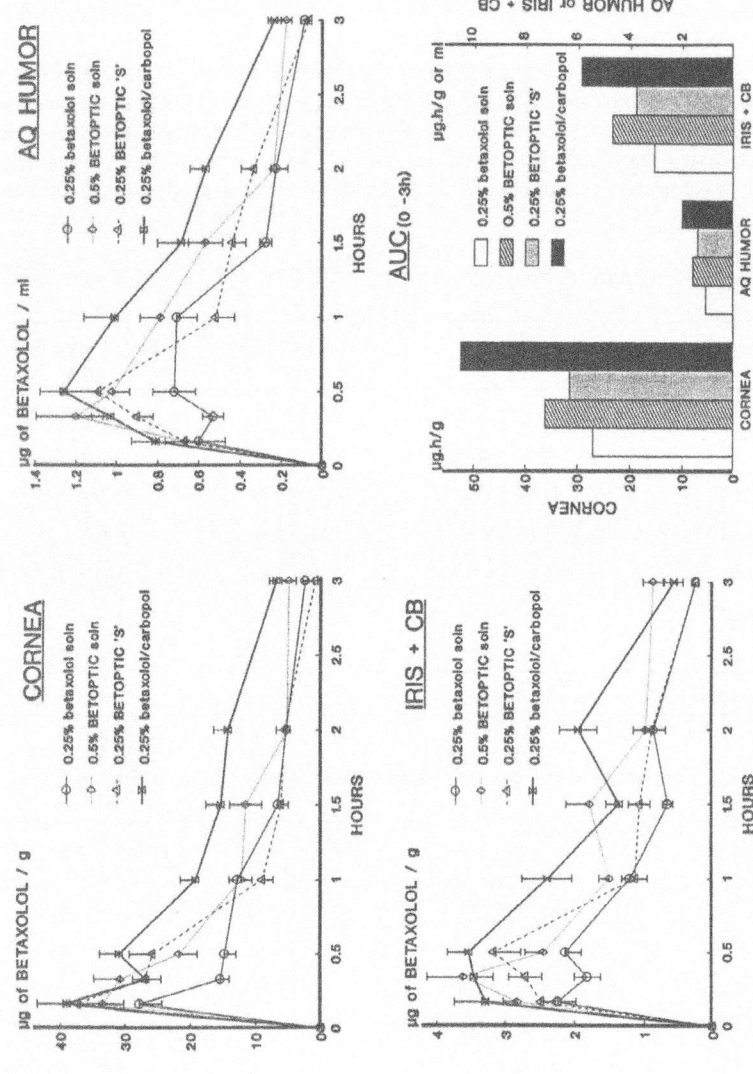

Figure 1. Mean concentrations and $AUC_{(0-3h)}$ values for three ocular sites of the albino rabbit eye following installation of 30μL of each betaxolol formulation.

We have presented evidence that ocular bioavailability in the rabbit increases concomitantly with increase in the viscosity of the vehicle (Grove et al, 1990). In agreement with others, we observed a two-fold increase in the bioavailability of the beta-blocker L-653,328 between an aqueous solution (0 cps) and a viscous hydroxyethyl cellulose solution of 100 cps. Similar two-fold increases had previously been reported for pilocarpine in methyl cellulose, (Chrai & Robinson, 1974), pilocarpine in polyvinyl alcohol (Patton & Robinson, 1975) and tropicamide in polyvinyl alcohol (Saettone et al, 1982). The present data confirm this two-fold increase for another compound, betaxolol, and another viscous vehicle, Carbopol 934P. Thus, for the 0.25% betaxolol solution, $AUC_{(0 - 3h)}$ values in the cornea, aqueous humor and iris + ciliary body were 27.0, 1.14 and 3.10 µg.h/g or ml, respectively. In contrast, the corresponding values for solution D (0.25% betaxolol with Carbopol 934F, 97 cps) increased two-fold to 52.6, 2.12 and 5.94 µg.h/g or ml. Bioavailability was not apparently dose-related, although the aqueous humor concentrations after administration of 0.5% Betoptic® are in good agreement with previous data (Jani et al, 1994). Furthermore, our results support the observations of these authors that 0.25% Betoptic 'S'®, (Solution C) delivers an ocular bioavailability equivalent to 0.5% Betoptic®, (Solution B).

Table 3. Concentrations of betaxolol following instillation of 30µL of Formulation C

Minutes	Cornea (µg/g)	Aqueous Humor (µg/mL)	Iris + Ciliary Body (µg/g)
10	37.33 + 3.85	0.67 + 0.10	2.48 + 0.21
20	26.98 + 2.46	0.90 + 0.08	2.71 + 0.24
30	25.76 + 3.53	1.09 + 0.18	3.18 + 0.40
60	9.03 + 1.71	0.52 + 0.09	1.13 + 0.18
90	6.13 + 1.13	0.44 + 0.06	1.07 + 0.15
120	5.59 + 1.31	0.34 + 0.06	0.89 + 0.16
180	0.94 + 0.33	0.07 + 0.01	0.26 + 0.05
AUC (µg.h/g or mL)	31.5	1.40	3.82

Table 4. Concentrations of betaxolol following instillation of 30µL of Formulation D

Minutes	Cornea (µg/g)	Aqueous Humor (µg/mL)	Iris + Ciliary Body (µg/g)
10	39.06 + 4.51	0.81 + 0.12	3.29 + 0.45
20	26.75 + 2.08	1.03 + 0.09	3.46 + 0.28
30	30.88 + 3.00	1.26 + 0.12	3.54 + 0.31
60	19.14 + 2.43	1.01 + 0.15	2.40 + 0.36
90	15.28 + 2.26	0.69 + 0.12	1.36 + 0.19
120	14.18 + 2.17	0.57 + 0.08	1.95 + 0.27
180	6.97 + 1.06	0.24 + 0.03	0.58 + 0.14
AUC (µg.h/g or mL)	52.6	2.12	5.94

Concentrations are Mean + SEM (n=12)

Greater than 90% of the betaxolol in the formulation is bound to the resin (Jani et al, 1994). Solution D consists essentially of the same ingredients as Betoptic 'S', (Solution C), without the suspended resin particles. Most of the improvement in ocular drug bioavailability with Betoptic 'S'® was probably due to the increased viscosity and mucoadhesion of the vehicle, Carbopol 934P. The presence in the formulation of the betaxolol bound to an anion-exchange resin did not appear to help ocular drug penetration since solution D (essentially C without resin) gave higher AUC values than those of C (Tables 3 and 4, Figure 1). $AUC_{(0-3h)}$ values for the cornea, aqueous humor and iris + ciliary body after instillation of solution D were, respectively, 1.89-, 1.5- and 1.5- fold higher than the corresponding values with the Betoptic 'S' suspension. Since the suspension does not prolong the time that ocular drug concentrations can be detected, and produces significantly lower concentrations than solution D, it would appear that addition of only a viscosifying agent would produce better bioavailability, at least in the rabbit.

Acknowledgements

The technical assistance of Annie Cerdeno, Paulette Chabrier, Gilles Faidit and Yvette Hodeau is gratefully recognized.

REFERENCES

Adler, C.A., Maurice, D.M. and Paterson, M.E., 1971, The effect of viscosity of the vehicle on the penetration of fluorescein into the human eye. *Exptl. Eye Res.* 11: 34

Blaug, S.M. and Canada, A.T., 1965, Relationship of viscosity, contact time and prolongation of action of methylcellulose-containing ophthalmic solutions. *Amer. J. Hosp. Pharm.*, 22: 662

Bungaard, H., Buur, A., Chang, S-C. and Lee, V.H.L., 1988, Timolol prodrugs: synthesis, stability and lipophilicity of various alkyl, cycloalkyl and aromatic esters of timolol. *Int J. Pharm.*, 46: 77

Chrai, S.S. and Robinson, J.R., 1974, Ocular evaluation of methylcellulose vehicle in albino rabbits. *J. Pharm.Sci.*, 63: 1218

Eriksen, S.P., Physiological and formulation constraints on ocular drug bioavailability. 1980, Ophthalmic Drug Delivery Systems. Amer. Pharm. Assoc. (Ed. J.R. Robinson), Amer. Pharm. Assoc., Washington, D.C., pp 55

Green, K. and Downs, S., 1975, Ocular penetration of pilocarpine in rabbits. *Arch. Ophthalmol.* 93: 1165

Grove, J., Durr, M., Quint, M-P., and Plazonnet, B., 1990, The effect of vehicle viscosity on the ocular bioavailability of L-653,328. *Int. J. Pharm.*, 66: 23

Jani, R., Gan, O., Ali, Y., Rodstrom, R. and Hancock, S., 1994, Ion exchange resins for ophthalmic delivery. *J. Ocular Pharmacol.*, 10: 57

Lee, V.H.L. and Robinson, J.R., 1986, Review: Topical ocular drug delivery: recent developments and future challenges. *J. Ocular Pharmacol.*, 2: 67

Li, V.H.K., Wood, R.W., Kreuter, J., Harmia, T. and Robinson, J.R., 1986. Ocular drug delivery of progesterone using nanoparticles. *J. Microencapsulation.* 3: 213

Maichuk, Y.F. 1975, Ophthalmic drug inserts. *Invest Ophthalmol.*, 14: 87

Niesman, M.R., 1992, The use of liposomes as carriers in ophthalmology. *Crit Rev. in Therap. Drug Carrier Systems.* 9: 1

Orhan Vaizoglu, M. & Speiser, P.P., 1986, Pharmacosomes- a novel drug delivery system. *Acta Pharm. Suec.*, 23: 163

Patton, T.F. and Robinson, J.R.,1975, Ocular evaluation of polyvinyl alcohol vehicle in rabbits. *J. Pharm.Sci.*, 64: 1312

Rozier, A., Grove, J., Mazuel, C. and Plazonnet B., 1989, Gelrite solutions : Novel ophthalmic vehicles that enhance ocular drug penetration. *Proc. Interntl. Symp. Control. Rel. Bioacti. Mater.*, 16: 109

Park, H. and Robinson, J.R., 1987. Mechanisms of mucoadhesion of poly(acrylic acid) hydrogel. *Pharm Res.*, 4: 457

Saettone, M.F., Giannaccini, B., Barattini, F. and Tallini, N., 1982, The validity of rabbits for investigations on ophthalmic vehicles: a comparison of four different vehicles containing tropicamide in humans and rabbits. *Pharma Acta Helv.*, 57: 47

Sugrue, M.F., Gautheron P., Grove, J., Mallorga, P., Viader, M-P., Baldwin, J.J., Ponticello, G.S. and Varga, S.L., 1988, L-653,328: An ocular hypotensive agent with modest beta-blocking activity. *Invest. Ophthalmol. Vis. Sci.*, 29: 776

Thermes, F., Rozier, A., Plazonnet, B. and Grove, J., 1992, Bioadhesion: The effect of polyacrylic acid on the ocular bioavailability of timolol. *Int. J. Pharmac.*, 81:59

CONTINUOUS FLOW CONTACT LENSES DELIVERY OF DICLOFENAC TO RABBIT CORNEA AND AQUEOUS HUMOR

V. Montoya[1], M.A. Company[2], M. Palmero, and A. Orts[2]

Departments of Pharmacology[2] and Therapeutics and Ophthalmology[1]
School of Medicine, Universtiy of Alicante, Alicante, Spain

INTRODUCTION

Although satisfactory therapeutic results are obtained with usual topical ophthalmic drug (topical ocular solutions and ointments) they present some inconveniences: 1st. Bioavailability is poor, requiring high doses and repeated applications. 2nd. Diffusion of the drug into the bloodstream across de nasal mucosa which is continuous with the conjuntival sac, represents an additional risk of systemic toxicity. (Chang and Lee, 1987, Salminen,1990).

Several drugs were investigated for delivery in different types of contact lens: pilocarpine (Hillman, 1974; Hilman et al., 1975; Krohn and Breitfeller, 1975; Podos et al., 1972; Rubin and Watkins, 1975), chloramphenicol and tetracycline (Praus et al., 1972), prednisolone (Hull et al.,1974), bacitracin and polimyxin (Brettscheneider et al., 1975), carbenicillin, gentamicin and cloramphenicol (Jain and Lal, 1983), gentamicin (McCarey et al., 1984; Busin and Spitznas, 1988) acetazolamide (Friedman et al., 1985), disodium cromoglicate (Iwasaki et al., 1988). Controlling the drug delivery in a constant way is usually the main problem in these studies. Anyway, this type of drug administration could be useful in acute treatment.

The purpose of this study is to determinate in the rabbits the absorption of diclofenac Na into the cornea, aqueous and vitreous humor delivered by contact lens, previously soaked in a sodium diclofenac solution.

MATERIAL AND METHODS

Materials

Male New Zealand rabbits of 2.2-2.7 Kg. were used. Contact lenses were applied onto the right eye and the contra lateral eyes were used as control.

Vifilcon A contact lens (Vifilcon A: 45%; water: 55%) were soaked during 72 hr in a diclofenac saline solution (0.1%); temperature: 22-25°C. and pH 6.9-7.2.

Diclofenac sodium assay

Samples from cornea, aqueous and vitreous humors were obtained and diclofenac concentrations were measured by HPLC (Wavelength 228-254 nm; absorbance: 0.032);

Ocular Toxicology, Edited by I. Weisse *et al.*
Plenum Press, New York, 1995

Column: C-18; 25 mm; Phosphoric acid 0.03 M. and acetic acid in methanol 0.2% (38/62, respectively) were used as eluyent. The flow was isocratic (1.5 ml/min). The injected volume was 20 μl.

Procedure

Contact lenses previously soaked in a diclofenac solution (0.1%) during 72 hr were applied onto the right cornea of the rabbit. Tarsorrhaphy was performed. Contra lateral eyes were used as control.

At the 30 min, 60 min, 2 hr and 6 hr, rabbits were sacrificed (Sodium pentobarbital i.v. 200 mg/Kg) and cornea aqueous and vitreous humors were removed from both eyes. Corneal tissue (in 10 ml of deionized water) and vitreous humor samples were homogenized with a politron and then centrifuged (20 min at 10000 rpm).

A total of 10 rabbits were used in each experimental group.

RESULTS

Several previous experiments were made to determine the time of immersion of contact lenses with the diclofenac concentration. Groups of ten contact lenses were soaked in different diclofenac solutions for 24, 48 and 72 hours. Then the contact lenses were immersed in distillated water during 4 hours. The water released concentration of diclofenac was then measured (Table 1).

Table 1. Mean values and standard deviation of diclofenac delivered by contact lens (μg DCFN/CL). The contact lenses were soaked during 24, 48 and 72 hours in diclofenac solutions (0.025%, 0.050%, 0.075% and 0.10%).

	24 hours	48 hours	72 hours
0.025%	5.00 ± 1.02	6.18 ± 1.77	7.12 ± 1.56
0.05%	8.43 ± 2.56	8.87 ± 1.78	10.11 ± 1.27
0.75%	11.56 ± 1.87	10.93 ± 1.57	15.31 ± 6.48
0.10%	13.03 ± 2.56	12.81 ± 2.13	20.93 ± 6.23

At the end of 4 hours the lenses were removed and homogenized to determine diclofenac levels. (Table 2). The percentage of retained diclofenac is low when contact lenses were placed 72 hours in 0.1% diclofenac solution (3.14%).

Table 2. Mean values of diclofenac retained into contact lens (μg DCFN/CL), standard deviation (s.d.) and percentage of total absorbed (%).

	24 hours			48 hours			72 hours		
	DCFN	s.d	%	DCFN	s.d.	%	DCFN	s.d.	%
0.025%	0.15 ± 0.06		2.91	0.21 ± 0.11		3.28	0.58 ± 0.05		7.53
0.05%	0.31 ± 0.11		2.68	0.15 ± 0.06		1.66	0.34 ± 0.10		3.25
0.75%	0.31 ± 0.07		2.61	0.31 ± 0.21		2.75	0.53 ± 0.23		3.34
0.10%	0.52 ± 0.27		3.83	0.37 ± 0.27		2.80	0.68 ± 0.12		3.14

Mean values and standard desviation of sodium diclofenac in cornea and aqueous humor are shown in Fig. 1.

Diclofenac concentrations in cornea (38.1, 108.4, 71.7 and 10.0 $\mu g/g$) are ten folds higher that in aqueous humor (3.3., 9.4, 5.7 and 1.5 $\mu g/ml$) at all time points. Concentrations of diclofenac in both tissues, cornea and aqueous humor, show the same pattern, achieving peak values when contact lenses were applied during 60 minutes.

Diclofenac was never found in vitreous humor.

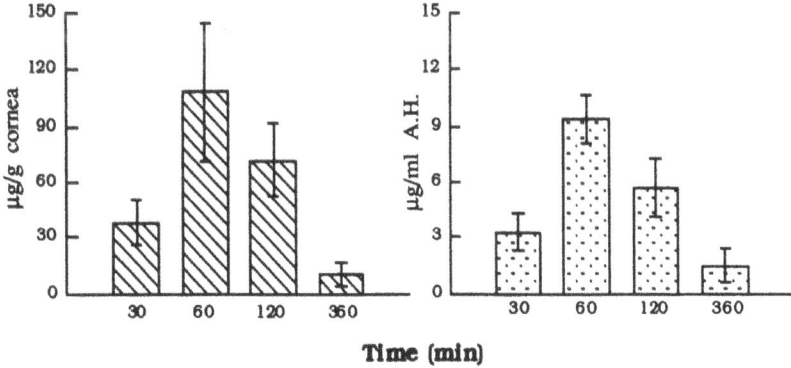

Figure 1. Diclofenac sodium levels in rabbit cornea ($\mu g/g$ cornea) and aqueous humor ($\mu g/ml$). Rabbits were wearing the contact lenses during 30, 60 minutes, 2 and 6 hours.

DISCUSSION

Although the release velocity from the soft hydrogel is not known, we demonstrated that corneal and aqueous absorption of diclofenac is clearly higher when contact lenses are used as delivery system, compared to levels obtained by topical application of a single 50 μl drop of 0.1% diclofenac eye drops in rabbits. (Internal Report B 4, 1983) (Table 3).

Table 3. Diclofenac concentration in cornea ($\mu g/g$) and aqueous humor ($\mu g/ml$) at different times. C.L.: Diclofenac was delivered from contact lenses previously soaked in 0.1% diclofenac solution in saline. Drops: one 50 μl drop of 0.1% diclofenac (50 μl at 0.1%) was instillated onto cornea.

	Cornea		Aqueous humor	
	C.L	Drops	C.L	Drops
30 min.	38.11	8.36	3.32	-
60 min.	108.38	3.45	9.39	0.16
120 min.	71.71	-	5.66	-
180 min.	-	1.12	-	0.05
360 min.	9.96	2.12	1.50	-

Similar results were obtained by Agata et al., (1983) in rabbits using diclofenac drops (50 μl; 0.1%). Peak values in aqueous humor appeared at 90 minutes after instillation (0.6 $\mu g/ml$). At 360 minutes values had decreased to 0.06 $\mu g/ml$.

These results offer another example that high-molecular-weight drugs which are soluble in water, may be more effective if administered in a hydrogel lens delivery system than eye drops (Robinson and Eriksen, 1978).

Moreover, keeping in mind that the real content of diclofenac in a contact lens represents less than the 50% of the content in a drop (29.93 μg/CL versus 50 μg/drop) the above statement becomes even more relevant.

Certainly, the systemic absorption of diclofenac and its possible systemic toxicity is lesser when the drug is applied onto cornea by contact lens.

Acknowledgments: partially suported by Ciba-Vision Ophthalmics. Bulach, Switzerland.

REFERENCES

Agata, M.,Abe, T and Kon, M.,1983. Effect of topical diclofenac sodium, a non steroidal anti-inflamatory drug onvarious ocular inflammatory models in animals. *Acta. Soc. Ophthalmol. Jap.* 87:19.

Brettschneider, L., Prauss, R., Kreja, L. and Havranek, M.,1975. Intraocular penetration of bacitracin and polimyxin B after administration by means of hydrophilic gel contact lenses. *Ophthalmol Res.* 7: 296.

Busin, M and Spitznas, M.,1988. Sustained gentamicin release by presoaked medicated bandage contact lenses. *Ophthalmology* 95: 796.

Chang, S.C. and Lee, V.H.L.,1987. Nasal and conjuntival contribution to the systemic absorption of topical timolol in the oigmented rabbit: implications in the design of strategies to maximize the ratio of ocular to systemic absorption. *J. Ocular Pharmacol.* 3:159.

Friedman, Z, Allen, R.C. and Ralph, S.M.,1985. Topical acetazolamide and methazolamide delivered by contact lenses. *Arch. Ophthalmol.* 103: 963.

Hillman, J.S.,1974. Managementof acute glaucome with pilocarpine spaked hydrophilic lens. *Br. J. Ophthalmol.* 58: 674.

Hillman, J.S. Marsters, J.B. and Broad, A.,1975. Pilocarpine delivery by hydrophilic lens in management of acute glaucoma. *Trans. Ophthalmol. Soc. UK* 95:79.

Hull, D.S. Edelhauser, H.F. and Hyndiuk, R.A.,1974. Ocular penetration of prednisolone and the hydrophilic lens. *Arch. Ophthalmol.* 92:413.

Iwasaki, W., Kosaka, Y., Momose, T. and Yasuda, Y.,1988. Absorption of topical Disodium Cromoglicate and its preservatives by soft contact lenses. CLAO J. 14/3:155.

Jain, M.R. and Lal, S., 1983. Intraocular penetration of carbenicillin, gentamicin and chloramphenicol with Sauflon 85 soft contact lenses. *Ind. J. Ophthalmol.* 31: 645.

Krohn, D.L. and Breitfeller, J.M.,1975. Quantification of pilocarpine flux across isolated rabbit cornea by hydrogel polimer lenses. *Invest. Ophthalmol. Vis. Sci.* 14: 152.

McCarey, B.E., Schmidt, F.M., Wilkinson, K.D. and Baum, J.P.,1984. Gentamicin diffusion across hydrogel bandage lenses and its kinetic distribution on the eye. *Curr. Eye Res.* 5:977.

Podos, S.M., Becker, B., Asseff, C. and Hartstein,J.,1972. Pilocarpine therapy with soft contact lenses. *Am. J. Ophthalmol* 73:336.

Praus, R., Brettscheider, L., Kreja, L. and Kalvadora, D., 1972. Hydrophilic contact lenses as a new therapeutic approach for topical use of chloramphenicol and tetracycline. *Ophthalmologica* 165:62.

Report B 4 / 1983. Diclofenac-Na: Distribution in the rabbit eye. Pharma Research and Development Pharmacological Chemistry. Ciba-Geigy limited. Basle. 1983.

Robinson, J.R. and Eriksen, S.P., 1978. Drug delivery from soft contact lens materials. In: "Soft Contact Lenses: Clinical Applied Technology." M. Ruben,ed. London Balliere-Tindall. pp. 265-280.

Rubin, M. and Watkins, R.,1975. Pilocarpine for the soft hydrophilic contact lens. *Brit. J. Ophthalmol.* 59: 455.

Salminen, L. Review:, 1990. Systemic absorption of topically applied ocular drugs in humans. *J. Ocular Pharmacol.* 6:243.

ONE-YEAR OCULAR TOXICITY STUDY OF OFLOXACIN OPHTHALMIC SOLUTION IN BEAGLE DOGS

Kenjiro Sawa, Mitsushi Hikida, Hiroyuki Mibu, Eiich Shirasawa, Kenji Takase and Hiroshi Suda

Santen Pharmaceutical Co., Ltd.
9-19, Shimoshinjo 3-chome Higashiyodogawa-ku Osaka 533, Japan

ABSTRACT

Ocular toxicity and systemic adverse effects of 0.3% ofloxacin ophthalmic solution (0.3%OFLX) which was administered 3 times daily for one year were studied in dogs.

In general conditions, food intake, behavior and body weights, no significant difference was observed between the non treated group and 0.3%OFLX treated group throughout the experimental period. Signs for ocular toxicity such as anterior ocular irritation, abnormality of cornea and lens opacity, as well as fundus abnormality were no observed during ophthalmological examination in either group. Electroretinogram showed no abnormality by administration of 0.3%OFLX. Hematological examinations and blood chemistry resulted in normal values in any test item. Autopsy, organ weight, histopathology of ocular tissues and systemic organs showed no change due to ofloxacin.

It is concluded from these results that one year application of 0.3%OFLX ophthalmic solution to dogs causes neither ocular toxicity nor systemic adverse effect.

INTRODUCTION

Ofloxacin, a fluoroquinolone derivative as an antibacterial agent, has a potent anti-bacterial activity due to inhibition of DNA-gyrase in bacteria[1]. Because ofloxacin easily penetrates into tissues and has a broad spectrum against common gram-positive and negative bacteria, ofloxacin ophthalmic solution and eye ointments is frequently used for the therapy of ocular infections, such as blepharitis, hordeolum, dacryocystitis and conjunctivitis etc[2-6]. On the other hand, ofloxacin has an affinity to melanin pigment and is highly distributed to iris/ciliary body and retina/choroid by topical application to pigmented rabbit eyes[7]. It was reported that this agent has a possibility to affect the central nerve system if a high dose was administered systemically[8]. Therefore ofloxacin may also affect the visual function or central nerve system in long term topical application.

In the present study, we examined ocular toxicity of ofloxacin ophthalmic solution (3 times daily for one year application) in beagle dogs with pigmented eyes. In order to investigate the effects of melanin-bound ofloxacin on retinal function and the effect of ofloxacin on central nerve system, electroretinogram (ERG) was recorded and behavior of dogs was observed during test periods.

MATERIALS AND METHODS

Ophthalmic Solution

Ofloxacin synthesized by Daiichi Pharmaceutical Co.,Ltd (Tokyo, Japan). was made into 0.3% ophthalmic solution (0.3%OFLX). 0.3%OFLX used had been confirmed to be stable for more than 3 years at room temperature. The vehicle for the above 0.3%OFLX was used as the negative control.

Animals and Accommodation

Male beagle dogs (3-month-old) were purchased from Nihon Nosan (Tokyo, Japan). The animals were acclimatized to an electroretinography for about 3 months before the experiment. The animals were housed individually in bracket cages (Clea Japan, Tokyo, Japan) in the room regulated to temperature 23°C, humidity 55±10%, ventilation 16 times/hour and 12-hour light and 12-hour dark cycle (on 7:00 a.m., off 7:00 p.m.). They were fed about 300 g of a food (DS, Oriental Yeast, Tokyo, Japan) a day. This study conformed to the ARVO Resolution on the Use of Animals in Research.

Treatment

As in clinical use, the ophthalmic solution was applied to the eyes at the concentration of 0.3%, 1 drop (about 50 μl) a time, three times daily (9:00, 12:00 and 15:00).
Ten dogs with normal eyes and well acclimatized to ERG were selected and assigned to 2 groups with no biased distribution of body weight. The negative control, the vehicle for ofloxacin ophthalmic solution, and the test ophthalmic solution, 0.3%OFLX, were applied topically to the conjunctival sac bilaterally for 12 months (instillation for 5 days weekly) in the respective groups.

General Condition

Animal conditions were observed at the first and third application on each treatment day (5 days weekly) and once a day on each nontreated day (2 days weekly). The food intake was checked at new supply only on each treated day. To know the details for animal condition, spontaneous movement, posture, gait, extremity tone, pain reaction and ocular change (ex. ptosis) were observed before, and 1.5, 3, 6 and 12 months after initiation of application.

Body Weight

The animals were weighed before application and once every month during application.

Observation of Anterior Segment

Anterior ocular irritation was observed before the start and once every month of application, and scored by the grades for ocular reaction according to the modified Draize's method, the criteria shown in Table 1. Observation of the nictitating membrane was omitted because the membrane is degenerated and hard to examine in dogs. Observation was made one hour after the third dose (15:00).

Observation of Aqueous Flare

Aqueous flare was mainly observed using a slitlamp biomicroscope (SL-2, Kowa, Tokyo, Japan) before the start and in the 1st, 3rd, 6th and 12th month of application.

Table 1. Grades for ocular reaction

CORNEA
 A) Opacity
  0 = No opacity
  1 = Scattered or diffuse areas of opacity (details of iris clearly visible)
  +2 = Easily discernible translucent areas of opacity (details of iris slightly obscured)
  +3 = Areas of opacity, no details of iris visible, size of pupil barely discernible
  +4 = Complete corneal opacity, iris not discernible
 B) Size of opacity
  +1 = Involving 0 - 1/4 of cornea
  +2 = Involving 1/4 - 1/2 of cornea
  +3 = Involving 1/2 - 3/4 of cornea
  +4 = Involving 3/4 - entirety of cornea

IRIS
  0 = Normal
  +1 = Markedly deepened folds, congestion, swelling, circumcorneal injection
    (any of these or combination of any thereof), iris still reacting to light
    (sluggish reaction is positive)
  +2 = No reaction to light, hemorrhage, gross destruction (any or all of these)

CONJUNCTIVA
 A) Redness of palpebral conjunctiva
  0   = No congestion
  +0.5 = Mucous membranes with slight flush, slight dilation of perilimbal vessels
  +1   = Definite congestion above normal, mucous membranes with definite flush,
      marked dilation of vessels
  +2   = Mucous membranes with crimson red, individual vessels not easily discernible
  +3   = Diffuse beefy red
 B) Chemosis of palpebral conjunctiva
  0   = No swelling
  +0.5 = Swelling tendency of conjunctiva
  +1   = Any swelling above normal
  +2   = Obvious swelling with partial eversion of lids
  +3   = Swelling with lids about half closed
  +4   = Swelling with lids about half closed to completely closed
 C) Redness of bulbar conjunctiva
  0   = No congestion
  +0.5 = Slight dilation of pericorneal vessels
  +1   = Definite dilation of vessels
  +2   = Marked dilation of vessels running toward palpebral conjunctiva or marked
      congestion
 D) State of nictitating membrane
  0   = No congestion
  +0.5 = Dilating tendency of vessels and swelling tendency of membranes
  +1   = Definite dilation of vessels, perilimbal congestion
  +2   = Marked dilation of vessels, congestion of membranes

 E) Discharge
  0 = No discharge
  +1 = Any amount different from normal (dose not include small amount observed in
    inner canthus of normal eyes)
  +2 = Discharge with moistening of the lids and hairs just adjacent to the lids
  +3 = Discharge with moistening of the lids and considerable area around the eye

---

Observation of Corneal Epithelium

Corneal epithelial damage was evaluated by a slitlamp biomicroscope with a cobalt filter (SL-2, Kowa), according to the criteria shown in Table 2, by fluorecein staining of the cornea before, and in the 1st, 3rd, 6th and 12th month of application.

Table 2. Classification and criteria for evaluation of fluorescein staining of the cornea

Grade of fluorescein staining of the cornea	Score
No staining	0
Slight staining (visible only with cobalt filter and magnification)	0.5
Moderate staining (visible with normal light and magnification)	1
Heavy staining (visible without magnification)	2
Staining area of cornea	
Greater than one quarter but less than half	3
Greater than half	4

Observation of the Lens

Observation of lens was done by slitlamp biomicroscope (SL-2, Kowa) after mydriasis with Midrin-P^R (0.5% tropicamide, 0.5% phenylephrine)(Santen, Osaka, Japan) one hour after the third dose in the 6th and 12th month of application.

Funduscopy

Funduscopy was performed with a fundus camera (R2, Kowa) after mydriasis with Midrin-P before application, and one hour after the third dose in the 1st, 3rd, 6th and 12th month of application.

Electroretinography (ERG)

ERG was recorded before, and in the 1.5th, 3rd, 6th and 12th month of application. The animals were dark-adapted for more than one hour in a shielded dark room. A contact lens electrode (Kyoto Contact lens Co.,Ltd, Kyoto, Japan) for picking-up ERG was put on the left eye anesthetized with instillation of Benoxil^R 0.4% solution (0.4% oxybuprocaine hydrocloride) (Santen, Osaka, Japan). The animals was grounded by a needle electrode picked in the hind foot. Photostimuli with an intensity of 20 joules were given with a Xenon flash tube controlled by a photostimulator (Model 3G22, NEC San-ei Inc., Tokyo, Japan) at a distance of 30 cm from the eye. The ERGs were amplified by a Polygraph (Model 366, NEC San-ei Ltd., Tokyo, Japan) in which the high frequency cut off was set at 1 KHz and the time constant at 0.3 sec and 0.003 sec.

The sum of amplitudes Aa and Ab of waves a and b and their peak latencies La and Lb were calculated from the wave pattern with a time constant of 0.3 sec (Figure 1-1). The sum of amplitudes AO1, AO2 and AO3 of oscillatory potentials O1, O2 and O3, their peak latencies LO1, LO2 and LO3, the peak interval T1 between O1 and O2, the peak interval T2 between O2 and O3 were then calculated from the wave pattern with a time constant of 0.003 sec (Figure 1-2).

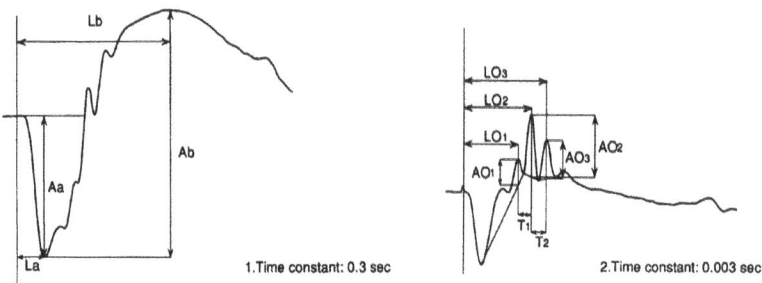

Figure 1. Wave pattern of ERG

Hematological Examinations

The following examinations were made with blood collected from the cephalic vein of forefoot in a tube containing EDTA-2K before and 12 months after application. Red blood cell (RBC) and platelet, white blood cell (WBC) and differential leukocyte count, hemoglobin and hematocrit were determined by Technicon H6000 system, calculated mean corpuscular volume (MCV), mean corpuscular hemoglobin (MCH) and mean corpuscular hemoglobin concentration (MCHC).

Blood Chemistry

Before the start and 12 months after application, blood was collected from the cephalic vein of forefoot, then it was centrifuged at 3000 rpm for 15 min to obtain the serum. The serum was used for the following determinations. Glutamic-oxalacetic transaminase (GOT), glutamic-pyruvic transaminase (GPT), alkaline phosphatase (ALP), lactate dehydrogenase (LDH), creatinine phosphokinase (CPK), total cholesterol (T cholesterol), triglyceride, phospholipid, total protein (T protein), albumin, albumin/globulin ratio (A/G), glucose, urea nitrogen (BUN), creatinine, inorganic phosphate, calcium, uric acid and sodium and potassium were determined by an autoanalyzer (Technicon, Model RA1000, SSR system).

Autopsy and Organ Weight

The animals were sacrificed by exsanguination under pentobarbital anesthesia on the next day of the last application and the brain, pituitary, eyeballs, thyroids, submaxillary glands, thymus, heart, lungs, liver, spleen, adrenals, kidneys, testes and prostate were removed and weighed. The relative organ weights to 1 kg of body weight were calculated respectively.

Histopathological Examinations

The tongue, trachea, esophagus, aorta, pancreas, stomach, duodenum, jejunum, ileum, cecum, colon, lymph nodes (cervical, hilar and mesenteric), bladder, vertebra, femur, rib, sternum, larynx, epiglottis, skin, skeletal muscle and sciatic nerve in addition to the above organs weighed were dissected and fixed in 10% neutral buffered formalin. The eyeballs and its appendages (extraocular muscle, bulbur conjunctiva, palpebral conjunctiva, optic nerve) were fixed in glutaraldehyde-formalin and then postfixed in 10% neutral buffered formalin. Hematoxilin-eosin stained preparation was made by the standard procedure for routine paraffin embedding and used for histopathological observation.

Statistical Analysis

F-test was used for body weight, ERG parameters, hematological and blood chemistry data, and Student's t-test was used when variances between the two groups were homogeneous at $p < 0.05$; otherwise Aspin-Welch's t-test was used. Mann-Whitney's U-test was used for differential leukocyte count.

RESULTS

General Conditions

Abnormal findings of general conditions were not observed during the experiment period.

Body Weight

Results of body weight measurement are shown in Figure 2. The body weights of the animals increased satisfactorily during the study period. No significant difference was noted between 0.3%OFLX group and the control group.

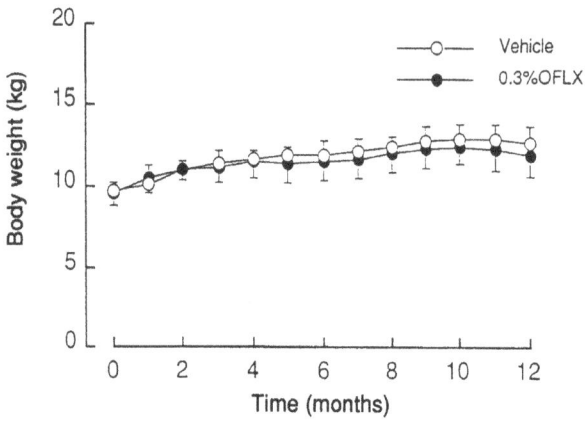

Figure 2. Body weight of beagle dogs

Anterior Ocular Irritation

Results of anterior ocular observation are shown in Table 3. Slight hyperemia in the bulbar conjunctiva was occasionally observed in each group. However, the intensity of hyperemia did not increase in treatment duration dependently.

Table 3. Score of ocular lesions after topical application of ofloxacin

Group	Month												
	0	1	2	3	4	5	6	7	8	9	10	11	12
(Redness of palpebral conjunctiva)													
Vehicle	0	0	0	0	0	0	0	0	0	0	0	0	0
0.3%OFLX	0	0	0	0	0	0	0	0	0	0	0	0	0
(Chemosis of palpebral conjunctiva)													
Vehicle	0	0	0	0	0	0	0	0	0	0	0	0	0
0.3%OFLX	0	0	0	0	0	0	0	0	0	0	0	0	0
(Redness of bulbar conjunctiva)													
Vehicle	0	0	0	0	0	0.1	0	0	0	0	0	0.1	0.1
0.3%OFLX	0	0	0.1	0	0	0.1	0.1	0.1	0.1	0.1	0.1	0	0.1
(Chemosis of bulbar conjunctiva)													
Vehicle	0	0	0	0	0	0	0	0	0	0	0	0	0
0.3%OFLX	0	0	0	0	0	0	0	0	0	0	0	0	0
(Discharge)													
Vehicle	0	0	0	0	0	0	0	0	0	0	0	0	0
0.3%OFLX	0	0	0	0	0	0	0	0	0	0	0	0	0

Each value represents the mean score of 5 eyes

Aqueous Flare

No abnormality was noted in the cornea or anterior chamber in each group.

Corneal Epithelial Damage

Very faint stained spots were found in some eyes of each group in the 1st, 3rd, 6th and 12th month (Table 3). However, the appearance of stained spots was sporadic and transient.

Table 4. Corneal epithelial damage after topical application of ofloxacin

	Month			
	1	3	6	12
Vehicle	0.2±0.1	0.1±0.1	0.2±0.1	0.2±0.1
0.3%OFLX	0.2±0.1	0.1±0.1	0.2±0.1	0.3±0.1

Each value represents the mean±S.E. of 10 eyes

Funduscopy

No abnormality was noted among the funduscopic findings in either group.

Observation of Lens

Lens abnormality was not observed in either group.

Electroretinogram

The each parameter of ERG was calculated from the ERG pattern and statistically analyzed between the 0.3%OFLX group and the control group (Figures 3, 4). A statistically significant difference was found in the peak latency of A wave (La) and ratio of Lb and La (Lb/La) in only 1.5th month. However, no significant difference was found in other ERG parameters.

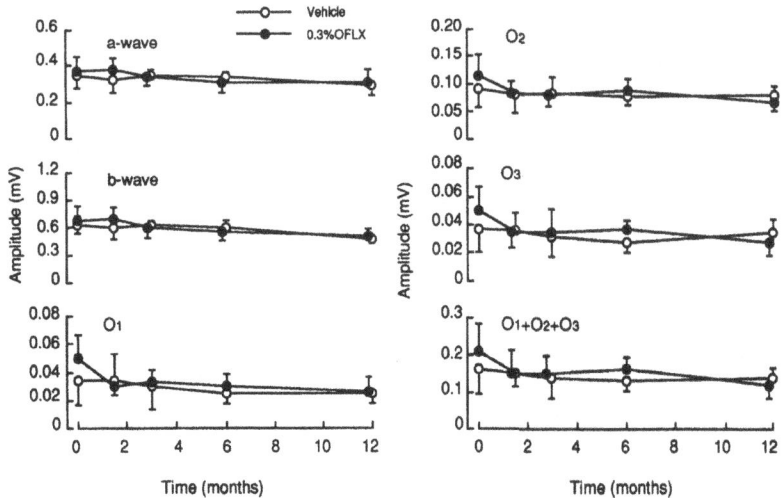

Figure 3. Effect of ofloxacin on amplitude of ERB

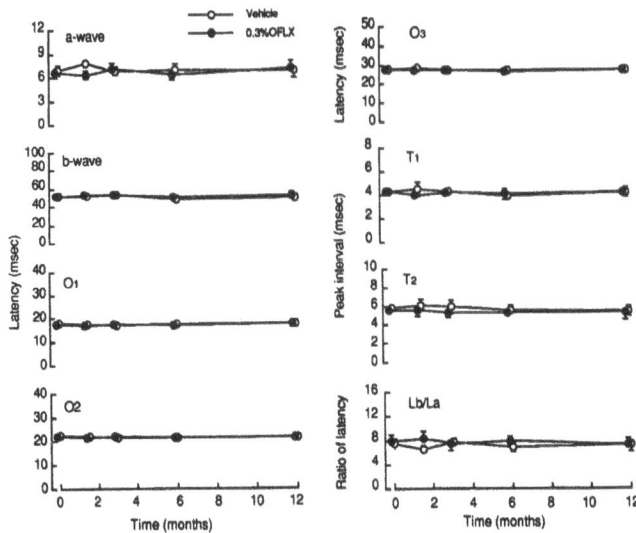

Figure 4. Effect of ofloxacin on latency of ERG

Hematological Examinations

Table 5 shows the results before and during the 12th month of application. Significant differences were noted in some test items between 0.3%OFLX group and the control group in the 12th month. However, each variation was within a normal range.

Blood Chemistry

Table 6 shows the results before and during the 12th month of application. Significant differences were noted in some test items between 0.3%OFLX group and the control group in the 12th month. However, each variation was within a normal range.

Autopsy

Adhesion of the pulmonary pleura to the throracic wall and nodules in the lung were found in one animal each. No abnormal changes were seen in the other organs.

Organ Weight Measurement

Table 7 and 8 show the absolute organ weight and relative organ weight, respectively. The relative weight of the thyroid slightly increased, within the normal range, in the 0.3%OFLX group. No noticeable change was found in the other organs.

Histopathology

No changes ascribable to the instillation of 0.3%OFLX were found in any organ. However, the following incidental changes, often observed in beagles, were noticed. Mild cysts in the pituitary, slight periportal cell infiltration in the liver and mild cellular infiltration in the zone surrounding the lobes of the liver were found in 1 animal in the 0.3%OFLX group. Slight vacuolation in the proximal renal tubules, cellular infiltration in the prostate and calcium deposition in the bladder were found in 1 animal in the control group. In the lung, dilatation of the alveolus, thickening in the alveolar wall, hyperplasia of the bronchial epithelium and granuloma, though slight, were observed in a few animals in each of the 0.3%OFLX and control group. In addition, slight deposition of hemosiderin in the spleen was found in all animals.

Table 5. Hematology in beagle dogs treated with ofloxacin

Group	RBC (10^6/mm^3)		Hb (g/dl)		Ht (%)		MCV (femto l)	
	0M	12M	0M	12M	0M	12M	0M	12M
Vehicle	6.75 ±0.22	7.62 ±0.24	14.8 ±0.7	17.3 ±0.3	44.0 ±1.9	49.1 ±0.9	65.3 ±3.9	64.5 ±1.3
OFLX	6.96 ±0.28	7.66 ±0.43	15.4 ±0.7	17.0 ±0.9	46.0 ±1.8	48.6 ±2.3	66.1 ±1.0	63.4 ±1.7

Group	MCH (pg)		MCHC (%)		WBC (10^3/mm^3)		PLT (10^3/mm^3)	
	0M	12M	0M	12M	0M	12M	0M	12M
Vehicle	22.0 ±1.4	22.8 ±0.4	33.6 ±0.4	35.3 ±0.1	18.54 ±4.45	14.56 ±2.82	360 ±27	343 ±32
OFLX	22.2 ±0.4	22.2 ±0.7	33.5 ±0.2	35.1 ±0.4	13.97 ±3.95	12.17 ±3.79	333 ±49	391 ±53

Differential leukocyte count (%)

Group	Baso		Eos		Neutro		Lymph		LUC		Mono	
	0M	12M	0M	12M	0M	12M	0M	12M	0M	12M	0M	12M
Vehicle	0.1 ±0.0	0.1 ±0.0	2.9 ±1.8	3.1 ±0.3	61.4 ±6.6	63.7 ±4.8	25.7 ±5.4	25.4 ±5.0	0.9 ±0.4	0.6 ±0.1	8.9 ±1.1	6.8 ±1.3
OFLX	0.1 ±0.0	0.1 ±0.0	5.2 ±2.1	5.3 ±3.2	50.5 ±3.5*	56.9 ±5.8	34.8 ±3.2*	30.6 ±4.7	1.2 ±0.3	0.6 ±0.2	7.9 ±1.2	6.3 ±1.6

Differential leukocyte count (10^3/mm^3)

Group	Baso		Eos		Neutro		Lymph		LUC		Mono	
	0M	12M	0M	12M	0M	12M	0M	12M	0M	12M	0M	12M
Vehicle	0.02 ±0.01	0.01 ±0.01	0.53 ±0.35	0.46 ±0.13	11.43 ±3.43	9.29 ±1.92	4.73 ±1.33	3.69 ±0.90	0.17 ±0.06	0.09 ±0.01	1.64 ±0.44	1.00 ±0.27
OFLX	0.02 ±0.00	0.01 ±0.00	0.78 ±0.39	0.68 ±0.62	7.05 ±2.10*	7.05 ±2.64	4.83 ±1.30	3.60 ±0.73	0.16 ±0.04	0.07 ±0.01	1.10 ±0.34	0.73 ±0.13

N=5, *:$p < 0.05$ vs Vehicle, M: Month, Baso: Basophil, Eos: Eosinophil, Neutro: Neutrophil, Lymph: Lymphocyte, LUC: Leukocyte, Mono: Monocyte, PLT: Plateret, Mean±S.D.

Table 6. Blood chemistry in beagle dogs treated with ofloxacin

	GOT (U/l serum)		GPT (U/l serum)		ALP (U/l serum)		LDH (U/l plasma)		CPK (U/l plasma)	
	0M	12M	0M	12M	0M	12M	0M	12M	0M	12M
Vehicle	42	31	34	45	86	29	88	41	214	88
	±8	±5	±5	±11	±15	±9	±29	±9	±41	±14
OFLX	44	32	35	54	97	36	93	40	205	95
	±3	±5	±6	±24	±39	±10	±19	±10	±43	±14

	T cholesterol (mg/dl serum)		Triglyceride (mg/dl serum)		Phospholipid (mg/dl serum)		T protein (g/dl serum)		Albumin (g/dl serum)	
	0M	12M	0M	12M	0M	12M	0M	12M	0M	12M
Vehicle	155	144	40	36	325	312	6.0	6.4	3.2	3.3
	±20	±15	±11	±4	±32	±21	±0.3	±0.2	±0.1	±0.1
OFLX	173	138	40	32	358	302	6.5	6.5	3.5	3.3
	±16	±20	±11	±11	±23	±19	±0.2*	±0.3	±0.2*	±0.1

	A/G [ALB/(TP-ALB)]		Glucose (mg/dl serum)		BUM (mg/dl serum)		Creatinine (mg/dl serum)		Uric acid (mg/dl serum)	
	0M	12M	0M	12M	0M	12M	0M	12M	0M	12M
Vehicle	1.1	1.1	107	103	13.3	14.0	0.88	1.21	0.8	0.5
	±0.1	±0.1	±20	±10	±2.8	±1.9	±0.05	±0.08	±0.3	±0.2
OFLX	1.1	1.0	103	113	12.2	14.4	0.91	1.23	0.8	0.5
	±0.1	±0.2	±13	±7	±1.6	±4.0	±0.06	±0.09	±0.3	±0.1

	Phosphorus (mg/dl serum)		Sodium (mEq/l serum)		Potassium (mEq/l serum)		Calcium (mg/dl serum)	
	0M	12M	0M	12M	0M	12M	0M	12M
Vehicle	7.2	4.0	149.4	149.4	4.42	3.93	11.1	10.7
	±0.4	±0.2	±1.8	±1.0	±0.38	±0.09	±0.2	±0.1
OFLX	7.0	3.6	150.6	148.3	4.34	3.88	11.3	10.6
	±0.5	±0.3*	±1.3	±1.4	±0.34	±0.18	±0.4	±0.2

N=5, *:p<0.05 vs Vehicle, M: Month, Mean±S.D.

Table 7. Absolute organ weight in beagle dogs treated with ofloxacin

Group	Body weight (kg)	Brain (g)	Pituitary glands (mg)	Eye balls (g)	Thyroids (g)
Vehicle	12.7±1.1	77.8±6.9	76±9	13.04±0.32	0.84±0.07
OFLX	11.9±1.3	82.7±4.8	73±5	12.94±0.17	1.04±0.26

Group	Submaxillary glands (g)	Thymus (g)	Heart (g)	Lungs (g)	Liver (g)
Vehicle	14.37±2.20	9.42±5.39	100.8±7.5	97.7±9.9	279.4±23.4
OFLX	13.11±1.92	10.30±3.19	105.5±12.9	98.4±10.6	262.0±23.4

Group	Spleen (g)	Adrenals (g)	Kidneys (g)	Testes (g)	Prostate (g)
Vehicle	29.9±8.5	1.08±0.23	56.9±10.8	23.98±4.02	11.67±3.92
OFLX	24.8±2.3	1.20±0.13	56.5±3.8	26.28±4.12	9.57±2.28

N=5, M: Month, Mean±S.D.

Table 8. Relative organ weight in beagle dogs treated with ofloxacin

Group	Brain (g%)	Pituitary glands (mg%)	Eye balls (g%)	Thyroids (g%)
Vehicle	6.2±0.6	6.0±0.7	1.03±0.08	0.066±0.009
OFLX	7.0±0.8	6.2±1.0	1.10±0.12	0.087±0.016*

Group	Submaxillary glands (g%)	Thymus (g%)	Heart (g%)	Lungs (g%)	Liver (g%)
Vehicle	1.14±0.23	0.74±0.40	8.0±1.0	7.7±0.6	22.0±1.2
0.3%OFX	1.11±0.19	0.86±0.23	8.9±1.0	8.3±1.1	22.2±2.8

Group	Spleen (g%)	Adrenals (g%)	Kidneys (g%)	Testes (g%)	Prostate (g%)
Vehicle	2.4±0.6	0.085±0.018	4.5±0.9	1.89±0.24	0.94±0.40
OFLX	2.1±0.2	0.102±0.016	4.8±0.5	2.24±0.48	0.81±0.21

N=5, *:p<0.05 vs. Vehicle, M: Month, Mean±S.D.

DISCUSSION

0.3%OFLX has been generally used at 3 times daily for the therapy of ocular infection. Ocular irritability and damage with ofloxacin have been investigated by using 0.5% ofloxacin eye drops administrated 4 times a day (the dose was higher than clinically used dose) for 1 month in albino rabbits and no ocular toxicity with ofloxacin has been found[9]. From the facts described above, we supposed that 0.3%OFLX would not have ocular irritability and damage. However, it has been reported that ofloxacin has an affinity for melanin pigment[7] and oral administration of ofloxacin caused abnormal behavior, such as decreased spontaneous movement tripping gait in beagles at high dose[10]. In the present one year study, we examined the ocular toxicity test of 0.3%OFLX in dogs that have a melanin pigment in order to confirm the safety of 0.3%OFLX.

No abnormality was noted in animal health conditions and in body weights.In this study, we observed carefully the behavior of animals because ofloxacin caused abnormal behavior in beagles at a dose of 50 mg/kg/day or higher in a subacute toxicity study. However, no abnormal finding attributable to the instillation of 0.3%OFLX was observed during the study period. If the volume of 1 drop of an ophthalmic solution is estimated to be 50µl, the dose of ofloxacin in the present study corresponds to 0.09mg/kg/day (if a beagle weighs 10 kg), approximately 1/600 of the dose that caused abnormal behavior in subacute toxicity study. Therefore, it was assumed that the instillation of 1 drop of 0.3%OFLX three times daily for as long as 1 year would not develop any action which might have adverse influence on central nerve system.

Slight hyperemia in the bulbar conjunctiva was occasionally observed in 0.3%OFLX. This is, however, assumed not to be caused by the instillation of 0.3%OFLX, because the same finding was observed in vehicle group and intensity of hyperemia did not increase in treatment duration dependently. Very faint stained spots were found in a few animals in both groups. However, application of 0.3%OFLX is not the cause because even normal eyes generally show the stained spots because of physiological detachment of corneal epithelium[11,12] and because the spots were found both in the control group and 0.3%OFLX group in this study. No abnormality was noted in any observation of aqueous flare, lens and fundus. In this study, electroretinogram was recorded in order to show clearly the effects of OFLX on retinal function. A statistically significant difference (Student t-test) was found in the La and Lb/La in only 1.5 month. We conclude that the change of La was induced with accidental change of Lb/La because the time cause of Lb/La was correlated completely to change of La. The statistical change of La was found in only 1.5 month, with no particular tendency at the other time points (before and 3, 6 and 12 months after start of instillation). Therefore, it was assumed that the change might not reflect the influence of the 0.3%OFLX on ERG. Furthermore, because no abnormal change was found in retina and chorioid during histopathological examination, it was assumed that the instillation of 0.3%OFLX had no influence on visual function.

Hematological examinations, blood chemistry, autopsy, organ weight measurement and histopathology were made in order to examine the systemic influence of 0.3%OFLX. No abnormality ascribable to ofloxacin was found.

It seems reasonable to conclude from these results that long-term application of 0.3%OFLX for one-year causes neither eye irritation nor damage and affects neither visual functions nor the general health condition.

ACKNOWLEDGMENTS

The authors wish to thank Dr. S. Mita for valuable comments on the manuscript, Mr. T. Nakano, Mr. K. Matuno, Mr. T. Terashima, Mr. T. Ikuse, Mr. A. Okahara, Mr. M. Fukumoto for technical help, Ms T. Shirakami and Y. Doura for typing of this manuscript.

REFERENCES

1. J. T. Smith, 1991, Ofloxacin, a bactericidal antibacterial, *Chemotherapy*, 37:2.
2 K. Sato, 1982, In vitro and in vivo activity of DL-8280, a new oxazine derivative, *Antimicrobial Agents and Chemotherapy*, 22:548.

3 K. Sato, M. Inoue and S. Mitsuhashi, 1984, In vitro and in vivo antibacterial activity of DL-8280, *Chemotherapy*, 32:1.
4 M. Tsumura, K. Sato, T. Une and H. Tachizawa, 1984, Metabolic disposition of DL-8280 the first report: Comparison between absorption and excretion of DL-8280 in the dog and monkey by bioassay and HPLC methods, *Chemotherapy*, 32:1179.
5 M. Fukuda and K. Sasaki, 1986, Penetration of administered ofloxacin into ocular tissues, *Foli. Ophthalmol. Jpn.*, 37:823.
6 Y. Mitsui, S. Sakuragi, O. Tamura, M. Abe, I. Watanabe, M. Ueno, K. Choshi, H. Sakata, T. Suehiro, N. Ohoba, S. Fujita, Y. Miyazono, K. Sasaki, T. Yamamura, N. Watanabe, M. Uyama, K. Kanai, T. Tokuyama, H. Miyatani, M. Itoi, Y. Kodama, H. Tasaka, R. Manabe, Y. Ohashi, Y. Shimomura, K. Segawa, K. Nishiyama, K. Norose, S. Inoue, K. Matsumura, M. Ooishi, F. Sakaue, A. Oomomo, J. Hara, S. Harino, J. Tsutsui, H. Kimura, S. Inoue, M. Higashitsutsumi, M. Sakamoto, T. Miwatani and T. Onoda, 1986, Effect of ofloxacin ophthalmic solution in the treatment of external bacterial infections of the eye, *Foli. Ophthalmol. Jpn.*, 37:1115.
7 M. Fukuda and K. Sasaki, 1988, The influence of melanin on intraocular dynamics, *Acta. Soc. Ophthalmol. Jpn.*, 92:1839.
8 H. Kojima, M. Hirohashi, T. Sakurai, Y. Kasai and A. Akashi, 1984, General pharmacology of DL-8280, *Chemotherapy*, 32:1147.
9 H. Yamauchi, H. Mibu, M. Sasano, M. Hayashi, K. Takase, S. Nagamori, T. Terashima, A. Okahara, H. Kito, N. Ueno and T. Iso, 1985, Safety evaluation of ofloxacin in rabbits II. Ocular irritation test and systemic influences with topical application for four weeks, *Foli. Ophthalmol. Jpn.*, 36:2302.
10 H. Ohno, F. Inage, K. Akahane, K. Aihara, M. Yoshida and T. Onodera, 1984, Acute toxicity of a synthetic antimicrobial, DL-8280, in mice, rats and monkeys, *Chemotheraphy* 32:1084.
11 Y. Kikkawa, 1972, Normal corneal staining with fluorescein. *Exp. Eye Res.* 14:13.
12 T. E. Hickey, G. L. Beck and J. A. Jr. Botta, 1973, Optimum fluorescein staining time in ocular irritation studies. *Tox. Appl. Pharmacol.*, 26:571.

TOPICAL FLUCONAZALE: HIGH PENETRATION WITHOUT CORNEAL TOXICITY

Kayo Uchiyama[1], Naoko Asano[1], Masafumi Ogata[1], Toshiro Tanahashi[1], Makoto Torisaki[1], Kiyofumi Mochizuki[1], Kazuo Kawasaki[1], Masami Kojima[2], Kazuyuki Sasaki[2] Yasuhisa Ishibashi[3], Cheng-Chin Hsu[4], Tuguhisa Kaneko[4], and Hiroshi Yamamoto[4]

[1]Department of Ophthalmology, Kanazawa University School of Medicine
[2]Department of Ophthalmology, Kanazawa Medical University
[3]Department of Ophthalmology, Tokyo Women's Medical College
[4]Department of Biochemistry, Kanazawa University School of Medicine

13-1 Takara-machi, Kanazawa, Ishikawa 920, Japan

ABSTRACT

PURPOSE Fluconazole has been reported to effectively combat keratomycosis or *Acanthamoeba* keratitis. We investigated ocular penetration and corneal toxicity of topically administered fluconazole. **METHODS** Fluconazole (0.2%) was administered to albino rabbit eyes by instillations every 5 minutes for 1 hour, every 30 minutes for 12 hours, and by a single 0.3-ml subconjunctival injection. Control eyes received topical saline. Various ocular tissues and serum were sampled at various time points and assayed for fluconazole concentrations by high performance liquid chromatography (HPLC). Corneal epithelial and endothelial integrity after instillation was examined by specular microscopy and ultrasonic pachymetry. Lactate dehydrogenase (LDH) activity and protein concentration in the tears were determined by the methods of Wroblewski and of Bradford, respectively. Corneal epithelial healing rates in the fluconazole-treated and control eyes were examined by corneal photography after mechanical abrasion of the corneal epithelium. **RESULTS** 1) Fluconazole concentration was maximal in the conjunctiva, the cornea, the aqueous humor and the iris-ciliary body 15 to 30 minutes after the final instillation in the 1-hour regimen. 2) Fluconazole was detected in the conjunctiva, the cornea, the aqueous humor and the anterior lens cortex 1 hour after the 12-hour regimen. Corneal thickness, intraocular pressure, LDH activity or protein concentration in the tears were not significantly affected by fluconazole instillation. 3) Fluconazole was detected in the vitreous humor, the retinal pigment epithelium-choroid (RPE-choroid) and the sclera, except for the anterior ocular segments, after a subconjunctival injection. 4) The corneal epithelial healing rate did not significantly differ between the fluconazole-treated and control eyes. **CONCLUSIONS** The high intraocular concentrations and the lack of toxicity to the anterior ocular segments indicate that topical fluconazole is effective and safe for treating keratomycosis or *Acanthamoeba* keratitis.

INTRODUCTION

Fluconazole, a newly developed antifungal triazole compound (molecular weight: 306.3), selectively suppresses ergosterol synthesis by freely penetrating the cerebrospinal fluid[1,2]. Usefulness of fluconazole treat fungal endophthalmitis, keratomycosis and *Acanthamoeba* keratitis[3-5] and high intraocular penetration of systemically administered fluconazole[6-8] have been described. However, to the best of our knowledge, intraocular penetration of topical fluconazole and its effect on the ocular surface have not yet been reported. In the present study, we investigated intraocular penetration, corneal toxicity and corneal epithelial wound healing after topical fluconazole administration to rabbit eyes.

MATERIALS AND METHODS

Animals

Thirty-four male and female albino rabbits weighing 2.0 to 3.0 kg were used.

1) Intraocular Penetration of Fluconazole 1 Hour after Instillation

Twelve albino rabbits were administered one drop of $50\mu l$ of 0.2% fluconazole in the inferior cul-de-sac of both eyes every 5 minutes for 1 hour. The animals were anesthetized with an intramuscular injection of 0.5-1.0 ml/kg ketamine hydrochloride (100 mg/ml) / xylazine hydrochloride (20 mg/ml) mixture (7/1) on sampling at 15 and 30 minutes and 1, 2, 4 and 8 hours after the last instillation. Blood was obtained by cardiac puncture and centrifuged at 2,000 rpm for 20 minutes to separate the serum. After corneal anesthesia with oxybuprocaine hydrochloride, 5×30-mm samples of the upper conjunctiva were excised. The animals were sacrificed with an overdose of intravenous pentobarbital sodium, and the eyes were immediately enucleated. Aqueous humor specimens were obtained by paracentesis using a 27-gauge needle on a tuberculin syringe. The eyes then were dissected under an operating microscope to separate the cornea, the lens, the iris-ciliary body and the vitreous body. The cornea was trephinated using a 7-mm trephine yielding a central corneal button and a peripheral ring of corneal tissue. In addition, the lens was extirpated and the nucleus was removed leaving the peripheral cortical material and capsule using a 8-mm trephine. The central lens disks were sliced in three parts, anterior and posterior cortexes and the nucleus, according to Müller's method[9]. The sclera was opened by radial incision and the optic nerve removed. The sensory retina and the retinal pigment epithelium-choroid(RPE-choroid) were excised separately. All specimens were stored frozen at -20℃ in cryotubes until assayed by HPLC.

2) Intraocular Penetration of Fluconazole after Subconjunctival Injection

A 27-gauge needle on a 1-ml tuberculin syringe was inserted into the subconjunctival space just temporal to the superior rectus muscle. Three hundred microliters of 0.2% fluconazole were injected into both eyes of 12 albino rabbits. One, 2, 4 and 8 hours after the injection, the conjunctiva was resected in the temporal upper and nasal lower portions under general and topical anesthesia as described in 1). Then the serum, the aqueous humor, the central and peripheral cornea, the lens, the iris-ciliary body, the vitreous humor, the sensory retina, the RPE-choroid, the sclera and the optic nerve were obtained as described in 1). All specimen were kept frozen at -20℃ until assayed.

3) Intraocular Penetration and Ocular Toxicity of Fluconazole 12 Hours after Instillation

Six albino rabbits were administered one drop of 50μl of 0.2% fluconazole and normal saline, respectively, in the right and left inferior cul-de-sacs every 30 minutes for 12 hours. One hour after the last instillation, the serum and the ocular portions were obtained and processed as described in 1) and 2). The corneal epithelium and endothelium were examined by specular microscopy and ultrasonic pachymetry before and 1 hour after the instillations. Intraocular pressure (IOP) was measured by applanation pneumotonography. LDH activities and protein concentrations in tear fluids were determined by the methods of Wroblewski[10] and of Bradford[11], respectively.

4) Effect of Topical Fluconazole on Corneal Epithelial Wound Healing

Under the general and corneal anesthesia, the corneal epithelium in both eyes of four albino rabbits was lightly marked at the center with a trephine of 7 mm in diameter and abraded with a spatula. One drop of 50μl of 0.2% fluconazole or normal saline was instilled into the right and left eyes, respectively, every hour for 53 hours after the mechanical abrasion. Immediately after the abrasion and 3, 6, 9, 12, 15, 19, 23, 27, 33, 39, 47 and 53 hours postabrasion, the epithelial defects were observed by fluorescein staining and photographed with Medical Nikkor (Nikon). The photographs (magnification × 4.1) were scanned and put into a Macintosh computer (Apple). The areas of epithelial abrasion were then measured using an Adobe Photoshop program (Adobe), and the corneal epithelial wound healing rates calculated. Statistical analysis was performed using the Wilcoxon rank sum test.

5) Determination of Fluconazole Concentration

HPLC Analysis. The ocular concentrations of fluconazole were assayed by HPLC in a solvent of ammonium acetate / acetonitrile (3/1) using an ODS-M column (Shimadzu Co., Kyoto, Japan). Typical absorbance at 260nm having the retention time of 6.72 min was measured and standardized with that of authentic fluconazole.

Extraction. Aliquots of the samples were transferred into test tubes containing small amounts of internal standard, then homogenized with 0.5 M sodium hydroxide / ethyl acetate (1/1), and centrifuged. The ethyl acetate layer was transferred to a new tube and back-extracted with 1 M hydrochloric acid. After aspiration of the ethyl acetate layer, the hydrochloric acid was alkalinized by the addition of 5 M sodium hydroxide. The solution was extracted with ethyl acetate. The ethyl acetate layer was transferred to a new tube, and then evaporated to dryness under a flow of nitrogen gas. The resultant residue was reconstituted in the mobile phase for injection into the HPLC. The lowest measurable concentration was 0.1μg/ml (or μg/g wet tissue).

RESULTS

1) Intraocular Penetration of Fluconazole 1 Hour after Instillation (Figure 1)

The flucoanzole levels detected in the cornea, the aqueous humor and the iris-ciliary body were maximal 15-30 minutes after the final administration, then decreased gradually and fell to undetectable levels 8 hours after the last instillation. Fluconazole concentrations in the conjunctiva and the sclera at 8 hours averaged 3.4 μg/g and 4.3 μg/g, respectively. The fluconazole levels in the conjunctiva, the sclera and the vitreous humor changed in parallel, suggesting that fluconazole had penetrated into the vitreous humor from the conjunctiva and the sclera.

2) Intraocular Penetration of Fluconazole after Subconjunctival Injection (Figure 2)

The cornea, the conjunctiva, the aqueous humor, and the iris-ciliary body were well penetrated by subconjunctivally injected fluconazole when judged 1 hour after the injection. The fluconazole levels fell gradually and became undetectable after 8 hours. The posterior segments, including the sclera, the RPE-choroid and the vitreous humor, were also well penetrated. The fluconazole levels in these tissues declined in parallel.

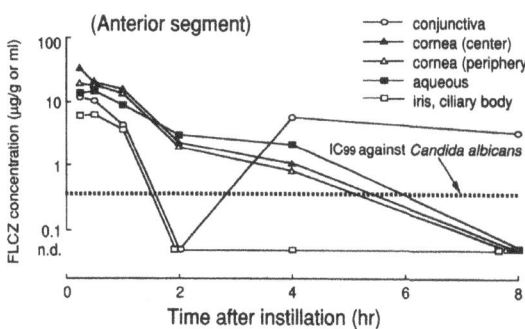

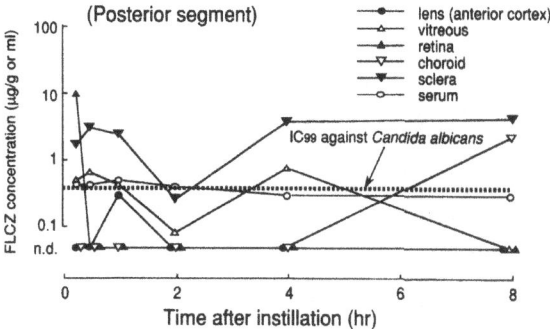

✳ lens (equator, posterior cortex, nucleus) and optic nerve < 0.1

Figure 1 Fluconazole concentrations in ocular tissues and serum after instillations every 5 minutes for 1 hour.

185

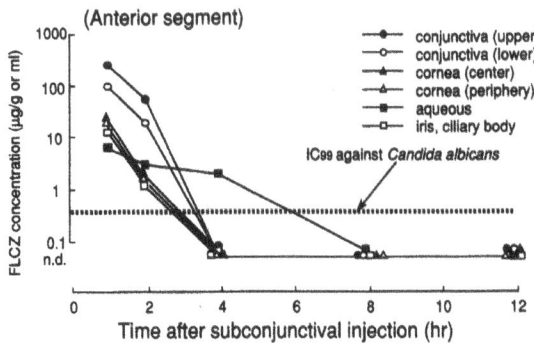

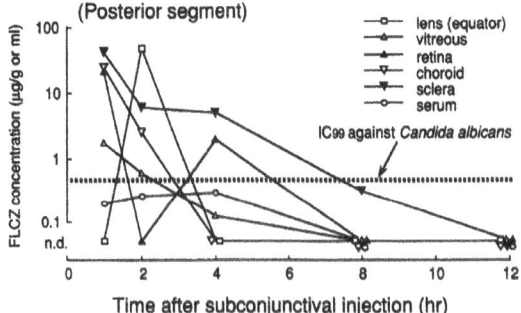

* lens (anterior cortex, nucleus, posterior cortex) and optic nerve < 0.1

Figure 2 Fluconazole concentrations in ocular tissues and serum after subconjunctival injection.

3) Intraocular Penetration and Ocular Toxicity of Fluconazole 12 Hours after Instillation (Figure 3)

Topical fluconazole (administered every 30 minutes for 12 hours) was found to have effectively penetrated into the conjunctiva, the cornea, the aqueous humor and the anterior lens cortex 1 hour after the last instillation. Only the cornea had fluconazole concentrations significantly greater than IC_{99} of *Candida albicans*. When compared with other regimens, fluconazole concentration in the cornea was lower than those after multiple instillations every 5 minutes for 1 hour or after subconjunctival injection. Fluconazole was not detected in the control fellow eyes even at 1 hour after the final instillation when the maximum serum level was observed.

No significant difference between pre- and post-instillation was observed in the corneal epithelium and endothelium, the corneal thickness, the IOP, and the tear fluid contents of LDH and proteins.

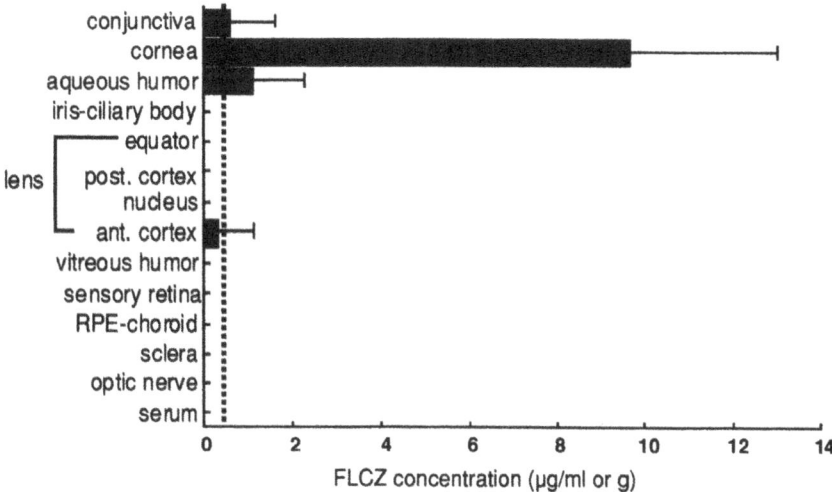

Fig. 3 Fluconazole (FLCZ) concentrations in ocular tissues and serum after instillations every 30 minutes for 12 hours.

4) Effect of Topical Fluconazole on Corneal Epithelial Wound Healing (Figure 4)

We determined the healing rates for the fluconazole-treated eyes and compared them with the control fellow eyes. The healing rates were expressed as the percentages of the denuded area over the initially abraded area in each rabbit. The healing process appeared to consist of two phases: a plateau phase within the first 12 hours, and a rapidly resurfacing phase. Matsumoto and Ishibashi[12] reported three phases in the healing process. However, the purported third phase with residual fluorescein staining was not observed in this study. In the first phase, no significant differences in the healing rate were found between the fluconazole-treatedand the control eyes, except for 3 hours after abrasion. The mean ratio of denuded / abraded areas was 103% in the fluconazole-treatedeyes, whereas it was 93% in the control eyes 3 hours after abrasion. The irregularity of the margin of the abraded area might account for this slight difference in the early phase healing rates. In the second phase, no significant differences were found in healing rates between the fluconazole-treatedand the control eyes: the values were 1.165 ± 0.074 mm^2/hr for fluconazole-treatedeyes and 1.264 ± 0.119 mm^2/hr for control eyes (mean $\pm$ standard deviation). Complete coverage of the corneal surface took place approximately 55 hours after the abrasion in both the fluconazole-treatedand control eyes.

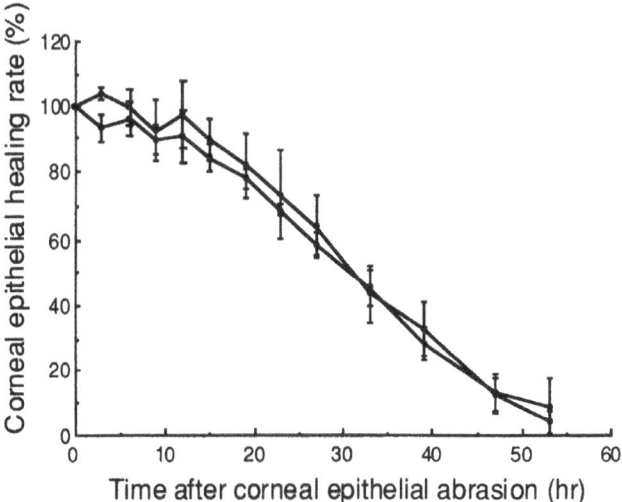

Figure 4 Corneal epithelial wound healing.
No significant differences were found between the fluconazole-treated eyes and the control eyes. ⎯•⎯ fluconazole,　　⎯▲⎯ saline　　(mean $\pm$ SD)

DISCUSSION

The present results demonstrate high intraocular penetration of topically administered fluconazole. Fluconazole concentrations reached maximum levels 15 to 30 min after the final instillationof the 1 hour regimen in the conjunctiva, the cornea, the aqueous humor and the iris-ciliary body. Fluconazole also penetrated well into the sclera and the vitreous humor. High fluconazole concentrations were achieved by the single subconjunctival injection in the RPE-choroid as well as in the sclera, except the anterior ocular segments. Because fluconazole is instilled every 30 min or 1 hour in usual clinical use, we investigated its intraocular penetration after administration every 30 min for 12 hours. Fluconazole was detected in the conjunctiva, the cornea, the aqueous humor and the anterior lens cortex 1 hour after the 12-hour regimen. The fluconazole tissue levels were low except in the cornea. The corneal fluconazole concentration 1 hour after the last instillation of the 12-hour regimen (9.5 μg/g) was lower than those 1 hour after the subconjunctival injection or 15 min to 1 hour after the final instillation in the 1-hour regimen. A combined use of multiple instillations and subconjunctival injection of fluconazole would seem to be most effective in treating keratomycosis or *Acanthamoeba* keratitis.

High intraocular penetration of systemically administered fluconazole has been reported by Savani et al.[6], O'Day et al.[7] and Yamashita et al.[8]. However, the systemic administration should require higher dosage and may cause anaphylaxis or systemic side effects. Possible adverse effects of topical fluconazole on the anterior ocular segment were also tested in this study. The cornea, the iris-ciliary body and the bulbar conjunctiva exhibited no abnormalities on slitlamp-microscopy examinations after instillations. Corneal thickness, IOP, and tear fluid LDH and protein determinations also disclosed any significant differences between pre - and post-instillations. Further, no significant difference was observed in the corneal epithelial healing rates between the fluconazole-treated and the control eyes. Fluconazole (0.2%) instillation was therefore considered nontoxic to the anterior ocular segment.

Our results indicate that topical fluconazole instillation may be useful to treat fungal and *Acanthamoeba* infections of the anterior ocular segment because it ensures sufficiently high ocular penetration of the drug without noticeable local toxicity.

REFERENCES

1. Morita, T. and Nozawa, Y., 1986, Selective inhibitory action of fluconazole, an antifungal agent of triazole-derivative, on sterol 14-C demethylation of *Candida albicans* cells. Jpn J Med Mycol 27: 190

2. Foulds, G., Brennan, D.R., Wajszcauk, C., Catanzaro, A., Grag, D.G., Knopf, W., Rinaldi, M. and Weildler, D.J., 1988, Fluconazole penetration into cerebrospinal fluid in humans. J Clin Pharmacol 28: 363

3. Van't Wout, J.W., Mattie, H. and van Furth, R., 1988, A prospective study of the efficacy of fluconazole (UK-49,858) against deep-seated fungal infections. J Antimicrob Chemother 21: 665

4. Laatikainen, L., Tuominen, M. and von Dickhoff, K., 1992, Treatment of endogenous fungal endophthalmitis with systemic fluconazole with or without vitrectomy. Am J Ophthalmol 113: 205

5. Fujii, T. and Inada, K., 1993, *Acanthamoeba* keratitis treated with fluconazole and miconazole -report of a case-. Folia Ophthalmol. Jpn. 44: 1434

6. Savani, D.V., Perfect, J.R., Cobo, L.M. and Durack, D.T., 1987, Penetration of new azole compounds into the eye and efficacy in experimental *Candida* endophthalmitis. Antimicrob Agents Chemother 31: 6

7. O'Day, D.M., Foulds, G., Williams, T.E., Robinson, R.D., Allen, R.H. and Head, W.S., 1990, Ocular uptake of fluconazole following oral administration. Arch Ophthalmol 108: 1006

8. Yamashita, Y., Mochizuki, K., Torisaki, M., Komatsu, M., Tanahashi, T. and Sakai, H., 1992, Intraocular penetration and effect of fluconazole on the retina. Atarashii Ganka 9: 1388

9. Müller, A., 1987, Profiles of enzyme activities in bovine lenses. Concepts Toxicology 4 (Hockwin O, editor), Basel, Karger, pp. 343-349.

10. Wroblewski, F. and LaDue, J.S., 1955, Lactic dehydrogenase activity in blood. Proc Soc Exp Biol Med 90: 210

11. Bradford, M.M., 1976, A rapid and sensitive method for the quantitaion of microgram quantities of protein utilizing the principle of protein-dye binding. Anal Biochem 72: 248

12. Matsumoto, Y. and Ishibashi, Y., 1984, Corneal epithelial wound healing. J Jpn Ophthalmol Soc 88: 1329

RELEVANCE OF CATARACT MODELS IN RODENTS AS A TOOL TO EVIDENCE A CO- OR SYNCATARACTOGENIC POTENTIAL OF DRUGS IN PRECLINICAL STUDIES

A. Wegener[1] and O. Hockwin[2]

[1]Dept. of Experimental Ophthalmology, University of Bonn
D-53105 Bonn, Germany
[2] Tulpenweg 4, D-53757 St. Augustin, Germany

ABSTRACT

Considerable experience has been gathered in the design and performance of drug side-effect and efficacy studies with cataract models. The spectrum of drugs tested for their potential cocataractogenic effects covered drugs from a wide range of medical applications, the compounds tested were administered systemically as well as topically. Animal models of primary importance for these studies were: the Streptozotocin-induced true diabetic cataract, naphthalene and the UV-A as well as UV-B cataract of the Brown-Norway rat. Less frequently used were galactose and X-ray cataracts. Rarely involved were the phenylketonuria (PKU), tryptophane deficiency or hereditary cataracts. Essential for the reliability of all models was their induction in young animals. Due to the variance in blood glucose levels in the diabetic cataract model, an appropriate selection of animals with an optimal blood glucose level is needed. Naphthalene and UV-B are less critical. Galactose cataract is the most easy to handle, but lacks clinical relevance and X-irradiation is suitable as additional noxa. Cocataractogenic effects have been found in all primary 4 models. They also proved to be useful to test cataract-preventive effects. Such statements were always based on data from objective transparency measurements in-vivo and post-mortem bio-chemistry results. In summary, these models proved to be the most reliable preclinical technique to elucidate a co- or syn-cataractogenic potential.

INTRODUCTION

The evaluation of undesired ocular drug side-effects has become an impor-tant issue in preclinical drug development and possible cataractogenic potentials are key issues in this respect (Hockwin and Wegener, 1987). A number of animal cataract models has been estab-lished in rodents, their suitability for toxicological research, however, varies considerably.

To select the most suitable among them, certain requirements had to be established: Clearly discernable and reproducible transparency changes as well as a typical morphology and location of onset are as essential as a development in a meaningful time-frame. Further more knowledge of an elucidated causative mechanism and means to interfere with it are of importance. Last but not least clinical relevance must not be neglected.

The heterogeneous group of cataract models can be divided into subgroups according to the origin of the noxious factors involved, i.e. internal versus external triggers (Wegener and Hockwin, 1987).

Internal triggers are either of genetic origin or reflect the effect of internal diseases on the transparency of the lens. The majority of cataract mutants proved not to be suitable for toxicological research because the genomic loci of their defects as well as their pathomechanisms are not elucidated. Among the few exceptions are the RCS-rat (Royal Coll. of Surgeons; Zigler and Hess, 1985) and the Scat mouse-mutant (Graw et al., 1989).

The external triggers subdivide again into physical and chemical triggers. Chemical triggers can originate from internal diseases or be chemicals and drugs. The physical triggers comprize non-ionizing radiation causing photo-chemical reactions or ionizing radiation, causing DNA-damage.

MATERIALS AND METHODS

Chemical Triggers

Sugar Cataracts. The formation of a juvenile diabetic cataract (comparable to human type 1 juvenile diabetic cataract) is induced by intravenous injection of Streptozotocin (STR) at a dosage of 70 mg /kg body weight, dissolved in citrate buffer (Sasaki et al., 1983). One or 2 injections are necessary to cause the formation of a stable diabetes that is present within a few days and remains stable for 6 or more weeks. Glucose concentrations in these animals can vary from 350 - 500 mg/100 ml blood, values below 300 mg/100 ml blood indicate an unstable diabetes. As the rapidness and intensity of formation of juvenile diabetic cataracts depends on the blood glucose levels, it is recommended to start an experiment with a larger set of animals than needed and select those in the range of 350 - 450 mg/100ml blood.

Galactose cataracts can easily be induced by feeding a diet containing 20% - 50% galactose. First signs of cataract development appear within days and a complete galactose cataract will be present within 3 weeks. It is the easiest cataract model in rodents, but cannot be compared directly to the human patho-physiological situation in sugar cataracts. Other sugars cause similar cataracts but are less relevant (Keller, 1979).

Spontaneous diabetic rats are less suitable for toxicological research, because the onset of a diabetes cannot be influenced. This reduces the repro-ducibility of cataract formation, because during aging, the lens becomes less sensitive to glucose due to an age-dependend decrease in activity of aldose-reductase. This slows down the formation of the diabetic cataract.

Oxidizing Agents. Naphthalene, dosed orally with a stomach tube every other day at 1g/kg body weight (in paraffin oil) is metabolized in several steps to naphthoquinone, a strong oxidizing agent. It causes the formation of a cortical zonular opacity, located in a ring of swollen fiber cells (van Heyningen and Pirie, 1968; Pirie and van Heyningen, 1968; Koch and Doldi, 1975). For compliance reasons the dosage of naphthalene can be reduced to 50% for the first 2 applications but then has to be kept constant to guarantee a reproducible cataract formation. The naphthalene cataract model in rats is most suitable for toxicologial research because of its reliability, it is less suitable in rabbits. The model is best established in young Brown-Norway rats, it is much less reliable in albino rats and cannot be induced in old animals.

Deprivation of nutritional compounds and induced metabolic defects. Tryptophane deficiency in the diet causes the rapid formation of a posterior subcapsular cataract (Buschke, 1943). The model has the disadvantage, however, that a concomittant corneal opacity is induced which prevents further lens observation. The corneal opacity disappears again when returning to normal chow, such that the deprivated diet and a normal chow have to be fed in intervals.

Calcium deficiency can be induced by treating rats with methoxy-ethanol which also leeds to the formation of a posterior subcapsular cataract.

Phenylketonuria (PKU) can be induced in rats by supplementing the diet with 1g/kg of DL-chloro-phenylalanin. This leeds to the formation of crystal-like deposits in the area of the posterior suture lines (Wegener et al., 1984).

Physical Triggers

Non-ionizing Radiation. Ultraviolet light of longer wave-lengths (UV-A, 315 - 400 nm, peak at 350 nm; 1 J/cm^2, irradiation in mydriasis every other day) for the initial period remains a subliminal noxious factor (Tuffs et al., 1987). After 4 weeks, however, a density increase of the anterior capsule and superficial cortex becomes measureable and continues to grow, although this area still is normal at the slitlamp microscope. Ultraviolet light of the shorter wavelengths (UV-B, 280 - 315 nm, 0,2 J/cm^2, irradiation in mydriasis every other day) directly damages the lenticular epithelium and causes the formation of an anterior polar cataract (Schmidt et al., 1992). First changes appear already after 2 irradiation sessions, after 8 weeks the density increase in the polar region reaches a plateau. The opacity as such remains restricted to the central sutural area with little progress into the sutural cleft.

Ionizing Radiation. X-irradiation directly damages proteins and the DNA in the lens. The dosages vary from 250 to 400 (anesthesia) with a direct relation to the latency period, but generally this noxa suits best as additional factor in a study with other cataract models. Further details on the methodology can be found in Hockwin et al., 1992.

DISCUSSION OF MODEL COMBINATIONS

When designing a drug side-effect study with cataract models, the choice of 1 or 2 appropriate models and the involvement of the relevant measurement techniques in-vivo (Wegener et al., 1990) and post-mortem (Hockwin et al., 1992) are of utmost importance. Each model on its own has to be combined with drug application in a meaningful dose range. It depends entirely on the type of the drug to be tested whether model combinations, i.e. naphthalene + diabetes to drug, are also included into the study or not. Apart from this, certain model combinations on their own proved to be meaningful: Diabetes and UV-B lead to an enhancement of the diabetic cataract; diabetes and naphthalene also lead to the enhancement of diabetic cataract formation with absence of visible naphthalene damage, but this combination proved to be to harmful to the animal; galactose cataract formation can be enhanced with X-irradiation; UV-A + UV-B lead to an enhancement of the visible UV-B effects; tryptophane deficiency and PKU provoque an enhancement of the PKU-cataract.

Among the genetically triggered cataracts, 2 models could be identified recently, that seem to allow a certain interaction with UV-B as external physical trigger: The formation of the anterior sutural cataract of the Scat-mouse mutant can be enhanced by additional UV-B irradiation; preliminary experiments with the RCS-rat did not yet show an enhancing effect but it can be expected that the UV-light stress promotes the destruction of the retina thus enhancing the formation of the posterior subcapsular cataract, which is typical for this mutant. Therefore, this could be the first animal model, where an intraocular cataractogenic pathomechanism can be influenced by an external noxious factor (O'Keefe et al., 1990).

Apart from the cataract model combinations, the individual interactions of drugs with these models has been studied in detail. We could indentify drugs or chemicals that interacted specifically with the diabetic, naphthalene or UV-B cataract models. These interactions lead to promotions or retardations of the model in question, that could be demonstrated with Scheimpflug photography and post-mortem biochemistry of the lens. None of the drugs or chemicals tested, however, interacted with more than one model = pathomechanism, which underlines the specificity and relevance of cataract models in regard to the evaluation of a potential co- or syncataractogenic effect.

CONCLUSION

The cataract models presented and discussed offer a choice of pathophysio-logical mechanisms, known to be causative for cataract induction, such that a test drug could interact with an appropriate selection of them. All those presented are easy to handle and do not require special equipment for cataract induction. We could identify drugs or compounds for each model that showed an undisputable interaction, positively or negatively. An exceptional case has been observed with triparanol which caused the formation of anterior and posterior subcapsular cataracts, independent but parallel to the lenticular expression of the cataract models involved (Henseler, 1992). The spectrum of rodent cataract models combined with the optical monitoring and measurement techniques in-vivo (Wegener et al., 1987) and the regional biochemical analyses of the lens with the Freeze Sectioning Technique (Kojima, 1992) have proven to be an indispensable tool for preclinical drug side-effect testing for potential co- or syn-cataractogenicity.

REFERENCES

Buschke, W., 1943, Classification of experimental cataracts in the rat. Recent observations on cataract associated with tryptophane deficiency and with some other experimental conditions, Arch. Ophthal. Chicago 30, 735 - 762.

Graw, J., Kratochvilova, J., Löbke, A., Reitmeir, P., Schäffer, E. and Wulff, A., 1989, Characterization of Scat (Suture Cataract), a dominant cataract in mice. Exp. Eye Res. 49, 469 - 477.

Henseler, W.,1992, Untersuchung der kataraktogenen oder cokataraktogenen Wirkung des Cholesterinbiosynthese-Inhibitors Triparanol an durch Streptozotocin-induzierten Diabetes, Naphthalinapplikation und UV-B-Bestrahlung vorgeschädigten Linsen bei Brown-Norway Ratten. Diss. Bonn.

Heyningen, R.v. and Pirie, A., 1968, Naphthalene cataract (1), in: "Biochemistry of the eye, Symposium Tutzing", M.U Dardenne and J. Nordmann eds., 407 - 409, Karger, Basel.

Hockwin, O.and Wegener, A., 1987, Syn- and cocataractogenesis. A system for testing subliminal lens toxicity, in: "Drug-induced ocular side effects and ocular toxicology", O. Hockwin ed., Concepts Toxicol. 4, 241-249, Karger, Basel.

Hockwin, O., Wegener, A., Bessems, G., Bours, J., Korte, I., Müller-Breitenkamp, U., Schmidt, J. and Schmitt, C., 1992, Models and methods for toxicity testing: Lens, in: "Manual of Oculotoxicity Testing of Drugs", O. Hockwin, K. Green, L. F. Rubin eds., 255 - 317 Gustav Fischer Verlag, Stuttgart.

Keller, H., 1979, Biochemische und tierexperimentelle Untersuchungen der kataraktogenen Wirkung von L-Arabinose. Diss. Med. Fak. Bonn.

Koch, H.-R. and Doldi, K., 1975, Naphthalene cataracts in rats of differently pigmented strains, Exp. Eye Res 20, 180.

Kojima, M., 1992, Enzymatic distribution patterns of rat lenses and the changes that occur during naphthalene cataract development, Ophthalmic Res. 24, 73 - 82.

O'Keefe, T.L., Hess, H.H., Zigler, J.S., Kuwabara, T., Knapka, J.: Prevention of cataracts in pink-eyed RCS rats by darl rearing. Exp. Eye Res. 51, 509 - 517 (1990)

Pirie, A., Heyningen, R.v., 1968, Naphthalene cataract (2), in: "Biochemistry of the eye, Symposium Tutzing", M.U Dardenne and J. Nordmann eds., 410 - 412, Karger, Basel.

Sasaki, K., Kuriyama, H., Yeh, L. and Fukuda, M., 1983, Studies on diabetic cataracts in rats induced by streptozotocin. I. Photodocumentation of lens opacities. Ophthalmic Res. 15, 185 - 190.

Schmidt, J., Schmitt, C., Kojima, M. and Hockwin, O., 1992, Biochemical and morphological changes in rat lenses after long-term UV-B irradiation, Ophthalmic Res. 24, 317 - 325.

Tuffs, A., Wegener, A. and Hockwin, O., 1987, Pilot study on cataractogenesis by UV irradiation, in: "Drug-induced ocular side effects and ocular toxicology", O. Hockwin ed., Concepts Toxicol. 4, 276-284, Karger, Basel.

Wegener, A. and Hockwin, O., 1987, Animal models as a tool to detect the subliminal cocataractogenic potential of drugs, in: "Drug-induced ocular side effects and ocular toxicology", O. Hockwin ed., Concepts Toxicol. 4, 250-262, Karger, Basel.

Wegener, A., Laser, H. and Hockwin, O., 1987, Measurement of lens transparency changes in animals. Comparison of the Topcon SL-45 combined with linear micro-densitometry and the Zeiss SLC system, in: "Drug-induced ocular side effects and ocular toxicology", O. Hockwin ed., Concepts Toxicol. 4, 263-275, Karger, Basel.

Wegener, A., Laser, H. and Hockwin, O., 1990, Reproducibility studies with the Zeiss SLC system and animal cataract models. Ophthalmic Res. 22(1), 18 - 23.

Wegener, A., Münch, C., Byrd, D.J., Jaeger, W., Hockwin, O. and Bours, J., 1984, Die Morphologie von Linsenveränderungen bei experimentell phenylketonurischen Ratten mit und ohne Tryptophanmangeldiät. Fortschr. Ophthalmol. 81, 626-628.

Zigler, J.S. and Hess, H.H., 1985, Cataracts in the Royal College of Surgeons rat: Evidence for initiation by lipid peroxidation products. Exp. Eye Res. 41, 67 - 76.

INFLUENCE OF PHAKAN[R] ON THE TOXICITY OF NAPHTHALENE IN RAT LENSES, ANALYZED BY ISOELECTRIC FOCUSING OF SINGLE LENS LAYERS

J. Bours, M.H.J. Ahrend, and A. Wegener

Department of Experimental Ophthalmology
University of Bonn, D-53105 Bonn, F.R.G.

INTRODUCTION

The concentration of reduced glutathione (GSH) in the eye lens decreases with increasing age. During the onset of an opacity and during later stages of cataract development, the concentration of glutathione was found to decrease further (Korte et al., 1986). Parallel to this observation a loss of activity of the enzymes necessary for the synthesis of glutathione was found to be associated with human cataract formation (Rathbun et al., 1993). Toa et al. (1991) determined diminishing concentrations of glutathione during the development of naphthalene cataract. In this model, glutathione acts as a protective agent for protein-SH groups by scavenging oxidative products that can impair lens metabolism (Korte et al., 1986). Phakan[R] shall act against this impairment by stimulating the synthesis of glutathione in the lens. This shall be achieved by additional administration of the GSH precursors glutamic acid, cysteine and glycine (Hockwin et al., 1982), present in Phakan[R] (Chauvin, 1982).

Phakan[R] (Chauvin, 1982) has been designed as a medication to slow down the progression of such lens opacities as spokes and water clefts and is composed of a mixture of essential amino acids and vitamines (Table 1; Hepp, 1979; Weigelin and Hockwin, 1982; Hockwin et al., 1982; Weigelin, 1985).

To investigate the possible beneficial influence of Phakan[R] on the naphthalene cataract model in rats, Brown-Norway rats were orally dosed with Phakan[R] in 2 concentrations in combination with the naphthalene cataract model. With this model, it is possible to examine a supposed retarding effect of the compound on the development of zonular cataracts. The cataract developes in the lenses of rats that are regularly dosed with naphthalene within a period of 4-6 weeks due to the action of naphthoquinone which is formed in the pigmented iris. This model of oxidative stress is frequently used in cataract research, together with Scheimpflug photography (Hockwin et al., 1984; Wegener and Hockwin, 1987a) as the documentation technique of choice to monitor changes in transparency of the lens precisely.

Ocular Toxicology, Edited by I. Weisse *et al.*
Plenum Press, New York, 1995

After an appropriate in-vivo dosing and documentation period, regional biochemical analyses were performed in specific layers of the lens utilizing the frozen-sectioning technique (Bours et al., 1987, 1990, Bours and Ahrend, 1993). The lens crystallins in these layers were analysis with isoelectric focusing in thin-layer agarose/polyacrylamide gels.

MATERIALS AND METHODS

One daily dose of Phakan^R (for composition see Table 1) consists of two galenic forms: one glass ampoule with 10ml solution and one gelatin capsule. Before dosing the animals, the contents of one capsule was dissolved in 10ml solution derived from one ampoule, diluted with 40ml 0.9g NaCl/l. The final 50ml contained 1200mg of active ingredients. The solution was freshly prepared every day.

Female Brown-Norway (BN) rats, 8 weeks old, which were chosen for this experiment, were assigned to the following treatment scheme:
- Group 1, control, no treatment, 6 rats;
- Group 2, 1g/kg body weight (BW) of naphthalene dissolved in paraffin oil, dosing every other day, 7 rats;
- Group 3, pretreatment for 4 days with 400mg Phakan/kg body weight and subsequent treatment with 400mg Phakan^R daily and 1g/kg BW of naphthalene every other day (Wegener et al., 1987b), 6 rats;
- Group 4, 800mg Phakan^R daily and 1g/kg BW of naphthalene, 6 rats.

Phakan^R was administered orally with a metal stomach tube.
During the in-vivo dosing period, the density of all lenses was documented with Scheimpflug photography using the Topcon SL-45 camera and subsequently measured with microdensitometry (Wegener et al., 1987).

Table 1. Composition of Phakan^R, as certified by Laboratoire Chauvin

One glass ampoule contains:		
glycin	100.0 mg	1.33 mmol
L-glutamic acid	200.0 mg	1.36 mmol
L-arginine	250.0 mg	1.44 mmol
myo-inositol	250.0 mg	1.39 mmol
pyridoxin.HCl	25.0 mg	0.12 mmol
One capsule contains:		
L-cystein	199.5 mg	1.65 mmol
ascorbic acid	173.5 mg	0.99 mmol
Total:	1198.0 mg	

After an in-vivo dosing period of 4 weeks, the animals were sacrificed, their lenses dissected, weighed and separated into 10 layers with the frozen-sectioning technique (Bours et al., 1987, 1993). The layers were homogenized in distilled water and centrifuged in a Heraeus Christ Biofuge B at 11,630 x g for 30 min at 4°C. The sediments were washed 3 times with distilled water, until all WS-crystallins were removed which has been controlled by a negative protein reaction (Bradford, 1976). The WI-crystallins were prepared in absence of denaturing agents, e.g. urea. For each layer the WS- and WI-crystallin content were measured by weight, following lyophilization. The dry weight (DW ≡ WS+WI) and the Ratio ≡ WS ÷ WI were then calculated (Bours et al., 1987).

The crystallin profiles of the WS- and WI-crystallins were obtained by using 1% agarose/0.5% linearly polymerized acrylamide gel isofocusing plates (IEF), specially designed to detect high-molecular weight proteins (Ahrend et al., 1987). The isofocusing and staining procedure has been published in detail by Ahrend et al. (1987). After staining with 0,05% Serva Blue W, the gels were photographed and used as they were for densitometry in a Joyce-Loebl Chromoscan 200, equipped to measure transmitted light. The WI-crystallins were solubilized in 100% formamide (Haff, 1978) just before application on the gel plate and lateron evaluated with the Chromoscan 200 as well.

RESULTS

To demonstrate the effect of Phakan treatment on the development of naphthalene cataracts in rats, the cortical peak heights from all Scheimpflug images was evaluated, because the cortex is the site of zonular cataract formation in this model. Immediately after enucleation, the wet weights of the lenses were determined. Thereafter, the lenses were frozen-sectioned and the crystallin patterns analyzed by IEF (Bours and Ahrend, 1992).

The densitometric data from Scheimpflug photography did not demonstrate any positive effect of the compound on the development of the naphthalene cataract, neither with pretreatment nore with the double dosage of Phakan[R].

The lens wet weights (LWW) of the naphthalene-cataractous lenses were: 27.23 ± 0.71mg (in groups 2 - 4) and those of the normal lenses: 27.30 ± 0.65mg (Group 1).

The WS and WI crystallin contents expressed in % of the lens fraction dry weight of all groups 1-4 were measured after sectioning perpendicular to the optical axis. They are displayed in Figure 1. The WS-crystallins showed u-shaped distribution curves (Figure 1a), whereas the WI-crystallins were characterized by an inversed u-curve (Figure 1b). The highest concentrations of WS-crystallins were detected in the anterior and posterior cortices, whereas the lowest concentrations were measured in the nucleus (Figure 1a). Furthermore the concentrations of WS- and WI-crystallins were expressed as ratio R (R = WS ÷ WI) which also provides characteristic curves (Figure 1c). In comparing the lenses of Phakan-treated naphthalene-cataractous rats versus those lenses, treated with naphthalene and not with Phakan[R], it is obvious that the concentration of the WS-crystallin fraction in the posterior supranuclear cortex is higher and the WI-crystallin fraction is lower in those lenses that were dosed with Phakan[R] and naphthalene simultaneously. However, in the nucleus and in the anterior supranuclear cortex this ratio is inversed (Figures 1a-c).

Densitometric evaluation of the isoelectric focusing patterns of WS- and WI-crystallins gave the percent distribution displayed as %DW in Figures 2 and 3. The WS α-, ß- and γ-crystallins displayed highest concentrations in anterior and posterior cortices and lowest in the nucleus (Figures 2a-f). The WS- HM_T-, α_L- and α_T-crystallins of the Phakan[R]-treated naphthalene-cataractous rats are lower than in the cataractous lens, and also lower than normal values. The same holds true for $ß_S$, pre-α- and γ-crystallins (Figures 2a-f). However, the lenses of Phakan[R]-treated naphthalene-cataractous rats showed, in contrast to the nucleus and anterior cortex, in the posterior supranuclear cortex an increased concentration of WS- $ß_S$-, pre-α-, $ß_T$- and γ-crystallins (Figures 2c,e,f).

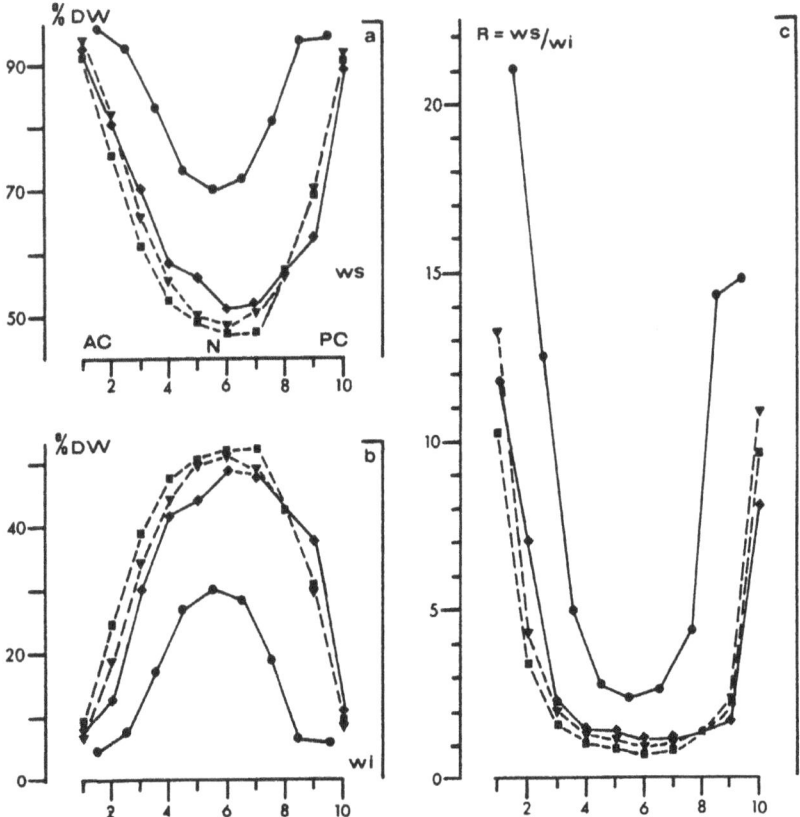

Figure 1. a) The water-soluble crystallin content (WS) in % from the lens fraction dry weight (DW), b) the water-insoluble protein content (WI) in % from the lens fraction dry weight and c) the crystallin ratio's R = WS ÷ WI of ▼--------▼ the naphthalene-cataractous lens, treated once a day with Phakan[R], ▲————▲ the naphthalene-cataractous lens, treated twice a day with Phakan[R], ■--------■ the napththalene-cataractous lens, ●————● the untreated lens (control experiment). AC = anterior cortex, N = nucleus, PC = posterior cortex. No. 1-10 are layer or fraction numbers.

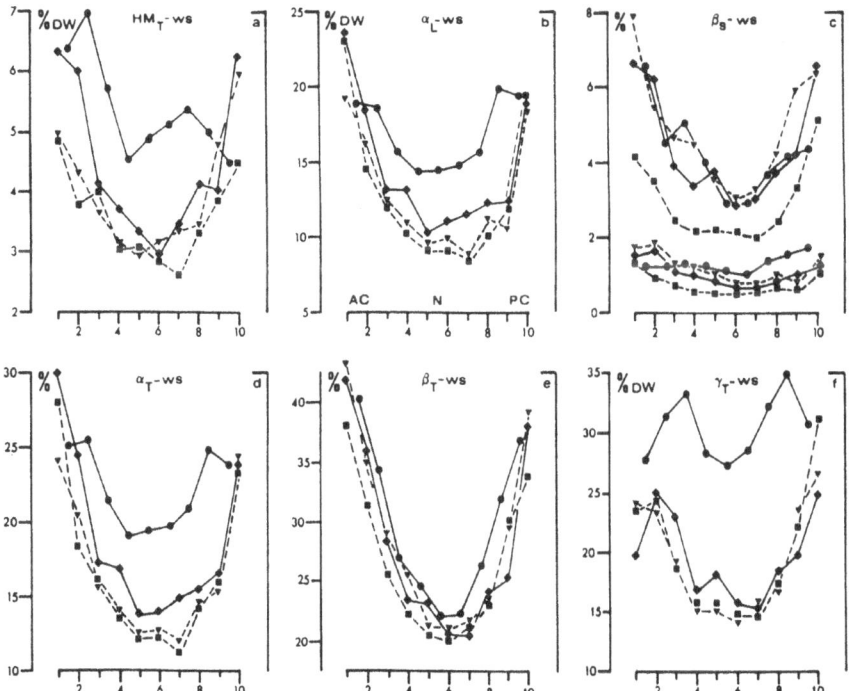

Figure 2. The % water-soluble (WS) HM-, α-, ß- and γ-crystallins from the lens fraction dry weight (DW): a) total high MW α-crystallins (HM$_T$), b) α-crystallins of low MW (α$_L$), c) ß-slow -crystallins (ß$_S$), pre- α-crystallins (pα), d) total α-crystallins (α$_T$ = HM$_T$ + α$_L$), e) total ß-crystallins (ß$_T$), f) total γ-crystallins (γ$_T$). See the legend of Figure 1 for further explanations.

The high MW crystallin complex, known as WI-crystallins consists for its greater part of HM- and α-crystallins (Figures 3a,b,d). The WI- HM$_T$-, α$_L$- and α$_T$-crystallin concentrations of the Phakan^R-treated cataractous lenses were generally higher than those values in the cataractous and normal lenses (Figures 3a-d). Phakan^R-treated naphthalene-cataractous lenses showed a tendency towards normal values in the anterior cortex and the nucleus, as compared to the controls, but do not reach those values entirely (Figures 3c,d,e). Incorporation of γ-crystallins in the high MW WI-complex is prevented by the administration of Phakan (Figure 3f). The high MW WI α-crystallin complex is higher concentrated than in the normal and cataractous lens (Figures 3a,b,d).

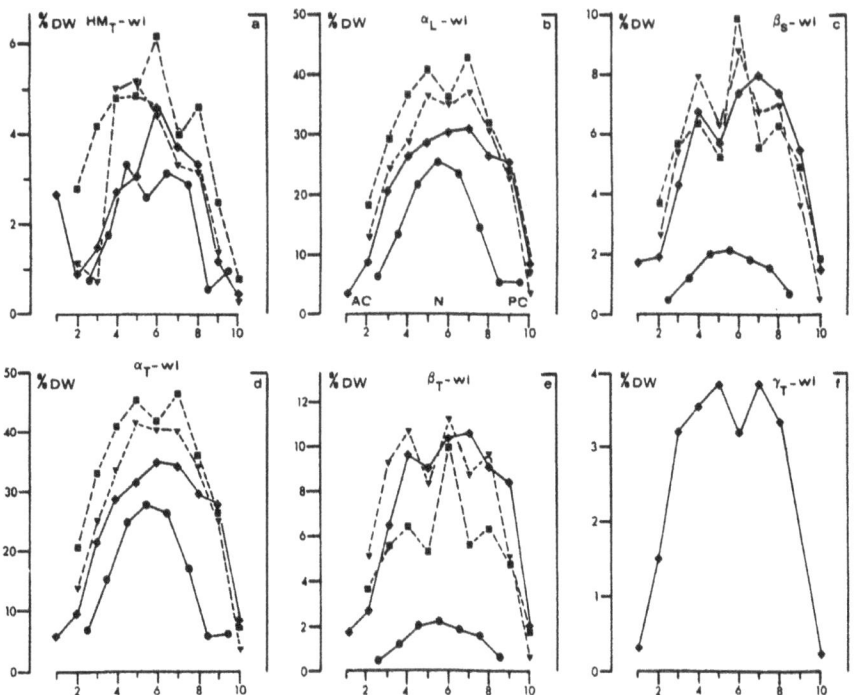

Figure 3. The % water-insoluble (WI) HM-, α-, ß-. and γ-crystallins from the lens fraction dry weight (DW): a) total high MW α-crystallins (HM_T), b) α-crystallins of low MW (α_L), c) ß-slow crystallins (β_S), d) total α-crystallins (α_T), e) total ß-crystallins (β_T), f) total γ-crystallins (γ_T). See the legends of Figures 1 and 2 for further explanations.

DISCUSSION

The Brown-Norway rat is the animal of choice to induce naphthalene cataracts in rats. The association of eye pigmentation and the presence of phenol oxidase in pigmented animals, contrary to its absence in albino rats, is the reason that naphthalene cataracts develop fast and regular in BN rats, as compared to albino rats (Murano et al., 1993).

The development of cataracts is characterized by a strong augmentation of the WI-moiety of the lens crystallins. In Figures 1(a-c) a higher % of WS-crystallins has been observed in the posterior cortex of the Phakan[R]-treated cataractous lenses. Also in Figures 2(c,e,f) there was a tendency of ß- and γ-crystallin concentrations towards normal values. In Figure 3f it has been shown that the incorporation of γ-crystallins into the WI-moiety can be influenced by the administration of Phakan[R]. The results presented here, are from the end of the dosing period. As the naphthalene cataract is based on a strong oxidative damage, the beneficial effect of Phakan[R] could have been more pronounced, if a few samples would have been collected already at half of the dosing period.

Our results concerning the effects of Phakan[R] in the posterior cortex of the lens are in agreement with the data of Kojima (1994, this volume). He could demonstrate that drug penetration is highest in the posterior cortex of the lens, if the administration is per oral route. A beneficial effect of Phakan[R] on the anterior cortex of the lens might have been found during earlier stages of naphthalene cataract development.

REFERENCES

Ahrend, M.H.J., Bours J., Hockwin, O.: Water-soluble and -insoluble crystallins of the developing human fetal lens, analyzed by agarose/polyacrylamide thin-layer isoelectric focusing, Ophthalmic Res.19:150 (1987).

Bours, J., Ahrend, M.H.J.:The effect of Phakan[R] treatment on the crystallin composition of the naphthalene-cataractous rat lens. Abstract, 32th AER Congress, Århus (DK). Documenta Ophthalmol. 80:259 (1992).

Bours, J., Ahrend, M.H.J.: Crystallin and water content of the aging bovine lens: Cross-sectional view by microsectioning perpendicular to the optic axis, Progr. in Veterinary & Comparative Ophthalmol. 3:141 (1993).

Bours, J., Födisch, H.J., Hockwin, O.: Age-related changes in water and crystallin content of the fetal and adult human lens, demonstrated by a micro-sectioning technique, Ophthalmic Res. 19:235 (1987).

Bours, J., Wegener, A., Hofmann, D., Födisch, H.J., Hockwin, O.: Protein profiles of microsections of the fetal and adult human lens during development and ageing, Mechanisms of Ageing and Development 54:13 (1990).

Bradford, M.M.: A rapid and sensitive method for the quantification of microgram quantities of protein utilizing the principle of protein-dye binding, Analyt. Biochem. 72:248(1976)

Chauvin, B.: PHAKAN[R] - Theoretische Grundlagen, vorklinische Prüfungen, klinische Anwendung, Verträglichkeit, Nebenwirkungen, in: "Symposium über die Augenlinse, Strasbourg", ed. O. Hockwin, Integra, Mayr, D-83174 Miesbach, 175-182 (1982).

Haff, L.A.: Fractionation of water-insoluble protein using Sephacryl S-200 in formamide. Preparat. Biochem. 8:99 (1978)

Hepp, R.: Einfluß einer Phakan[R]-Behandlung auf die Röntgenkatarakt von Ratten. Dissertation, University of Bonn (1979).

Hockwin, O., Dragomirescu, V., Shibata, T., Laser, H., Wegener, A.: Long-term follow-up examination of experimental cataracts in rats by Scheimpflug photography and densitometry, Graefes Arch. Clin. Exp. Ophthalmol. 222:20 (1984).

Hockwin, O., Weigelin, E., Baur, M., Boutros, G.: Controlled clinical study on the efficacy of Phakan[R] as an anti-catarakt treatment, Fortschr. Ophthalmol. 79:179 (1982).

Kojima, M.: Drug distribution studies in single lens layers through the application of a sectioning technique. Fourth Congress of the International Society of Ocular Toxicology, Annecy, France (1994).

Korte, I., Hockwin, O., Brass, M.: Attempts to increase the glutathione content in the lens, In: Modern Trends in Aging Research. Colloque INSERM-EURAGE/John Libbey Eurotext, 147:397 (1986).

Murano, H., Kojima, M., Sasaki, K.: Differences in naphthalene cataract formation between albino and pigmented rat eyes, Ophthalmic Res. 25:16 (1993).

Rathbun, W.B., Schmidt, A.J., Holleschau, A.M.: Activity loss of glutathione synthesis enzymes associated with human subcapsular cataract, Invest. Ophthalmol. Vis. Sci. 34:2049 (1993).

Tao, R.V., Holleschau, A.N., Rathbun, W.B.: Naphthalene-induced cataract in the rat. II. Contrasting effects of two aldose reductase inhibitors on glutathione and glutathione redox enzymes. Ophthalmic Res 23:272 (1991).

Wegener, A., Hockwin, O.: Animal models as a tool to detect the subliminal cocataractogenic potential of drugs; in Hockwin, O. (Ed): Drug-induced ocular side effects and ocular toxicology. Concepts Toxicol. Basel, Karger, 4, 250-262 (1987) a.

Wegener, A., Laser, H., Hockwin, O.: Measurement of lens transparency changes in animals. Comparison of the Topcon SL-45 combined with linear microdensitometry and the Zeiss SLC system. In: O. Hockwin (ed.): Drug-induced ocular side effects and ocular toxicology, Concepts Toxicol. 4, 263-275, Karger, Basel (1987) b.

Weigelin, E.: Results of clinical studies on the efficacy of drugs intended to halt the progression of lens opacities, Klin. Mbl. Augenheilk. 186:462 (1985).

Weigelin, E., Hockwin, O.: Bericht über eine zufallsverteilte, kontrollierte klinische Studie mit PHAKAN[R]/PHAKOLEN[R], in: "Symposium über die Augenlinse, Strasbourg", ed. O. Hockwin, Integra, Mayr, D-83174 Miesbach, 183-199 (1982).

INVESTIGATIONS INTO THE CATARACTOGENIC POTENCY OF A NON-TRICYCLIC ANTIDEPRESSANT

A. Wegener[1], K. Krauser[2], H.-J. Zechel[2], W. Jahn[2], and
D. Perrissoud[3]

[1]Department of Experimental Ophthalmology, University of Bonn,
D-53105 Bonn, Germany
[2]Institute of Toxicology, ASTA Medica AG, D-33790 Halle/
Westfalen, Germany
[3]ASTA Medica AG, D-60314 Frankfurt/Main, Germany

ABSTRACT

During the preclinical development of a non-tricyclic antidepressant, lens changes were observed in a 13-week subacute toxicity study. They consisted of radial striations, a prominent anterior suture and focal opacities in the posterior lens cortex. No such lens changes were observed in beagle dogs during the same study period. To get an insight into the dose-response characteristics of this cataractogenic potential of the compound during 26-week chronic toxicity studies, Scheimpflug photography has been performed in albino rats and beagle dogs. Parallel to slit lamp examinations, changes in lens density were recorded with the SL-45 on 2 occasions, at baseline and end of the study. The images were recorded on T-Max 400 (BW) film, developed and evaluated according to standard procedures. The density data of the capsular region of the rat lens evidence a significant increase in density in group 4 (highest dose) in male and female animals at the last examination, as compared to group 1 (control) and group 2 (lowest dose). As there were no visible cataracts in a majority of lenses of group 4 yet, the data evidence a subliminal cataractogenic potential, on the borderline of being direct. The other 2 groups did not show a density increase, as compared to group 1. No animal of the beagle dog study did have an increase in lens light scattering over the study period. The data from the chronic toxicity studies evidence a cataractogenic potential in rats present at toxic respectively even lethal dosage levels. The 2 lower dosages were free of this potential. The clinical observations support these data.

INTRODUCTION

Slit lamp biomicroscopy in many cases has become an instrument for routine eye inspections in preclinical drug development and side effect testing in animals. It allows precise localization of opacities and morphological abnormalities in the anterior eye segment of all animal species that are standardly involved in preclinical drug toxicity studies (Wegener and Hockwin, 1990). The instrument does, however, not permit precise density measurements in the lens. For this purpose, Scheimpflug photography has become the method of choice, as it allows to document and evaluate reproducibly density changes of all transparent media of the anterior eye segment as well as changes in their biometrical characteristics (Wegener et al., 1990). The accuracy of the measurement is independent of the size of the eye.

During the preclinical development of a non-tricyclic antidepressant, lens changes were observed in a 13-week subacute toxicity study in albino rats. These changes consisted of water-clefts in the anterior superficial cortex and a widening of the anterior suture system, parallel to the occurance of focal opacities in the posterior subcapsular cortex. The changes, however, were present only in a few animals of the highest (toxic) dosage group and could not be found in a comparable study in beagle dogs. Therefore the question was brought up, whether the other animals of the same dosage group are perhaps in a precataractous stage and if so, whether the lower dosages are free of such a potential or not. To answer these questions, Scheimpflug photography with subsequent densitometric image analysis was introduced into two 26-week chronic toxicity studies of the compound in question in albino rats and beagle dogs, parallel to regular and detailed slit lamp examinations.

MATERIAL AND METHODS

The design of the chronic toxicity studies in each species comprized 3 dosed groups and a vehicle-treated control. In the rat study the highest dosage was 4 times higher than the middle dosage. All optical examinations have been performed in a dark room of the animal facilities. Mydriasis was induced by instillation of tropicamide 0.5%, 10 - 15 minutes prior to examination or photography, respectively. The routine ophthalmological examinations were performed in regular intervals (weeks 0, 12, 25, 31) with a slit lamp microscope (Zeiss 30 SL/M). Examplary cases were photographed on Agfachrome 1000 RS Professional colour slide film. Parallel to these, two Scheimpflug examinations with the Topcon SL-45 were performed, one at baseline, prior to any treatment and the other at the end of the treatment period, prior to sacrifice. Two images per eye and examination were recorded on Kodak T-max 400 black-and-white film. The films were standardly processed in D-76 and lateron multilinear microdensitometry was performed in the optical axis and 1 mm above and below, respectively (Wegener et al., 1987). The peak heights (mm) of the cornea, anterior capsule and subcapsular layer, cortex and nucleus of the lens were evaluated and compared statistically between the different treatment groups within one examination. Those animals that had already visible opacities were excluded from the statistical evaluation, because these would only increase the standard deviation thus decreasing the possibility to detect significant differences in light scattering, before a visible opacity appears.

RESULTS

The slit lamp micrograph of the rat lenses shows circumferrential water-clefts that indicate bundles of swollen lens fibers in the superficial lenticular cortex (Figure 1). They cause a widening of the anterior suture system. Independent of these features, focal opacities could be found in the posterior lens cortex, that might represent maldifferentiated fiber cells.

The density data of the anterior capsular and subcapsular layer derived from the chronic toxicity study in rats show a significant increase between group 1 (control) and group 4 (highest dosage) at the second examination. This effect is found in both sexes but appears to be more pronounced in females (Figure 3) than in males (Figure 2). The low and middle dosage groups do not show such a density increase in comparison to the control group. At the highest dosage marked toxic symptoms and even death occurred.

In the dog study, slit lamp microscopy did not demonstrate any changes in morphology or transparency of the lens. The density data for the lens capsule show some variations between the different treatment groups in both sexes within and between the examinations (Figures 4, 5). There are, however, no significant differences between the treated groups and the control.

In both chronic toxicity studies, the density data from the cortical and nuclear lens region do not show treatment related differences as compared to the control groups. Also the comparison of relative density changes between the first and the second examination do not evidence other trends or effects. It confirms, however, the significant difference in capsular density between groups 4 and 1 of the rat study at the final examination.

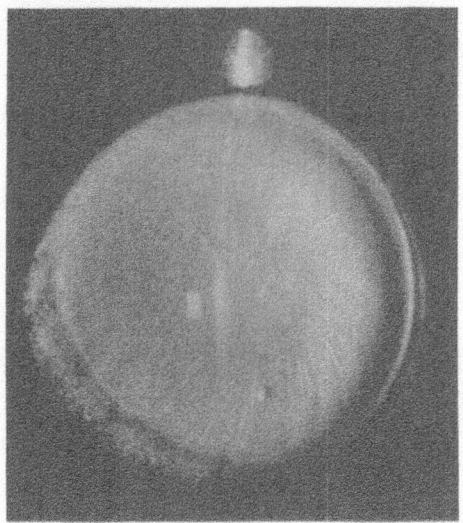

Figure 1. Slit lamp micrograph from a rat of group 4 at the final examination; waterclefts (radial striations) and a swollen, dilated suture (arrow head) are clearly discernible.

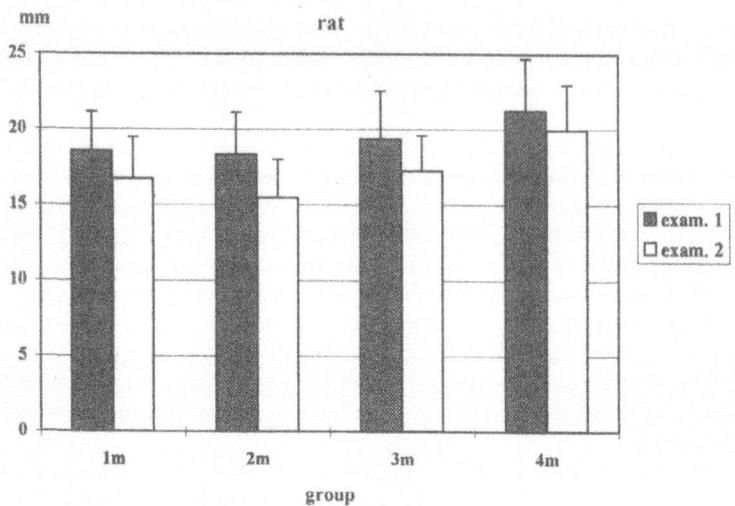

Figure 2. Mean capsular density values (mm) and standard deviations of the male (m) rats at the basic (1) and final (2) examination.

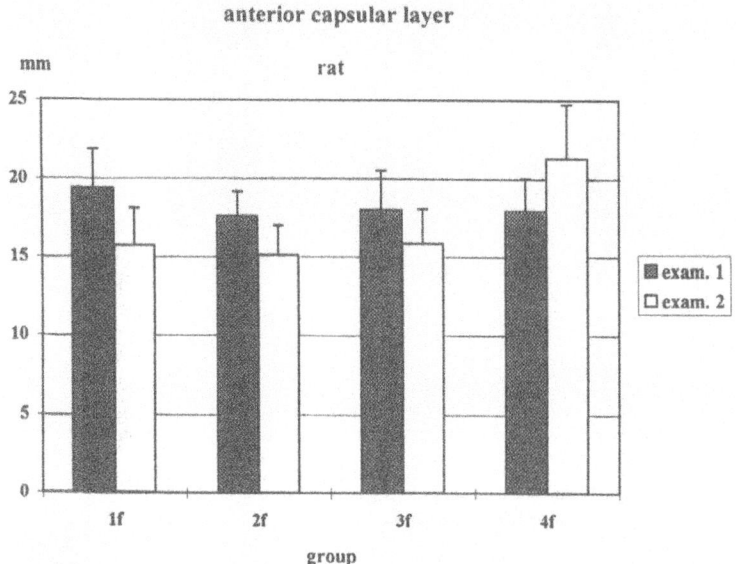

Figure 3. Mean capsular density values (mm) and standard deviations of the female (f) rats at the basic (1) and final (2) examination.

208

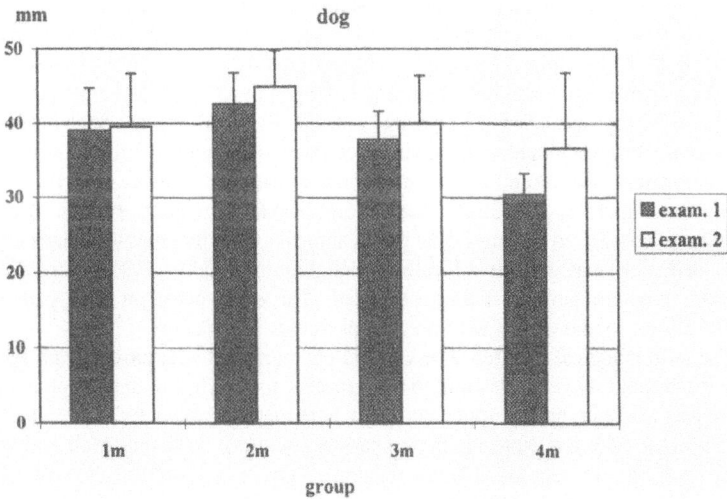

Figure 4. Mean capsular density values (mm) and standard deviations of the male (m) dogs at the basic (1) and final (2) examination.

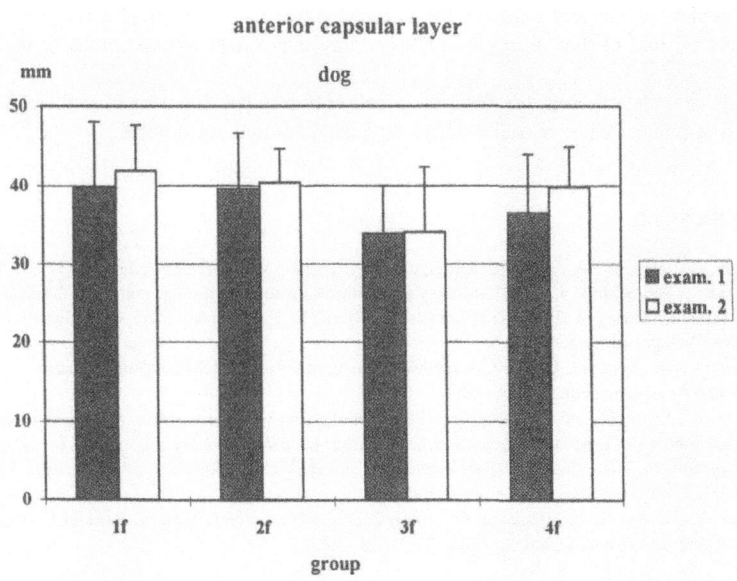

Figure 5. Mean capsular density values (mm) and standard deviations of the female (f) dogs at the basic (1) and final (2) examination.

DISCUSSION

The results of the two chronic toxicity studies presented here highlight the importance of involving two relevant optical examination techniques in such studies. Slitlamp biomicroscopy as the monitoring technique to follow-up the dynamics of changes in the tissues of the anterior eye segment and Scheimpflug photography as the measurement technique for changes in density and biometry (Hockwin et al., 1992). However, Scheimpflug photography should only be included in studies when there is an indication for lens changes from preliminary trials. Therefore, it is of importance to examine as many animals as possible in ophthalmological investigations during e.g. subacute toxicity studies. This should especially be considered for high dose group animals. Only by doing this, lens changes of low incidence or changes which develop slowly with only few animals affected after e.g. 13 weeks, are detectable as treatment-related. The early detection of a cataractogenic potential allows to plan subsequent preclinical studies adequately.

The morphological features observed and photographed with the slit lamp microscope during the chronic study in rats point to an unspecific toxic effect of the compound probably to those lens fibers in the superficial cortex that are metabolically very active, because they just underwent differentiation. As these changes could not be found in all animals of the highest dosage group, reproducible and reliable data were needed from all layers of the lens which could be provided by Scheimpflug photography. The density data for the capsular and subcapsular layers from the second and final examination clearly demonstrate that also those animals which are visually still normal at the slit lamp microscope do undergo changes that will lead to the appearance of cataracts. They are still beyond the threshold of visible opacities, but the light scattering values for the subcapsular layers in group 4 differ significantly from the control group and the two lower dosage groups. In extension to these findings it could also be documented with Scheimpflug photography that the two lower dosage groups are unaffected, the dosages thus being safe with respect to alterations of the transparency of the lens. During the chronic toxicity study in beagle dogs it could be documented that neither dose group showed any indications of cataractous change of the lens.

The data and observations from the preclinical drug development fit to the experiences from first clinical phase 1 trials, where no lens alterations were noted.

REFERENCES

Hockwin, O., Wegener, A., Bessems, G., Bours, J., Korte, I., Müller-Breitenkamp, U., Schmidt, J. and Schmitt, C., 1992, Models and methods for toxicity testing: Lens, in: "Manual of Oculotoxicity Testing of Drugs",O. Hockwin, K. Green, L. F. Rubin eds., 255 - 317 Gustav Fischer Verlag, Stuttgart.

Wegener, A. and Hockwin, O.,1990, Arzneimitteltestung und Risikoabschätzung am Tierauge, Deutsche Apothekerzeitung 130, 61-70.

Wegener, A., Laser, H. and Hockwin, O., 1987, Measurement of lens transparency changes in animals. Comparison of the Topcon SL-45 combined with linear microdensitometry and the Zeiss SLC system, in: "Drug-induced ocular side effects and ocular toxicology", O. Hockwin ed., Concepts Toxicol. 4, 263-275, Karger, Basel.

Wegener, A., Laser, H. and Hockwin, O., 1990, Reproducibility studies with the Zeiss SLC system and animal cataract models. Ophthalmic Res. 22(1), 18 - 23.

COMPARATIVE INVESTIGATIONS ON THE CATARACTOGENIC EFFECT OF A
TRIAZIN-DERIVATIVE IN ALBINO AND PIGMENTED RATS:
I. EFFECTS DETECTED WITH A SLIT LAMP*)

R. Eiben[1] and A. Wegener[2]

[1] Institute of Industrial Toxicology, Bayer AG,
   42096 Wuppertal, Germany
[2] Dept. of Experimental Ophthalmology, University of Bonn,
   53105 Bonn, Germany

ABSTRACT

Cataracterogenesis of a newly developed chemical of the
triazin class was studied in male albino (Wistar) and pigmented
(FB 30) rats to examine possible influences of pigmentation on
eye lesions. 10 animals per group were treated with 0, 400, 500
or 625 ppm triazin in their diet up to 15 weeks. Eyes of all
animals were monitored in vivo with a ZEISS photo slit lamp in
four investigations (week 0, 4, 8 and 15). Onset and
morphological pattern of cataract formation were recorded.
Cataracts induced by triazin occurred in posterior and anterior
parts of the lens. At first, focal turbidities were detected in
the area of lens fissures of the posterior subcapsular region.
Later these opacities progressed and were followed by opacities
in anterior lens parts. After 15 weeks mature cataracts in the
whole lens were apparent in some cases. In pigmented rats such
lens lesions were seen earlier, more frequently and at a higher
degree than in albinos. Pigmented but not albino rats
developed opacities in the cornea, too. The effects on the
lens indicate a lower sensitivity of Wistar rats to this
cataractogen compared to pigmented rats. This assertion is in
accordance with density measurements of Scheimpflug photographs
(WEGENER and EIBEN, 1992) performed on the same lenses. The
autors stress the importance of considering strain-specifity
and pigmentation of eyes, when a no-effect-level for eye
lesions is established in toxicity studies.

---

*) Results were presented on the third ISOT congress in 1992
   (Sedona, USA)

INTRODUCTION

Recent toxicological investigations with a newly developed chemical of the triazin class (called "triazin" in the following) revealed that this compound induces lens opacities, when administered to Wistar albino rats at a toxic dose (625 ppm) in their diet for 3 months. In more detailed experiments, this type of cataract was investigated ophthalmologically in pigmented and albino rats using a ZEISS photo slit lamp. These two strains were used in order to compare onset and development of cataracts induced by triazin because a pilot study had revealed a higher sensitivity of pigmented animals to this cataractogen. Male rats were used because in recent studies males were shown to be more sensitive to this ocular effect than females.

MATERIALS AND METHODS

Groups of nominally 10 male albino (Wistar) or pigmented (FB 30 black hooded) rats were treated with triazin in dietary concentrations of 0 or 625 ppm (83 mg/kg body weight per day) over a period of 15 weeks. In addition, two groups of 10 pigmented FB 30 males received 400 or 500 ppm triazin. All animals were about 8 weeks old at start of dosing. The diet fed ad-libitum was Altromin®1321. Animals were kept singly housed under conventional conditions. Detailed quantitative and qualitative examinations of cornea and lens were performed using a ZEISS photo slit lamp before application as well as in week 4, 8 and 15. At the same dates (except in week 4) all animals were additionally photographed with a Scheimpflug camera (WEGENER and EIBEN, 1992). All pupils were dilated with Roche Mydriaticum®eye drops 10 minutes prior to photography. Slit lamp photos were evaluated using three classifications of the findings: N.a.d. (no alteration detected), slight or moderate/severe cataract.

RESULTS

I. Formation of Subcapsular Cataracts in the Posterior Part of the Lens

Pigmented Rats. In pigmented eyes of dose group 625 ppm slight subcapsular turbidities occurred in the area of the posterior lens fissures already after 4 weeks (Figures 1-2, for the number of animals affected see Figure 9). Four weeks later more pigmented rats were affected (Figure 10). In some animals diffuse opacities occurred in a area around the fissures (Figures 1a-4a), others showed turbidities mainly along lens suture lines (Figures 1b-4b).
In week 8, slight subcapsular opacities were detected in the anterior lens, too. Up to week 15, these posterior lens opacities progressed rapidly to moderate or severe cortical and nuclear cataracts (Figures 3-4) in all animals (Figure 11). By then a dose dependence of this lesion was apparent (Figures 15-17).

Albino Rats. 625 ppm dosed albino rats first showed slight subcapsular turbidities around the suture area in week 8 (Figures 5-7, for frequency see Figure 13). The number of rats affected increased more slowly than that of pigmented rats. After a period of 15 weeks, a smaller number of albinos had developed severe cataracts (Figure 8), as compared to the pigmented animals (compare Figures 11 and 14).

II. Cataracts Formed in the Anterior Lens Part

In addition to posterior cataracts, 625 ppm dosed rats have also formed mature opacities in the anterior cortex and nucleus (Figures 21 and 25).
In pigmented rats, these lesions were preceded by wedge-shaped cataracts (Figures 18 and 19) whereas albinos first developed cortical water clefts (Figures 22 and 23) over the whole lens. Most of the albino eyes showed swollen cortical zones in the lens cortex (Figures 22 and 23). With regard to onset and frequency of anterior cortical cataracts, pigmented rats proved to be more sensitive than albinos (Figure 26).

III. Effects on the Cornea

From week 8 onwards, focal or diffuse opacities were observed in the cornea (Figures 27 and 28) of most pigmented rats treated with triazin. These lesions remained unchanged up to week 15. Albinos were not affected in this way.

DISCUSSION

As already established in recent toxicity studies with rats, a triazin-derivative has shown a direct cataractogenic potential.
In a special study over 15 weeks, triazin induced cataract formation has been studied in pigmented and albino rats receiving 0, 400, 500 or 625 ppm in their diet. Onset, development, dose dependence and possible differences with respect to pigmentation were the main points of interest in these ophthalmological investigations.
Treated and untreated rats were investigated ophthal-mologically prior to the first triazin application and after 4, 8 and 15 weeks of treatment using a ZEISS slit lamp.
Within a relatively short time triazin-treated albino and pigmented rats first developed cataracts in the posterior lens (suture) region. These lesions, which were rarely observed spontaneously, transformed dose-dependently into mature cataracts in the anterior cortex and whole lens in many cases.
The comparison of slit lamp photographs revealed that lens opacities occurred earlier and more frequently in pigmented rats than in albinos. In pigmented animals opacities progressed more quickly to severe cataract forms, as compared to albinos. Moreover, pigmented but not albino rats showed turbidities in the cornea, too. These results demonstrate that pigmented rats are more sensitive to such a cataractogen than albinos treated in the same way with a triazin.
This assertion is in accordance with results of density measurements performed on Scheimpflug photographs (WEGENER and EIBEN, 1992) of the same animals where pigmented rats have proved to be the more sensitive strain, too.

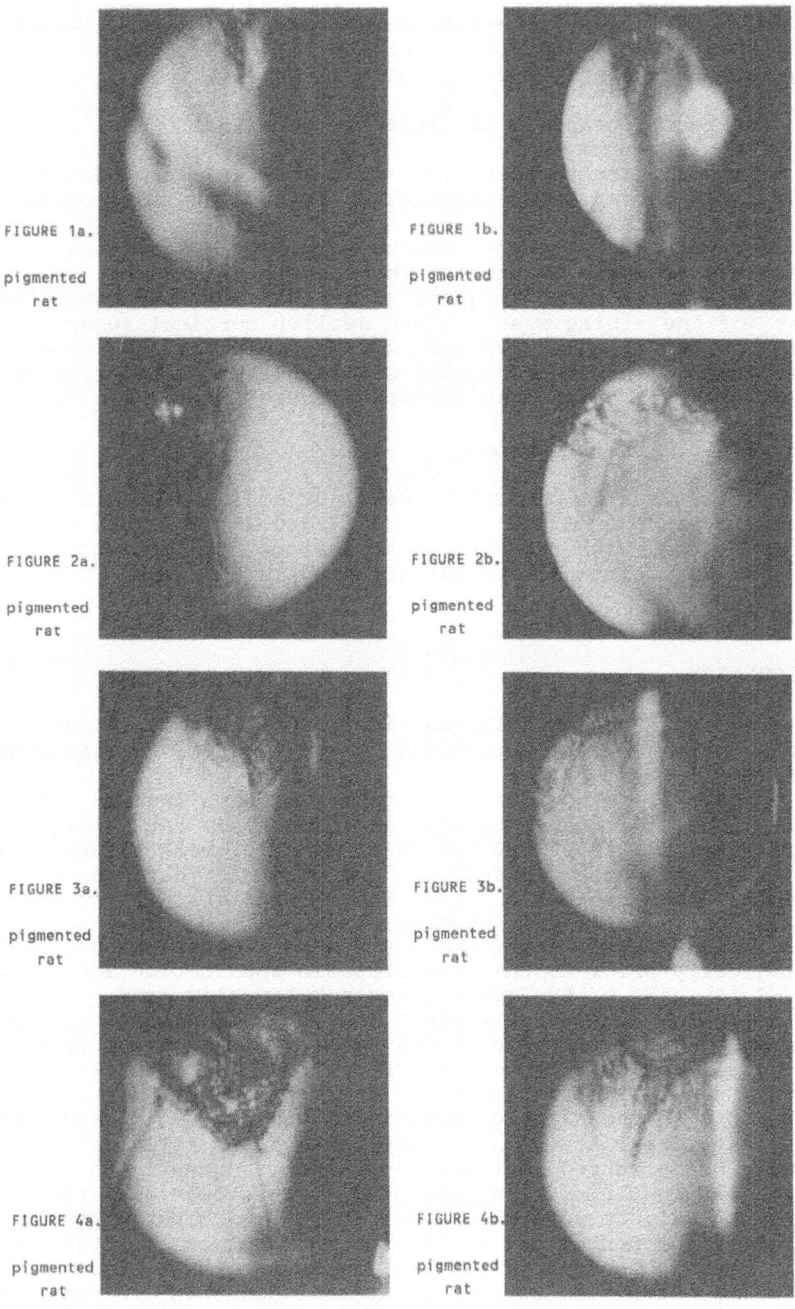

FIGURE 1a.
pigmented
rat

FIGURE 1b.
pigmented
rat

FIGURE 2a.
pigmented
rat

FIGURE 2b.
pigmented
rat

FIGURE 3a.
pigmented
rat

FIGURE 3b.
pigmented
rat

FIGURE 4a.
pigmented
rat

FIGURE 4b.
pigmented
rat

Figures 1-4: Stages of cataract formation in the posterior lens of pigmented rats receiving 625 ppm triazin up to 15 weeks in their diet. Subcapsular opacities occurred in the posterior lens region _around_ the suture area (Figures 1a, 2a, 3a, 4a) or predominatly _along_ lens fissures (Figures 1b, 2b, 3b, 4b). These lesions were graded as slight (Figures 1a+b, 2a+b), moderate (Figures 3a+b), or severe (Figure 4a+b).

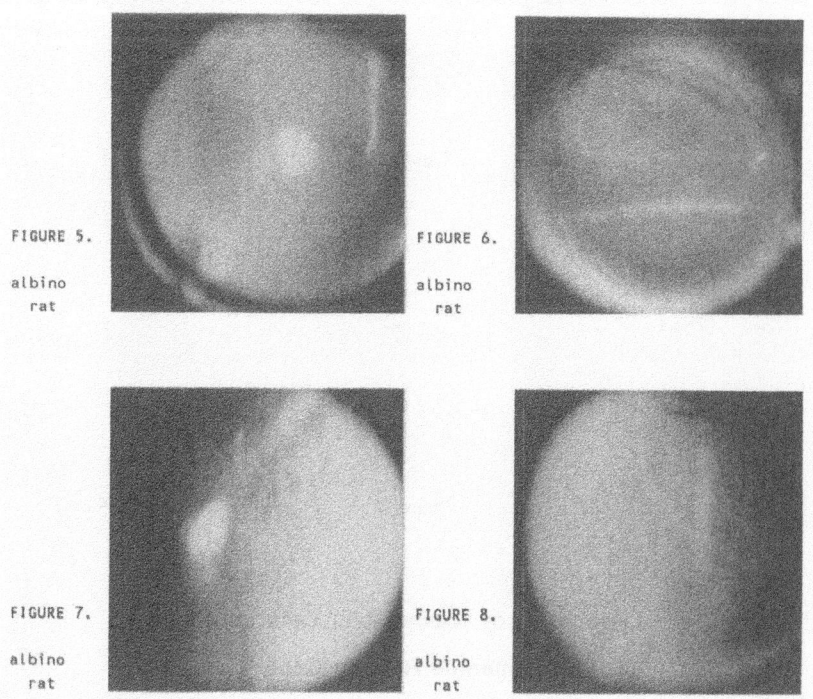

FIGURE 5.

albino
rat

FIGURE 6.

albino
rat

FIGURE 7.

albino
rat

FIGURE 8.

albino
rat

Figures 5-8: Stage of cataract formation in the posterior lens of albino rats receiving 625 ppm triazin up to 15 weeks in their diet. Subcapsular turbidities were graded as slight (Figures 5-7) or severe (Figure 8) cataracts.

In general, pigmentation-dependent differences must be considered, if cataractous effects of chemicals or drugs are investigated in rats.

To document the appearance and progression of precataractous lesions in different lens regions, slit lamp and Scheimpflug photography have proved to be sensitive and indispensable tools in toxicity studies also with reference to determine a no-effect-level with respect to lens toxicity.

215

Formation of Subcabsular Cataracts in Pigmented
and Albino Rats by Time

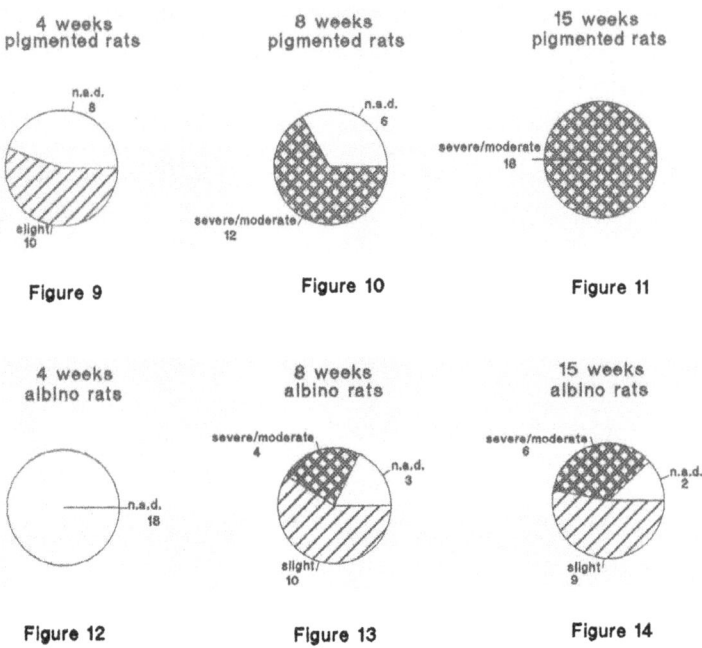

Figure 9   Figure 10   Figure 11

Figure 12   Figure 13   Figure 14

Formation of Subcapsular Cataracts in
Pigmented Rats by Dose

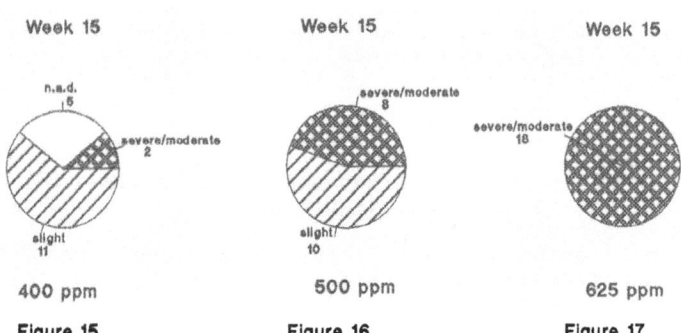

400 ppm   500 ppm   625 ppm

Figure 15   Figure 16   Figure 17

Figures 9-17: Quantitative evaluation of subcapsular cataracts in the posterior lens by time (Figures 9-14) or dose (Figures 15-17). Stages of development were classified by the following grades: n.a.d. (= no alteration detected), slight or moderate/severe (see Figures 1-4). In all figures numbers of eyes are given.

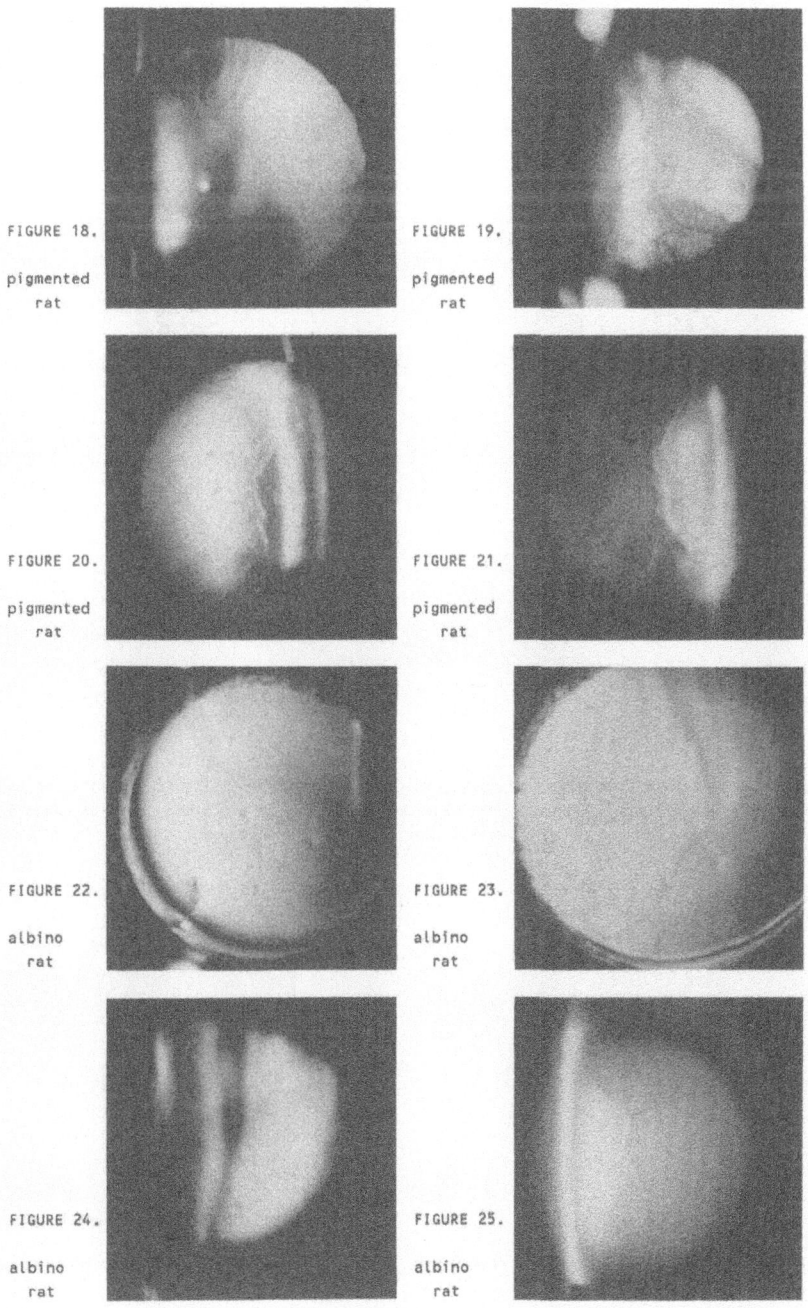

FIGURE 18.
pigmented
rat

FIGURE 19.
pigmented
rat

FIGURE 20.
pigmented
rat

FIGURE 21.
pigmented
rat

FIGURE 22.
albino
rat

FIGURE 23.
albino
rat

FIGURE 24.
albino
rat

FIGURE 25.
albino
rat

Figures 18-25: Stages of cataract formation in anterior lens parts of pigmented (Figures 18-21) and albino (Figures 22-25) rats receiving 625 ppm triazin up to 15 weeks in their diet. In pigmented rats mature cataracts (Figures 20 and 21) were preceded by wedge-shaped opacities (Figures 18 and 19) whereas in albino rats water clefts occured in the whole lens cortex (Figures 22 and 23) first.

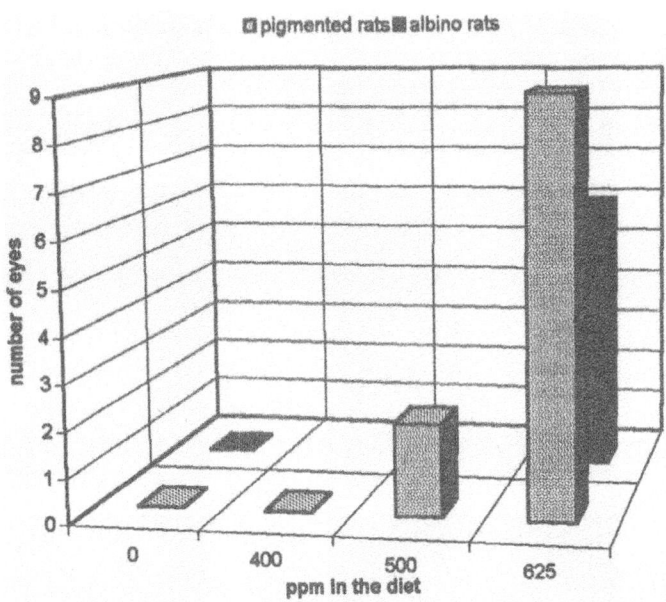

Figure 26: Given is the number of eyes, which had developed cataracts in anterior lens parts up to 15 weeks independently of their degree. Pigmented and albino rats of group 625 ppm are compared. For pigmented animals a dose-dependency was apparent.

FIGURE 27.

pigmented rat

FIGURE 28.

pigmented rat

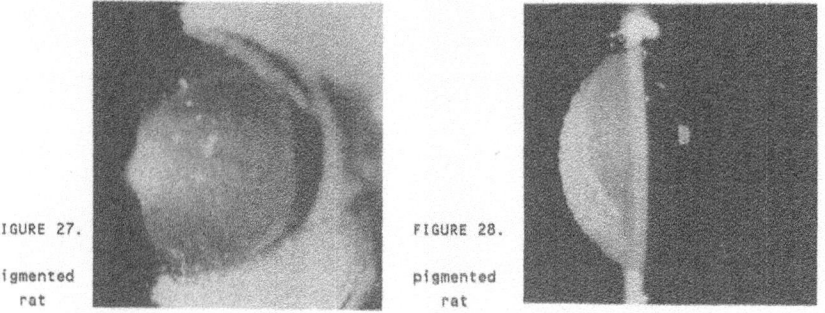

Figures 27 and 28: Focal or diffuse turbidities were detected in the cornea of all pigmented animals of group 625 ppm.

REFERENCES

WEGENER, A. and EIBEN, R., 1992, Lens and Eye Tox. Res. 9: 321.

REGIONALITY OF GLYCATED CALF LENS CRYSTALLIN SUBUNITS

DEMONSTRATED BY LECTIN STAINING

J. Bours, M.H.J. Ahrend and W. Breipohl

Department of Experimental Ophthalmology,
University of Bonn, D-53105 Bonn, F.R.G.

INTRODUCTION

Nonenzymatic glycation of lens crystallins involves a bimolecular condensation reaction between a reducing sugar and the ϵ-amino-group of a lysine residue[1-3]. Glycation[3-5] and a subsequent browning reaction[4,5] appear to be linked with age related protein aggregation and insolubilization[6,7]. Ageing of the bovine lens has specifically been attributed to the glycation of: HM-crystallins, ß-crystallins and nuclear γ-crystallins in the native form. In contrast, in the equator (EQ), anterior cortex (AC) and posterior cortex (PC) of bovine lenses younger than 10 years, α-crystallin was not glycated[8]. The various bovine lens crystallins in the unfolded subunit form appear to be increasingly glycated with increasing intrinsic age. Uptil now, it was not yet known which carbohydrate(s) are involved in crystallin glycation.

This study is to characterize the expression of different types of glycated crystallin subunits in calf lens sections of different localization i.e. intrinsic age.

MATERIALS AND METHODS

Calf lenses of 0.12 ± 0.08 years (n=15, lens wet weight: 1.02 ± 0.21g) were divided into inner cylinder (IC) and EQ with a trephine of a diameter of 11mm. The IC was cut into 9 sections of about 1mm each, from AC (S1,S2) to PC (S8,S9) through the nucleus (N) (S4-S6)[9]. Sections from the same region were pooled and homogenized. Crystallins were separated into water-soluble (WS) and water-insoluble crystallins. The WS-fraction was analyzed by 7M urea isoelectric focusing (IEF)[8]. Staining was done with Coomassie Brilliant Blue, western blotting and subsequent agglutination with a panel of four digoxigenin-labeled lectins: Concanavalin A (CON-A) from Canavalia ensiformis (Jack bean, Boehringer 1284 100), Wheatgerm lectin (WGA) from Triticum vulgaris (Boehringer 1284 118), a lectin (MAA) from a bean of Maackia amurensis (a Papilionaceae from S.E.

Asia and Mongolia, Boehringer 1206 826) and a lectin (SNA) from the bark of Elder (Sambucus nigra, Boehringer 1206 940)[10]. After densitometry of the Coomassie Blue stained bands (CBB, Fig. 1) and of the lectin stained bands (Fig. 2), densitometer values in arbitrary units were determined. A glycoprotein to protein ratio (G = LEC ÷ CBB) was calculated. This ratio G was taken as a measure for the intensity of glycation, which is characteristic for each purified protein, as will be shown for example by horseradish peroxidase (HRP).

RESULTS

IEF revealed up to 13 groups of protein bands with isoelectric points ranging from 3.5 to 9.5. Stained bands from groups 1-10 were assigned to a mixture of α- and ß-crystallin polypeptides. The bands of groups 11-13 were identified as γ-crystallin monomers. They had the highest isoelectric points (Fig. 1a-h). By comparison with earlier results from Kramps et al.[11], the following α-crystallin subunits could be traced in the patterns from EQ and sections S1-S9: αA_1-, αA_3-, αA_2-, αB_1- and αB_2-crystallins (single components indicated in groups 2, 3, 4, 8 and 10). Group 1 represents the HM-crystallins, whereas single bands from groups 2, 4, 5, 6, 7, 8 and 9 are the ß-crystallins. The γ-crystallin monomers (Groups 11-13) are higher concentrated in the supranuclear sections (S3,S7) and the nuclear sections (S4-S6) than in the anterior and posterior cortices (sections S1-S2 and S8-S9) (Fig. 1a-h). Specially in the nuclear sections S4-S6 the α-crystallin subunit A_2 generates subunit A_3 by deamidation, whereas bands right above the αA_1-subunit are duplicated by deamidation (Fig. 1d-f). The αB_1-crystallin subunit emerges in high concentrations in the supra-nuclear and nuclear sections (Fig. 1c-g).

Samples from Fig. 1 were blotted and subsequently agglutinated with CON-A, WGA, MAA and SNA, respectively. Specimen of lectin blotting are shown in Fig. 2a-d. The γ-crystallin monomers (groups 11-13) reacted well with Con-A, WGA and MAA, whereas with SNA only a weak staining of γ-crystallins was observed. The ß-crystallin groups (subunits $ß_6$ and $ß_7$) reacted strongly with all four lectins. The α-crystallin subunits αB_1 and αB_2 were stained by all four lectins, especially strong in the nucleus. The α-crystallin subunits αA_1, αA_2 and αA_3 were negative with WGA and MAA, whereas αB_1 and αB_2 were positive with all four lectins. Subunit αA_2 was positive with CON-A and SNA, whereas only αA_3 was positive with SNA. HM-crystallins were strongly positive with WGA in all sections, with CON-A only in EQ, AC and PC. They stained weakly positive with SNA in the N.

After densitometry, the intensity of glycation could be expressed as the glycation ratio G = LEC ÷ CBB. This ratio G was characteristic for HRP and used as reference: G = 3.87 ± 0.35 (n=2). G is equally taken as characteristic for lens crystallins. The glycation ratio G of the crystallin subunits in EQ and in AC, N and PC in 7 lens sections (Nrs 1, 3-7, 9) was determined and qualitatively shown in Table 1. HM- and γ-crystallins are highly glycated, which is expressed in G ratios between 0 and 4 (++++, +++), whereas the other crystallins show G ratios between 0.5 and 1 (+++, ++, +). With CON-A and WGA, the HM-crystallins display highest glycation in the AC and PC. The glycation of the αA_2 subunit is similarly high in AC and PC with CON-A and SNA (+++, ++). However, the αA_2 subunit glycation shows a minimum in the N (+), where αA_3 shows a distinct maximum (+++), due to deamidation of αA_2 which causes a loss of nuclear αA_2 and a similar gain in αA_3, together with a decrease in isoelectric point. The glycation of αB_1, αB_2, $ß_6$ and $ß_7$ crystallin subunits forms a maximum in the nucleus with the lectins CON-A, MAA and SNA (+++, ++). The γ-crystallin monomers show a high glycation in the N, with CON-A and MAA (++, +++) and a low glycation in the N for SNA and WGA (+). The total glycation (Σ) of all crystallin subunits, defined as the addition of the densitometer units, thus forming by division their

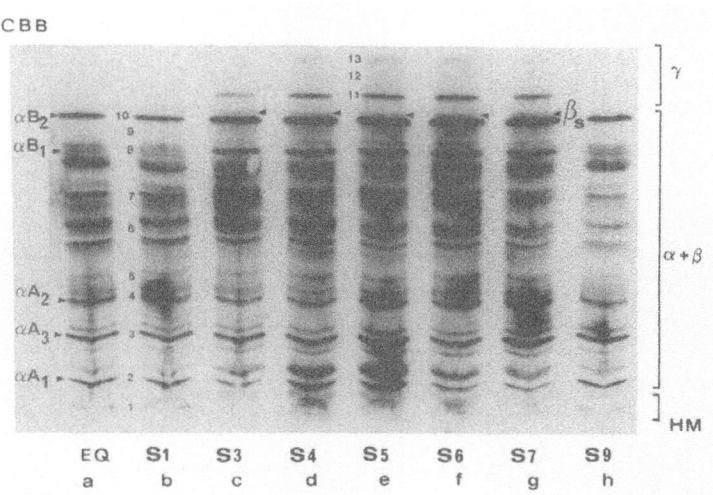

Fig. 1(a-h). Isoelectric focusing of the various subunits of calf lens WS-crystallins, after frozen-sectioning, separated into 13 component groups. A_1, A_2, A_3, B_1 and B_2 are α-crystallin sub-units. All other components in groups 1-10 are preferentially representing ß-crystallin subunits. Groups 11-13 are monomeric -crystallins. The ß$_S$-crystallin monomer is indicated by arrow heads. HM = high-molecular weight α-crystallin, EQ = equator, Nrs. S 1-S9 are the lens layer numbers. CBB = stained with Coomassie Brilliant Blue.

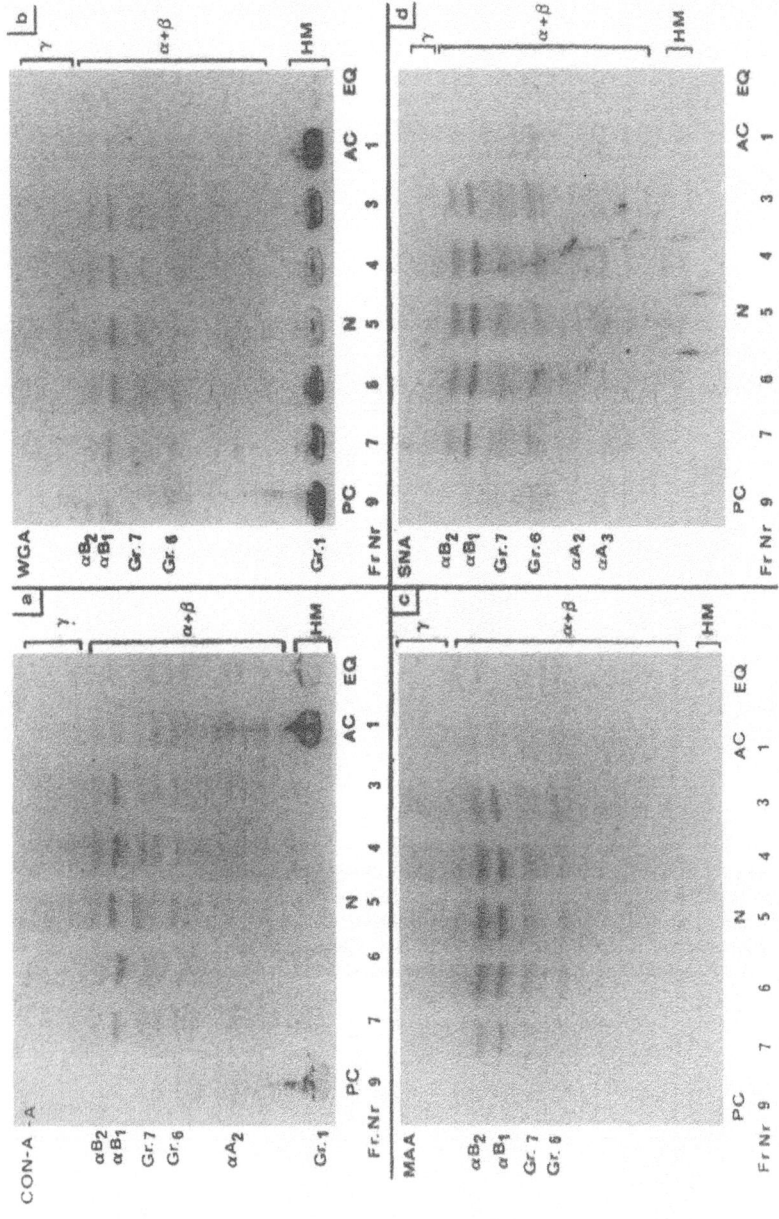

Fig. 2(a-d). Blotting after isoelectric focusing of the samples from calf lens from Fig. 1, and agglutination with the lectins CON-A, WGA, MAA and SNA. PC = posterior cortex, N = nucleus, AC = anterior cortex, EQ = equator. Fr.Nr. refers to the respective sections Nrs S9-S1 (reversal of numbers caused by the blotting process). A_2, A_3, B_1 and B_2 are glycated α-crystallin subunits. In a-d αA_1 is negative. Groups 6 and 7 are glycated β-crystallin subunits. HM = high-molecular weight α-crystallin. The region of Fr.Nr. 4 in 2d shows an unspecific streak, due to an artifact.

222

Table 1. Type of glycation of crystallin subunits in the anterior and posterior cortices, compared to the nucleus of the calf lens.

Glycated with Carbohydrate(s) →→			Man/Glc	GlcNAc	Gal (2-3-NANA)*	Gal (2-6-NANA)′
↓ Crystallin Subunit			CON-A	WGA	MAA	SNA
HM	HM	AC/PC	++++	++++	±/∅	∅
		N	+	+	∅	±
αA₂	αA₂	AC/PC	+++	∅	∅	++
		N	+	∅	∅	+
αA₃	αA₃	AC/PC	∅	∅	∅	+
		N	∅	∅	∅	+++
αB₁	αB₁	AC/PC	+	+	+	+
		N	+++	+	+++	+++
αB₂	αB₂	AC/PC	+	++	+	+
		N	++	+	++	++
ß₆	ß₆	AC/PC	+	++	+	+
		N	++	+	++	++
ß₇	ß₇	AC/PC	+	+	+	+
		N	++	+	++	++
γ		AC/PC	+	++	+	∅
γ		N	++	+	+++	+
Σ		AC/PC	+	++	+	+
Σ		N	++	+	++	++

Legend: AC/PC = anterior and posterior cortices, N = nucleus, Man/Glc = α-D-Mannose/α-D-glucose, GlcNAc = ß-D-N-acetyl-glucosamine, Gal = galactose. *MAA binds specifically to terminal N-acetyl-neuraminic acid, which is α(2-3) glycosidically linked to galactose. ′SNA binds specifically to terminal N-acetyl-neuraminic acid (NANA), which is α(2-6) glucosidically linked to galactose. ++++ = very strong reaction (Scale: 0-4), +++ = strong reaction (Scale 0-1 or 0-3, respectively), ++ = moderate reaction (Scale 0-0.5), + = weak, but positive reaction (Scale 0-0.3), ± = weak reaction (Scale below 0.1), ∅ = negative.

G ratios of all crystallins, shows maxima in the N with CON-A, MAA and SNA (++), and minima with WGA (+).

It has to be concluded that αB₁-, αB₂-, ß₆-, ß₇- and γ-Crystallins in the N were by preference glycated with Man/Glc, Gal(2-3-NANA) and Gal(2-6-NANA). These subunits were predominantly glycated with GlcNAc in the AC and PC. In all cases glycation of equatorial crystallin subunits was lower than in the N. This is due to the fact that the former fetal lens crystallins, positioned in the oldest part of the N were longer exposed to the glycation process, compared to the present cortices of the lens.

DISCUSSION

This study has shown regionality of calf lens crystallin glycation related to ageing. Crystallin glycoproteins, as detected by lectin staining with CON-A, WGA, MAA and SNA, apparently undergo regional age-related changes. Crystallin subunits, visualized by blotting experiments with lectins, can better be differentiated into a larger number of glycated components by the use of 7M urea, than after lectin binding with the carbohydrates of crystallins under native conditions.

Lectins bind to glycoproteins in the lens[10], even after the lens crystallins have been subjected to 7M urea isoelectric focusing (Fig. 2). Using this blotting method, an assignment of sugar residues on specific glycoprotein subunits (αA_2-, αA_3-, αB_1-, αB_2-, ß- and γ-crystallins) can be made. The subunit αA_1 was negative with all lectins. The finding that these subunits bands bound CON-A, WGA, MAA and SNA indicates that the sugars found on many of these crystallins had mannose/glucose, N-acetylglucosamine and galactose bound to N-acetylneuraminic acid (Table 1). This is consistent with the analysis of calf lens insoluble proteins by Broekhuyse and Kuhlman[12]. They found binding to the same lectins, with the insoluble crystallin moiety of the calf lens. Our results revealed high levels of glycation of γ-crystallins, specially in the N (Table 1). Due to nonenzymatic modifications of crystallins that produce anodic shifts (e.g. glycation, carbamylation, deamidation and addition of glutathione[13]), the α-crystallins were condensed to the HM-crystallins (high-molecular weight α-crystallins). These HM-crystallins incorporated glycated ß- and γ-crystallins to become the highly glycated HM-crystallin complex (Fig. 3). This is in accordance with the data of van Boekel and Hoenders[3]. They found also high levels of early glycation products in HM-crystallin. Our results show that αA-subunits were glycated to about the same extent on the scale, compared with αB-subunits (Figs. 2,3). This is in contrast to the results of van Boekel and Hoenders[3], who found a higher glycation for αA-subunits in the calf lens. Also Swamy et al.[14] found preferential glycation of αA-subunits, but in the human lens.

CONCLUSION

Sequential cutting of lens layers in combination with IEF in 7 M urea, polypeptide blotting and lectin binding studies are useful to differentiate region-related expression of lens protein glycation. The application of this method is of special interest for the characterization of carbohydrate types of cataract and age related differentiation processes (e.g. cortex versus nuclear layers).

REFERENCES

1. J.N. Lyang and L.T. Chylack Jr., Spectroscopic study on the effects of nonenzymatic glycation in human lens α-crystallin. *Invest. Ophthalmol. Vis. Sci.* 28:790(1987).
2. M.A.M. van Boekel and H.J. Hoenders, Glycation-induced crosslinking of calf lens crystallins. *Exp. Eye Res.* 53:89(1991).
3. M.A.M. van Boekel and H.J. Hoenders, In vivo glycation of bovine lens crystallins. *Biochim. Biophys. Acta* 1159:99(1992).
4. V.M. Monnier and A. Cerami, Nonenzymatic browning in vivo: Possible process for aging of long-lived proteins. *Science* 211:491(1981).
5. J. Bours and M.H.J. Ahrend, Crystallin and water content of the ageing bovine lens: Cross-sectional view by microsectioning perpendicular to the optic axis. *Progr.in Veterinary & Comparative Ophthalmol.* 3:141(1993).
6. J.N. Lyang and M.T. Rossi, In vitro non-enzymatic glyca-tion and formation of browning products in the bovine lens alpha-crystallin. *Exp. Eye Res.* 50:367(1990).
7. A. Kamei, Glycation and insolubility of human lens proteins. *Chem. Pharm. Bull. 40:* 2787(1992).
8. J. Bours, M.H.J. Ahrend and W. Breipohl, The presence of ß-, $ß_S$- and γ-crystallins in the water-insoluble crystallin complex of the ageing bovine lens, *in:* "Eye Lens Membranes and Ageing", G. Vrensen and J. Clauw-aert, eds., Topics in Aging Research in Europe 14:341(199).
9. J. Bours, A. Wegener, D. Hofmann, H.J. Födisch and O. Hockwin, Protein profiles of microsections of the fetal and adult human lens during development and ageing. *Mechanisms of Aging and Development* 54:13(1990).

10. P. Russell and S. Sato, A study of lectin-binding to the water-insoluble proteins of the lens. *Exp. Eye Res.* 42:95(1986).
11. H.A. Kramps, H.J. Hoenders and J. Wollensak, Protein changes in the human lens during development of senile nuclear cataract. *Biochim. Biophys. Acta* 434:32(1976).
12. R.M. Broekhuyse and E.D. Kuhlman, Lens membrane. IV. Preparation, isolation and characterization of membranes and various membrane proteins from calf lens. *Exp. Eye Res.* 26:305(1978).
13. J.J. Harding, Nonenzymic posttranslational modification of lens proteins in aging, *in:* "Presbyopy Research", G. Abrecht, L.W. Stark, ed., Chapter 7, Plenum Press, New York, (1991), pp. 57-60.
14. M.S. Swamy, A. Abraham and E.C. Abraham, Glycation of human lens proteins: Preferential glycation of αA subunits. *Exp. Eye Res.* 54:337(1992).

SPATIAL DISTRIBUTION OF ADENOSIN NUCLEOTIDES IN LENSES OF SPECIES WITH DIFFERENT ACCOMMODATIVE CAPACITIES

Alfred Wegener, Elke Thome, and Winrich Breipohl

Department of Experimental Ophthalmology
University of Bonn, D-53105 Bonn, Germany

ABSTRACT

It has been hypothesized that the lens actively participates in the accommodative process. This hypothesis is based on the presence of high ATP/ADP ratios found in total lens homogenates of accommodating lenses as opposed to non-accommodating lenses with a lower ATP/ADP ratio. To get an insight into physiological differences between lenses of high and low accommodative capacity respectively, we studied the spatial distribution of adenosin nucleotides in the lenses of species that differ with respect to their accommodative capacity. Lenses of species with a high accommodative range (chicken and turkey) and with low or no such capacity (calf, cow, rabbit and rat) were analysed. Each lens was deep frozen, separated into an equatorial ring and a central cylinder, the latter was sliced into 6 layers (anterior to posterior pole). Tissue samples were homogenized and processed for biochemical assays. The data obtained are in contradiction to the expectations: non-accommodating lenses from rats and rabbits had higher ATP ratios in the equatorial region and section 1 than accommodating lenses (chicken and turkey). In the deep cortical and nuclear region, however, the avian lenses have higher ATP ratios than the rodent and bovine lenses. This changes again in the posterior subcapsular layer.

INTRODUCTION

The accommodative capacity of vertebrate eyes, including primate and human eyes, varies considerably from 0 to over 20 diopters. Extreme cases among birds are reported to go up to 80 diopters (Duke-Elder, 1958). Differences in accommodative capacity have been linked to variations in morphology of the suspension apparatus and elasticity of the capsular bag of the lens, as well as lenticular shape and internal tissue architecture. Marine vertebrates with a low accommodative range for example, have spherical lenses that can be moved forwards and backwards with a retractor lentis muscle (Walls, 1963). Birds with the highest accommodative range, in contrast, have elipsoid lenses with an annular pad, formed by epithelial cells. This pad allows extreme changes of the anterior lenticular curvature through the squeezing action of the iris sphincter. Alternatively, differences in accommodative capacity have also been linked to variations in physiology. It has been hypothesized that the lenses of terrestrial species with a higher accommodative range participate actively in the accommodative process (Gullstrand, 1911; Kleifeld, 1956). Kleifeld could even support his hypothesis experimentally by demonstrating that electrical stimulation of the lens changes the shape of the lenticular fiber cell. Apart from an appropriate presence of (contractile) cytoskeletal proteins, the basis for such a process could be a high ratio of ATP/ADP in distinct regions of the lens. Investigations of adenosin nucleotide ratios in total lens homogenate seem to support this assumption and at the same time allow to distinguish between "energy type" lenses (rich in ATP; high accommodative range, **HAR**) versus "synthesis" type lenses (rich in ADP, AMP, low accommodative capacity, **LAR**; Korte et al., 1985). It has not been investigated so far, whether there is a correlation between the ATP/ADP ratio in distinct regions of the lenticular cortex and epithelium and the accommodative capacity of such a lens. Therefore it has been the intention of this study to investigate the distribution patterns of ATP, ADP and AMP concentration in lenses of vertebrates with varying degrees of accommodation.

MATERIAL AND METHODS

Freshly disected lenses of chicken, turkeys, rats, rabbits and cattle have been separated in 2 steps into 7 distinct lens parts with the Bonn Freeze Sectioning Device (Müller et al., 1987; Selzer et al., 1991): a) an equatorial ring (20% of equ. diameter) and a central cylinder (80% of the equ. diameter); b) the central cylinder has been sliced into 6 sections of identical thickness, section 1 being the anterior capsulo/epithelial complex with superficial cortex and section 6 the posterior capsule and superficial cortex (Figure 1). The frozen tissue samples were sonnicated (20 - 30 pulses, 10 W each) for homogenization and processed for spectrophotometric analysis according to Bücher (1974, ATP) and Jaworek et al. (1974, ADP/AMP). The enzymatic tests were modified to be suitable for analysis of small samples of lenticular tissue.

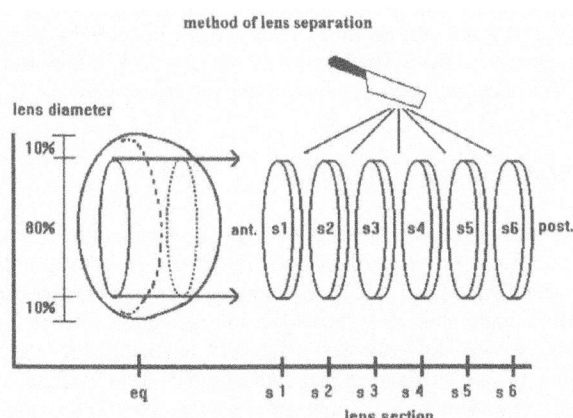

Figure 1: Schematic diagram of the lens separation into an equatorial ring (20% of diameter) and a central cylinder, the latter being separated into 6 sections of identical thickness (S1 - S6). Ant. = anterior pole; post. = posterior pole; eq. = equator. Further processing of the tissue samples as described by Selzer et al., 1991

RESULTS

The concentrations (expressed as μmoles / g sample wet weight, SWW) of ATP versus ADP and AMP differ remarkably between those lenses with high accommodative capacity (HAR) and those with medium or low such capacity (LAR). Turkeys and chicken have high ATP concentrations in the outer and inner layers of the lens, the concentrations in the equator and section 1 being even lower than those in the deeper cortex, nucleus and posterior subcapsular layer (Figure 2b). The ratio ATP / ADP + AMP evidences even more clearly that the ATP concentrations in sections 2 - 5 of the central cylinder are several folds higher than in the equator and section 1 (Figure 5b). Rats, rabbits, calf and cow lenses, however, have highest ATP concentrations in the equator, section 1 and 6 and medium or low concentrations in the deeper cortex and nucleus (Figures 2a, 5a). A further differentiation between rats and rabbit and bovine lenses can be found in that rats have higher absolute ATP concentrations in the equator and section 6 than the others (Figure 2a) In addition the ratio evidences that this is the case for all regions of the lens (Figure 5a). ADP concentrations are exceptionally high in the equator and section 1 of chicken lenses (Figure 3b) and among the LAR species they are highest in calf lenses (Figure 3a) but generally follow an u-shaped pattern in all HAR and LAR lenses. AMP concentrations are remarkably high in the equator, section 1 and 6 (not in chicken) of HAR lenses (Figure 4b). Among the LAR lenses, AMP follows an u-shaped pattern with little differences, a tendency can be seen, however, for higher values in sections 1, 2 and 6 of bovine lenses (Figure 4a).

DISCUSSION

The data reported here evidence a difference between bird lenses (energy type) and the non-avian species (synthesis type) investigated. Bird lenses have much higher ATP concentrations in the deeper cortical and nuclear layers than in the superficial regions. This is in contrast to rats, rabbits and cows which have higher ATP concentrations in the superficial layers. The rat data, however, are an astonishing exception: they have the highest ATP concentrations of all species investigated in the equator and superficial cortex and they still have quite high concentrations in the deeper cortical and nuclear layers. Furthermore the lenses of all non-avian species especially bovine seem to use ADP to form ATP, whereas bird lenses obviously use ADP in the outer lenticular regions but do use more ADP in the inner lenticular layers. The data confirm that there are at least two different metabolic types of lenses (Korte et al., 1985). The data do not yet provide a closer look into a possible active accommodative mechanism, postulated and also in a way demonstrated by Kleifeld in 1956. They seem to fit, however, to the observations reported by Rafferty and Scholz (1989), that the different types of actin fiber arrays point to an active internal resistence of the lenticular epithelium and the fiber cells to extension and compression by the zonular fibers. The data support the hypothesis that there are most probably 2 different metabolic types of active lenticular accommodation, a "muscle type" using higher levels of ATP for a working potential and a "liver type" using higher levels of ADP for synthesis purposes.

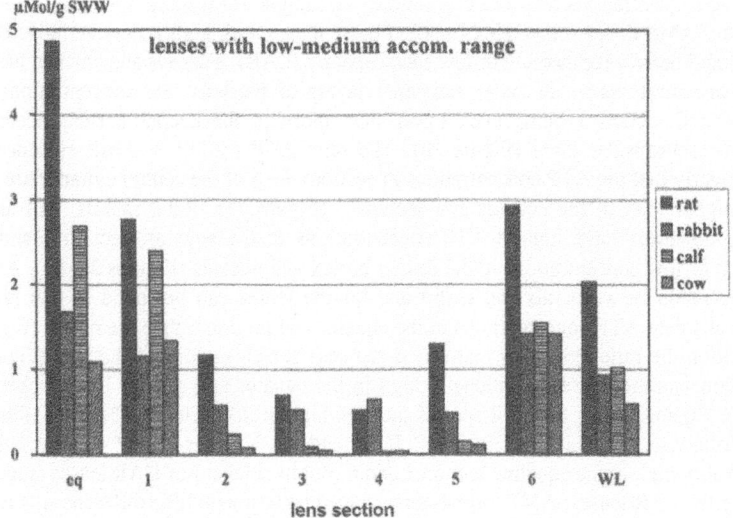

Figure 2a. ATP concentration (μmoles/g sample wet weight, SWW) in rat, rabbit, calf and cow lenses; Eq = equator; WL = whole lens. The WL data are arithmetic means of the data for equator and section 1 - 6 to demonstrate the importance of the sectioning approach.

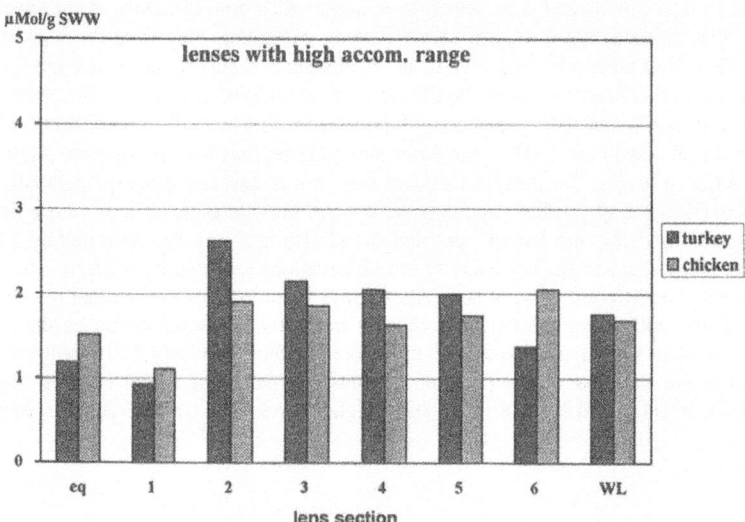

Figure 2b. ATP concentration (μmoles/g sample wet weight, SWW) in turkey and chicken lenses, Eq = equator; WL = whole lens. The WL data are arithmetic means of the data for equator and section 1 - 6 to demonstrate the importance of the sectioning approach.

ADP content

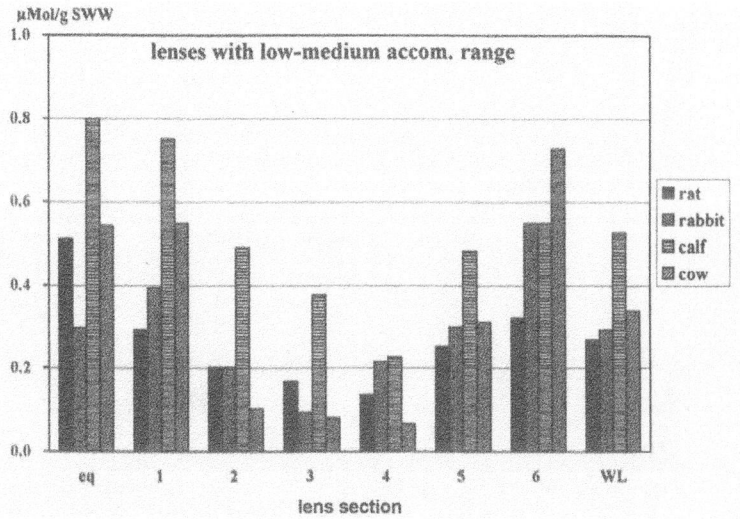

Figure 3a. ADP concentration (μmoles/g sample wet weight, SWW) in rat, rabbit, calf and cow lenses; See also legend of figure 2.

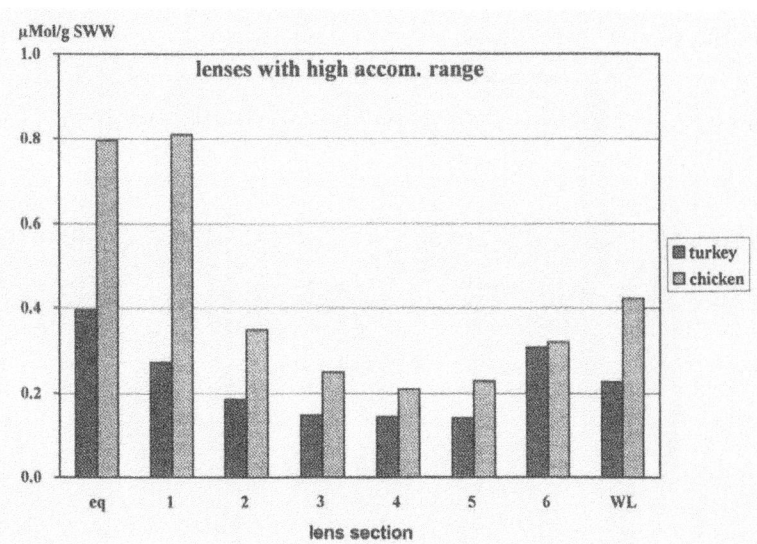

Figure 3b. ADP concentration (μmoles/g sample wet weight, SWW) in turkey and chicken lenses. See also legend of figure 2.

231

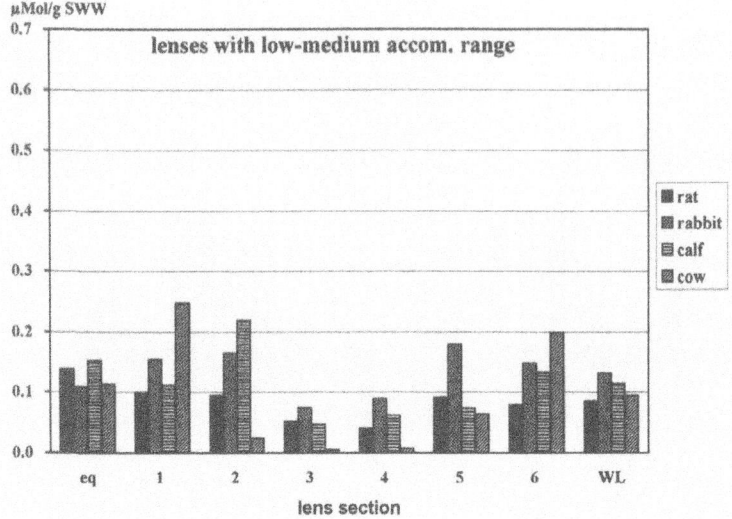

Figure 4a. AMP concentration (μmoles/g sample wet weight, SWW) in rat, rabbit, calf and cow lenses; b) AMP concentration (μmoles/g sample wet weight, SWW) in turkey and chicken lenses. See also legend of figure 2.

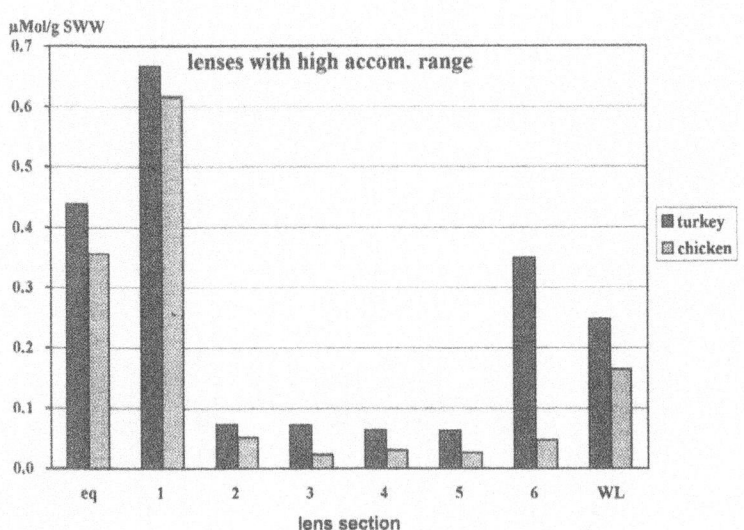

Figure 4b. AMP concentration (μmoles/g sample wet weight, SWW) in turkey and chicken lenses. See also legend of figure 2.

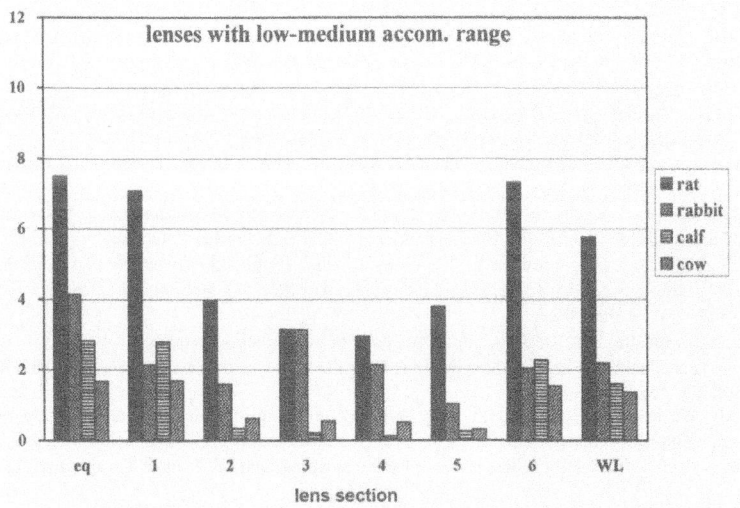

Figure 5a) Ratio of ATP / ADP + AMP in rat, rabbit, calf and cow lenses.

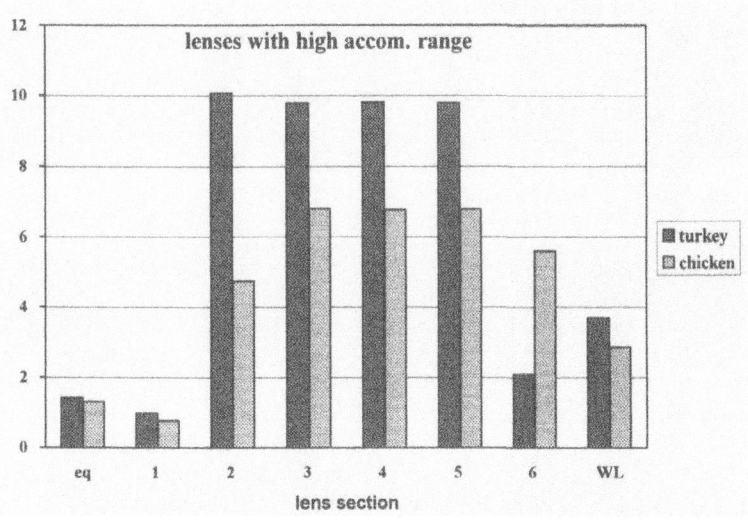

Figure 5 b) Ratio of ATP / ADP + AMP in turkey and chicken lenses.

233

REFERENCES

Bücher, Th., 1947, Über ein Phosphatübertragendes Gärungsferment. Biochim. biophys. Acta(Amst)1, 292 - 314.

Duke-Elder, S., 1958, "System of Ophthalmology", 1, The eye in evolution, Henry Kimpton, London.

Gullstrand, A., 1911, Der intrakapsuläre Akkommodationsmechanismus der Augenlinse, in: "Handbuch der Physiologischen Optik", H. v. Helmholtz ed., Voss, Hamburg, Leipzig.

Jaworek, D., Gruber, W., Bergmeyer, H.U., 1974, Adenosin-5'-triphosphat, in: "Methoden der enzymatischen Analyse", H.U. Bergmeyer ed., 2, 2020 - 2024 (1974).

Kleifeld, O., 1956, Beiträge zum intrakapsulären Akkommodationsmechanismus. Documenta Ophthalmologica 10, 132 - 168.

Korte, I., Bours, J., Weigelin, E., Hockwin, O., 1985, Ophthalmobiochemische Spezies-Unterschiede, in: "Biochemie des Auges", O. Hockwin ed., 261 - 273, Enke Verlag , Stuttgart.

Müller, P., Möller, B., Dragomirescu, V., Hockwin, O., 1987, Profiles of enzyme activities in bovine lenses, in: "Drug-induced ocular side effects and ocular toxicology", O. Hockwin ed., Concepts Toxicol. 4, 343 - 349, Karger Basel.

Rafferty, N.S., Scholz, D.L., 1989, Comparative study of actin filament patterns in lens epithelial cells. Are these determined by the mechanism of accommodation? Curr. Eye Res. 8, (6), 569 - 579.

Selzer, M., Wegener, A., Hockwin, O., 1991, Regional enzyme profiles in rabbit lenses with early stages of naphthalene cataract. Lens and Eye Toxicity Research 8(4), 415 - 430.

Walls, G.L., 1963, The vertebrate eye and its adaptive radiation, Haffner Publishing Company, New York.

HYPERBARIC OXYGEN THERAPY INDUCES A LENTICULAR MYOPIC SHIFT EVEN WITH SHORTER TREATMENT PROTOCOL: A PRELIMINARY REPORT

S.M. Johnson[1], P.J. Bryson[2], R. Clark[3], and R.C. Tripathi[1]

The University of South Carolina School of Medicine, Department of Ophthalmology[1], Richland Memorial Hospital, Department of Hyperbaric Medicine[2], Columbia, SC, U.S.A. and The South Western Hyperbaric Medical Centre, Devon, United Kingdom[3]

ABSTRACT

Hyperbaric oxygen (HBO) is currently a widely accepted treatment modality for a variety of disorders. Previous reports have shown that prolonged treatment with HBO induces a myopic shift in refraction. We evaluated the frequency, duration and reversibility of myopia in patients who were undergoing HBO with the current shorter protocols (up to 36 treatments). Patients were followed at two medical centers (South Carolina, USA and Devon, England). Four patients, analyzed retrospectively in South Carolina, had blurred vision after 8 to 15 treatments, and two were documented to have a myopic shift. Twenty-nine patients (5 in South Carolina and 26 in Devon) were followed prospectively. Eleven of the prospective group developed a myopic shift in refraction. Maximum shifts were -3.00 diopters. Of the 11 patients, 5 returned to baseline, and 6 were lost to follow-up. The duration of myopic shift has been less than 3 months. No other ocular changes have been noted during the course of HBO. Our findings from two separate institutions indicate that HBO therapy can induce a transient lenticular myopia even with shorter protocols.

INTRODUCTION

Hyperbaric oxygen therapy involves the delivery of 100% oxygen at pressures in excess of normal atmospheric conditions. The intermittent application of hyperbaric hyperoxia is associated with direct and indirect antibacterial effects,[1-9] angiogenesis in partially ischemic tissue,[10-15] tissue hyperoxygenation,[16-19] vasoconstriction without component hypoxia,[17,20-22] and direct pressure effects.[23-26] Clinically, these effects are exploited in the management of acute severe carbon monoxide intoxication,[27-30] clostridial myonecrosis,[1,2,5,31-33] decompression sickness,[34,36,37] cerebral arterial gas embolism[24,38,39] and osteoradionecrosis.[12,40-42] Additionally, HBO is an useful adjunct in the treatment of acute thermal burns,[43-45] crush injury/acute ischemia,[46-48] skin graft and skin flap support,[28,50,51] refractory wound healing,[52-55] chronic refractory osteomyelitis,[9,53,56,57] and necrotizing soft tissue infections.[59-62]

Hyperoxic-induced myopic shifts have been reported in patients undergoing extensive courses of HBO therapy, 100 hrs or more in one study, and 4 to 52 weeks daily for 2 hrs in another.[67,68] Anderson and associates[69,70] reported that patients undergoing treatment protocols of 80 hrs had detectable myopic shifts. Current protocols are shorter and patients typically receive 30 to 45 hrs total HBO treatment. We investigated whether the shorter protocols can induced a myopic shift in patients who underwent treatment for a variety of disorders.

MATERIALS AND METHODS

Patients were followed at the University of South Carolina, Department of Ophthalmology, USA or at the South Western Hyperbaric Medical Centre in Devon, England. At the South Carolina center, we initially evaluated retrospectively 4 HBO patients who complained of blurred vision. Subsequently, we followed 5 HBO patients prospectively. Prior to HBO, these patients received a complete baseline ophthalmologic examination that included refraction, slit-lamp biomicroscopy, measurement of intraocular pressure and axial length, keratometry, pupillary reaction, ocular motility and alignment, and dilated funduscopy. The patients were followed every ten treatments and then monthly, until their refraction returned to baseline. Follow-up examinations included refraction with a fogging technique, axial length, keratometry, slit lamp biomicroscopy and intraocular pressure. Patient age, sex, race, indication for HBO, and treatment protocol were recorded.

All patients received 90 minute HBO sessions at 2.0 or 2.5 ata (atmospheres absolute) for 19 to 36 sessions (mean of 28 ± 6). Five of the patients were diabetic. One eye was pseudophakic. Twenty-six patients were followed prospectively in Devon. Patients were examined pre-, mid-, and post-HBO which were at approximately one month intervals, and thereafter at 3 months after conclusion of therapy.

RESULTS

A total of 31 patients were followed prospectively (Table 1). In all patients examined, the myopic shifts ranged from none to a maximum of -3.00 diopters. Shifts were apparent by approximately one month after beginning HBO therapy and were resolved by 3 months after conclusion of the treatment regimen. The mean shift at one month was 1 diopter ± 0.6 for 20 eyes. The pseudophakic eye showed no myopic shift. No patient had a monocular myopic shift. However, 6 patients with a shift did not return for follow-up refraction after completion of HBO therapy.

DISCUSSION

Previous clinical studies have suggested that the etiology of hyperoxic myopia is lenticular,[67,69,70] because axial length and keratometry did not change as significantly as did the refractive error of the patients. Our study of patients undergoing shorter courses of HBO demonstrates that these patients remain at risk for a transient myopia, probably of lenticular origin. To prove this hypothesis, we included pseudophakic and aphakic patients as a control population. Prior studies of patients undergoing extended courses of HBO suggested a risk of cataract[68] which was not borne out in our study of patients who underwent the shorter HBO treatment. A study in Moscow indicated that the lens suture thickness and transparency of the lens decreased in patients exposed to HBO[71] and another study indicated an increased occurrence of nuclear vacuoles, some reversible.[72] These findings suggest that the induced myopia could be a pre-cataract state, possibly dose dependent and that the shorter protocols of HBO therapy may prevent permanent lens damage. Further study is required to follow larger series of patients to better define any incidence of cataract in this population and to elucidate whether their lifelong risk of cataract is increased. No correlation was found between age, sex, or race of the patients and the incidence of lenticular changes.

Table 1. Patients who received hyperbaric oxygen (HBO) therapy were examined for myopic shift (D.sph.) midway (mid-HBO) and after final treatment (post-HBO). NA-data not available. ND-not detectable. NFF- no further follow-up.

Patient No.	Age (yrs)	Diagnosis	# HBO R_x	Mid-HBO Shift	Post-HBO Shift	Post-HBO 1 month	Post HBO 3 months
1	52	Osteomyelitis	33	NA	-1.25	NA	ND
2	67	Osteomyelitis	26	NA	ND	NFF	NFF
3	49	Osteomyelitis	27	-1.00	Lost to follow-up		
4	78	Osteomyelitis	33	NA	ND	NA	NA
5	72	Wound healing	34	NA	ND	NFF	NFF
6	63	Radionecrosis	33	NA	NA	NA	NA
7	60	Radionecrosis	25	NA	ND	NFF	NFF
8	54	Pneumatosis	36	NA	-0.50	Lost to follow-up	
9	36	Macroembolism	20	NA	ND	NFF	NFF
10	67	Radionecrosis	35	NA	-0.25	Lost to follow-up	
11	58	Radionecrosis	32	NA	ND	NFF	NFF
12	59	Radionecrosis	32	NA	-0.50	Lost to follow-up	
13	51	Radionecrosis	35	NA	-1.75	Lost to follow-up	
14	60	Radionecrosis	30	NA	ND	NFF	NFF
15	73	Radionecrosis	30	NA	ND	NFF	NFF
16	60	Radionecrosis	25	NA	ND	NFF	NFF
17	36	Amputation	34	NA	ND	NFF	NFF
18	60	Skin Ulcer	27	NA	-1.00	Lost to follow-up	
19	31	Skin Ulcer	26	NA	ND	NFF	NFF
20	83	Skin Ulcer	26	NA	-2.00	Lost to follow-up	
21	48	Radionecrosis	30	NA	ND	NFF	NFF
22	46	Radionecrosis	15	NA	ND	NFF	NFF
23	68	Radionecrosis	28	NA	ND	NFF	NFF
24	68	Radionecrosis	20	NA	ND	NFF	NFF
25	71	Radionecrosis	30	NA	ND	NFF	NFF
26	76	Radionecrosis	33	ND	ND	NFF	NFF
27	62	Osteoradionecrosis	30	-1.62	-2.04	-1.65	NA
28	54	Osteoradionecrosis	23	-1.20	NA	Lost to follow-up	
29	33	Skin graft	19	ND	ND	NFF	NFF
30	69	Postradiation proctitis	20	ND	ND	-2.75	ND
31	61	Reconstructive surgery	20	ND	ND	NFF	NFF

The generation of free oxygen radicals is implicated to have a role in the formation of cataracts. Mice exposed to hyperbaric oxygen develop cataract.[73] Lens epithelial cells in vitro exposed to oxygen at increased pressures show a decreased mitotic activity.[74] Both decreased and unaltered levels of reduced glutathione, an oxygen radical scavenger, have been reported[74,75] and this loss has been localized to the nucleus rather than the lens cortex.[76] Correlative clinical and laboratory studies are warranted to establish the causal role of HBO in lenticular myopic shift of the eye.

ACKNOWLEDGMENTS

This study is supported by a grant from Research to Prevent Blindness, Inc., New York, Richland Memorial Hospital, SC, and Vision Research Foundation.

Address correspondence to: Prof. Ramesh C. Tripathi, M.D., Ph.D., F.A.C.S., Department of Ophthalmology, the University of South Carolina School of Medicine, South Carolina Eye Institute, 4 Richland Medical Park, Suite 100, Columbia, SC 29203.

REFERENCES

1. W.H. Brummelkamp, J. Hogendijk, and I. Boerema, Treatment of anaerobic-infections (clostridial myositis) by drenching the tissues with oxygen under high atmospheric pressure, *Surgery.* 49:299(1961).
2. W.H. Brummelkamp, Considerations on hyperbaric oxygen therapy at three atmospheres absolute for clostridial infections type welchii, *Ann NY Acad Sci.* 117:688(1965).
3. A.J.M. Van Unnik, Inhibition of toxin production in Clostridium in vitro by hyperbaric oxygen, *Antonie Van Leeuwenhoek.* 31:181(1965).
4. F.J. Demello, J.J. Haglin, and C.R. Hitchcock, Comparative study of experimental Clostridium perfringens infection in dogs treated with antibiotics, surgery, and hyperbaric oxygen, *Surgery* 73:936(1973).
5. D.J. Bakker, Clostridial myonecrosis, *in*: "Problem Wounds: The Role of Oxygen," J.C. Davis, and T.K. Hunt, eds., Elsevier, New York (1988).
6. G. Mandell, Bactericidal activity of aerobic and anaerobic polymorphonuclear neutrophils, *Infect Immun.* 9:337(1974).
7. T.K. Hunt, M. Linsey, G. Grislis, M. Sonne, and E. Jawetz, The effect of differing ambient oxygen tensions on wound infection, *Ann Surg.* 181:35(1975).
8. J.T. Mader, K.R. Adams, and T.E. Sulton, Infectious diseases, pathophysiology and mechanisms of hyperbaric oxygen, *J Hyperbaric Med.* 2:133(1987).
9. J.T. Mader, G.L. Brown, J.C. Guckian, C.H. Wells, and J.A. Reinarz, A mechanism for the amelioration by hyperbaric oxygen of experimental staphylococcal osteomyelitis in rabbits, *J Infect Dis.* 142:915(1980).
10. T.K. Hunt, and M.P. Pai, The effect of varying ambient oxygen tension on wound metabolism and collagen synthesis, *Surg Gynecol Obstet.* 135:561(1972).
11. D.R. Knighton, S. Oredsson, M. Bander, and T.K. Hunt, Regulation of repair: hypoxic control of macrophage mediated angiogenesis, *in*: "Soft and Hard Tissue Repair," T.K. Hunt, P.B. Heppenstall, E. Pines, and D. Rovee, eds., Praeger, New York (1984).
12. R.E. Marx, and R.P. Johnson, Problem wounds in oral and maxillofacial surgery: the role of hyperbaric oxygen, *in*: "Problem Wounds: The Role of Oxygen," J.C. Davis, and T.K. Hunt, eds., Elsevier, New York (1988).
13. D.R. Knighton, J.H. Silver, and T.K. Hunt, Regulation of wound healing/angiogenesis: effect of oxygen gradients and inspired oxygen concentration, *Surgery.* 90:262(1981).
14. D.R. Knighton, T.K. Hunt, H. Scheustuhl, Z. Werb, and M.J. Banda, Oxygen tension regulates the expression of angiogenesis factor of macrophages, *Science.* 221:1283(1983).
15. R.E. Marx, W.J. Ehler, P. Tayapongsak, and L.W. Pierce, Relationship of oxygen dose to angiogenesis induction in irradiated tissue, *Am J Surg.* 160:519(1990).
16. C.H. Wells, J.E. Goodpasture, D.J. Harriaan, G.B. Hart, Tissue gas measurements during hyperbaric oxygen exposure, *in*: "Proceedings of the Sixth International Conference on Hyperbaric Medicine," D. Smith, Ed., University Press, Aberdeen (1977).
17. A.D. Bird, and A.M.B. Tefler, Effect of hyperbaric oxygen on limb circulation, *Lancet.* 1;355 (1965).
18. E.H. Bergofskv, and P. Bertun, Response of regional circulations of hyperoxia, *J Appl Physiol.* 21;567(1966).
19. D. Jamieson, and H.A.S. VanDen Brenk, Measurement of oxygen tensions in cerebral tissues of rats exposed to high pressures of oxygen, *J Appl Physiol.* 18:869(1963).
20. M.B. Strauss, A.R. Hargens, D.H. Gershuni, D.A. Greenberg, A.G. Crenshaw, G.B. Hart, and W.H. Akeson, Reduction of skeletal muscle necrosis using intermittent hyperbaric oxygen in a model compartment syndrome, *J Bone Joint Surg.* 65A:656(1983).
21. G. Nylander, D. Lewis, H. Nordstrom, and J. Larsson, Reduction of the post-ischemic edema with hyperbaric oxygen, *Plast Reconstr Surg.* 76:596(1985).
22. B. Pelled, Y. Seki, F. Ramsey, C.J. Lambertsen, A.J. Davidson, and P.A. Trapp, eds., Effects of Hyperoxia on the Coronary Circulation and Myocardial Functions. Proceedings of the Fifth International Congress on Hyperbaric Medicine, Vol. 2, Simon Frazier University, British Columbia (1974).
23. G.B. Hart, Treatment of decompression sickness and air embolism with hyperbaric oxygen, *Aerosp Med.* 45:1190(1974).
24. E.C. Pierce, Cerebral gas embolism with special reference to iatrogenic accidents, *Hyperbaric Oxygen Review.* 1:161(1980).
25. J.C. Davis, and D.H. Elliott, Treatment of decompression disorders, *in*: "The Physiology and Medicine of Diving and Compressed Air Work," P.B. Bennett, and D.H. Elliott, eds., Balliere-Tindall, London (1969).
26. J.J.W. Sykes, J.M. Hallenbeck, and D.R. Leitch, Spinal cord decompression sickness, a comparison of recompression therapies in an animal model, *Aviat Space Environ Med.* 57: 561(1986).
27. J.S. Smith, and S. Brandon, Morbidity from acute carbon monoxide poisoning at three year old follow-up. *Br Med J.* 1:318(1973).

28. S.R. Thom, Experimental carbon monoxide-mediated brain lipid peroxidation and the effects of oxygen therapy, *Ann Emerg Med.* 17:403(1988).
29. R.A.M. Myers, S.K. Snyder, S. Linbera, and R.A. Cowley, Value of hyperbaric oxygen in suspected carbon monoxide poisoning, *J Am Med Assoc.* 246:2478(1981).
30. D.M. Norkool, and J.N. Kirkpatrick, Treatment of acute carbon monoxide poisoning with hyperbaric oxygen, a review of 115 cases, *Ann Emerg Med.* 23:315(1985).
31. G.B. Hart, R.C. Lamb, and N.M. Strauss, Gas gangrene, II. A 15-year experience with hyperbaric oxygen, *J Trauma.* 23:995(1983).
32. J.A. Holland, G.B. Hill, W.G. Wolfe, S. Osterhaut, H.A. Saltzman, and I.W. Brown, Jr., Experimental and clinical experience with hyperbaric oxygen in the treatment of clostridial myonecrosis, *Surgery.* 77:75(1975).
33. M. Hirn, J. Niinikoski, and O.P. Lehtonen, Effect of hyperbaric oxygen and surgery on experimental gas gangrene. *Eur Surg Res.* 24:356(1992).
34. D.H. Elliott, J.M. Hallenbeck, and A.A. Bove, Acute decompression sickness, *Lancet.* 1:1193 (1974).
35. D.R. Leitch, Treatment of air decompression illness in the Royal Navy, *in:* "Treatment of Serious Decompression Sickness and Arterial Gas Embolism," J.C. Davies, ed., Undersea Medical Society, Bethesda (1979).
36. P.D. Griffiths, Clinical manifestations and treatment of decompression sickness in divers, *in:* "The Physiology and Medicine of Diving and Compressed Air Work," P.B. Bennett, and D.H. Elliott, eds., Balliere-Tindall, London (1969).
37. J.C. Rivera, Decompression sickness among divers, an analysis of 935 cases, *Milt Med.* 129: 317 (1964).
38. C.L. Waite, W.F. Mazzone, M.E. Greenwood, and R.T. Larsen, Dysbaric cerebral air embolism. *in:* "Proceedings of the Third International Conference on Hyperbaric Medicine, T.W. Brown, and B.G. Cox, eds., National Academy of Sciences, Washington, DC (1966).
39. D.R. Leitch, L.J. Greenbaum, and J.M. Hallenbeck, Cerebral air embolism. I. Is there benefit in beginning HBO treatment at 6 bar? *Undersea Biomed Res.* 11:221(1984).
40. R.E. Marx, Osteoradionecrosis of the jaws, review and update, *Hyperbaric Oxygen Review* 5:48(1984).
41. R.E. Marx, A new concept in the treatment of osteoradionecrosis, *J Oral Maxillofac Surg.* 41:351(1983).
42. R.E. Marx, and R.P. Johnson, Problem wounds in oral and maxillofacial surgery, the role of hyperbaric oxygen, *in:* "Problem Wounds: The Role of Oxygen," J.C. Davis, and T.K. Hunt, eds., Elsevier, New York (1988).
43. C.H. Wells, and J.G. Hinton, Effects of hyperbaric oxygen on post-burn plasma extravasation, *in:* "Hyperbaric Oxygen Therapy," J.C. Davies and T.K. Hunt, eds., Undersea Medical Society, Bethesda (1977).
44. H.N. Kom, E.S. Wheeler, and T.A. Miller, Effect of hyperbaric oxygen on second degree burn wound healing, *Arch Surg.* 112:732(1977).
45. P. Cianci, H. Lueders, H. Lee, R.L. Shapiro, J. Sexton, C. Williams, and R. Sato, Adjunctive hyperbaric oxygen reduces the need for surgery in 40-80% burns, *J Hyperbaric Med.* 3:97 (1988).
46. G. Nylander, H. Nordstrom, L. Franzen, K.G. Hendrickson, and J. Larsson, Effects of hyperbaric oxygen treatment in post-ischemic muscle, *Scand J Plast Reconstr Surg.* 22:31(1988).
47. G. Nylander, H. Nordstrom, D. Lewis, and J. Larsson, Metabolic effects of hyperbaric oxygen in post-ischemic muscle. A quantitative morphological study, *Plast Reconst Surg.* 79:91(1987).
48. M.B. Strauss, and G.B. Hart, Crush injury and the role of hyperbaric oxygen, *Topics Emerg Med.* 6:9(1984).
49. P.N. Manson, M.J. Im, R.A.M. Myers, and J.E. Hoopes, Improved capillaries by hyperbaric oxygen in skin flaps, *Surg Forum.* 31:564(1980).
50. R.O. Gruber, F.B. Brinkley, J.J. Amato, and J.A. Mendelson, Hyperbaric oxygen and pedicle flaps, skin graft and burns, *Plast Reconstr Surg.* 45:25(1970).
51. P.M. Neniiroff, G.E. Mervin, T. Brant, and N.I. Cossisi, Effect of hyperbaric oxygen and irradiation on experimental skin flaps in rats, *Otolaryngol Head Neck Surg.* 93:485(1985).
52. G. Baroni, T. Porro, E. Faglia, G. Pizza, A. Mastropasqua, G. Oriani, G. Pedesini, and F. Favales, Hyperbaric oxygen in diabetic gangrene treatment, *Diabetes Care* 10:81(1987).
53. J.C. Davis, The use of adjuvant hyperbaric oxygen in treatment of the diabetic foot, *Clin Podiatr Med Surg.* 4:429(1987).
54. G. Oriani, D. Meazza, C. Sacchi, and A. Ronzio, Hyperbaric oxygen therapy in diabetic gangrene, *J Hyperbaric Med.* 5:171(1990).
55. N. Doctor, S. Pandya, and A. Supe, Hyperbaric oxygen therapy in diabetic foot, *J Postgrad Med.* 38:112(1992).
56. D.L. Hamblin, Hyperbaric oxygenation, its effect on experimental staphylococcal osteomyelitis in rats, *J Bone Joint Surg.* 5OA:1129(1968).

57. J.T. Mader, J.C. Gucklan, D.L. Glass, and J.A. Reinarz, Therapy with hyperbaric oxygen for experimental osteomyelitis due to Staphylococcal aureus in rabbits, *J Infect Dis*. 138: 312(1978).

58. J.C. Davis, Refractory osteomyelitis, *in*: "Problem Wounds: The Role of Oxygen," J.C. Davis, and T.K. Hunt, eds., Elsevier, New York (1988).

59. D.J. Bakker, Pure and mixed aerobic and anaerobic soft tissue infections with hyperbaric oxygen, *Hyperbaric Oxygen Review* 6:65(1985).

60. C.L. Zanetti, Necrotizing soft tissue infection and adjunctive hyperbaric oxygen, *Chest*. 92:670 (1988).

61. A. Ziser, Z. Girsh, D. Gozal, Y. Melamed, and M. Adler, Hyperbaric oxygen therapy for Fournier's gangrene, *Crit Care Med*. 13:773(1985).

62. P. Rieoels-Nielsen, J. Hesselfeldt-Nielsen, E. Ganz-Jensen, and E. Jacobsen, Fournier's gangrene. 5 patients treated with hyperbaric oxygen, *J Urol*. 132:918(1984).

63. A. Attar, W.G. Esmond, and R.A. Cowley, Hyperbaric oxygen in vascular collapse, *J Thorac Cardiovasc Surg*. 44:759(1962).

64. G.B. Hart, Exceptional blood loss anemia. Treatment with hyperbaric oxygen in exceptional acute blood-loss anemia, *J Hyperbaric Med*. 2:205(1987).

65. J.C. Davis, Hyperbaric medicine, patient selection, treatment procedures and side effects, *in*: "Problem Wounds: The Role of Oxygen," J.C. Davis, and T.K. Hunt, eds., Elsevier, New York (1988).

66. G.B. Hart, and M.B. Strauss, Central nervous system oxygen toxicity in a clinical setting, *in*: "Undersea and hyperbaric physiology IX," A.A. Bove, A.J. Bachrack, and L.J. Greenbaum, eds., Undersea and Hyperbaric Medical Society, Bethesda (1987).

67. A.J. Lyne, Ocular effects of hyperbaric oxygen, *Trans Ophthalmol Soc UK*. 98:66(1978).

68. B.M. Palmquist, B. Philipson, and P.O. Barr, Nuclear cataract and myopia during hyperbaric oxygen therapy, *Br J Ophthalmol*. 68:113(1984).

69. B. Anderson Jr., and D.L. Shelton, Axial length in hyperoxic myopia, *in*: 9th International Symposium on Underwater and Hyperbaric Physiology, Undersea and Hyperbaric Medical Society, Bethesda, (1987).

70. B. Anderson Jr., Hyperoxic Myopia, *Trans Am Ophthalmol Soc*. 76:116(1978).

71. G.S. Polunin, S. Fyodorov, and A.A. Ivanov, Influence of some factors on the sutures of lens, *Lens Eye Toxic Res*. 7:651(1990).

72. B.M. Palmquist, P.P. Fagerholm, and B.T. Philipson, Nuclear vacuoles in nuclear cataract. *Acta Ophthal Copenh*. 64:63(1986).

73. V. Padgaonkar, F.J. Giblin, J.R. Reddan, and D.C. Dziedzio, Hyperbaric oxygen inhibits the growth of cultured rabbit lens epithelial cells without affecting glutathione levels, *Exp Eye Res*. 56:443(1983).

74. F.J. Giblin, L. Schrimscher, B. Chakrapani, and V.N. Reddy, Exposure of rabbit lens to hyperbaric oxygen in vitro: regional effects on GSH level, *Invest Ophthalmol Vis Sci*. 29:1312 (1988).

75. V. Padgaonkar, F.J. Giblin, and V.N. Reddy, Disulfide cross-linking of urea-insoluble proteins in rabbit lenses treated with hyperbaric oxygen, *Exp Eye Res*. 49:887(1989).

POSTERIOR SUBCAPSULAR CATARACTS AND RAISED INTRAOCULAR PRESSURE ARE CAUSED BY PROLONGED ORAL CORTICOSTEROID THERAPY IN ADULT PATIENTS WITH INFLAMMATORY BOWEL DISEASE

Ramesh C. Tripathi,[1] Neri Malka,[2] Michael A. Kipp,[3] Stephen Hanauer,[4] and Brenda J. Tripathi[1,5]

Department of Ophthalmology, The University of South Carolina School of Medicine,[1] Cornell Medical Center, NY,[2] Department of Ophthalmology, University of Michigan, MI,[3] Department of Medicine, The University of Chicago Medical Center, IL,[4] and Department of Pathology, The University of South Carolina School of Medicine,[5] Columbia, SC 29208, U.S.A.

ABSTRACT

We examined 50 randomly-selected patients with inflammatory bowel disease (IBD) (ages 21-74 yrs; mean 38.5 yrs; 24 male, 26 female) who were treated with a total dose of 140 to 154,000 mg of oral prednisone for up to 24 years. We assessed their risk for posterior subcapsular cataract (PSC) and raised intraocular pressure (IOP). At the time of examination, 17 patients had not received prednisone for at least 6 months. Twenty four of the 50 patients (50%) had PSC. Fourteen patients had grade 1 PSC, 8 patients had grade 2 PSC, and 2 patients had grade 3 PSC in either eye. Four of the 24 patients with PSC had visual acuity between 20/40 and 20/100. One patient with grade 3 PSC complained of blurry vision (VA 20/70). The incidence of PSC correlated (p=0.03) with the number of days patients received high doses of prednisone ($\geq$ 25 mg). The average intraocular pressure (IOP) of the treated population was 13.64 $\pm$ 3.36 mm Hg. Four of the 50 patients (8%) had raised IOP (IOP $\geq$ 21 mm Hg in either eye; or difference in IOP of 6 mm Hg between the two eyes); one patient with normal IOP had cup/disk ratio of 0.5, and an additional 6 patients with normal IOP (one with a family history of glaucoma) had asymmetrical cup/disc ratios (0.2/0.4). Based on our study, we advocate careful ophthalmologic monitoring of IBD patients receiving corticosteroid therapy, and development of steroidal agents that will have ocular side effects.

INTRODUCTION

Inflammatory bowel disease (Crohn's disease and ulcerative colitis) occurs among all age groups but has peaks of incidence in the second and fourth decade of life.[1] Currently, corticosteroid therapy is the most effective treatment for moderate to severe cases of IBD. Ocular pathology in the setting of IBD may be related to inflammation of the gastrointestinal tract or secondary to corticosteroid treatment. The two major ocular side effects of systemic corticosteroid therapy are posterior subcapsular cataract (PSC) and raised intraocular pressure (IOP).[2] Recently, we reported that PSC was detected in 12 of 58 (20.7%) corticosteroid-treated pediatric IBD patients and that 21 patients of the same population (36.2%) had raised IOP.[3,4] Because pediatric IBD patients continue corticosteroid therapy into adulthood, we analyzed the prevalence of PSC and raised IOP in a series of adult IBD patients.

MATERIALS AND METHODS

We examined 50 randomly-selected IBD subjects (age range, 21-74 years, mean, 38.4 years; 24 male, 26 female) who attended the adult Gastroenterology clinic of the University of Chicago Medical Center during the summer of 1992. The patients had no history of inflammatory eye disorders, glaucoma, or risk factors for PSC, such as retinitis pigmentosa, diabetes mellitus, and radiation exposure. Thirty-two of the 50 patients had Crohn's disease and 18 had ulcerative colitis as confirmed by endoscopy, intestinal biopsy, and barium radiography. Most of the patients received oral prednisone but some were given additional hydrocortisone enemas and intravenous methyl prednisolone. Supplementary medications included azulfidine, metronidazole, 6-mercaptopurine, azocol, imuran, and dipentum.

Ocular history, current visual disturbances, and any family history of glaucoma and cataracts were obtained. Ocular examination included: visual acuity test, measurement of IOP with a Goldmann applanation tonometer and, after dilatation of the pupil, examination of the lens and fundus by slit-lamp biomicroscopy and ophthalmoscopy, respectively. The criteria for classifying PSC were those proposed by Crews:[5] Grade 1: occasional subcapsular opacities or vacuoles in the central region with or without polychromatic lustre and distortion of specular reflex; Grade 2: small clusters of opacities which remain discrete; Grade 3: multiple clusters of opacities which have mainly coalesced; Grade 4: extensive subcapsular opacities forming a plaque on the back of the lens that extended into the posterior cortex.

For each patient, we calculated the total amount of prednisone received over the entire treatment period, the duration of treatment, the number of days on a dose of prednisone ≥ 25 mg/day, and the average daily dose of prednisone over the entire treatment period as well as during the 30 days immediately before the eye examination. We performed statistical analyses to correlate the above parameters with the development of PSC and raised IOP. For those patients who received corticosteroids other than prednisone, we converted the nonprednisone dosages to a prednisone equivalent.

RESULTS

Each patient had received a total of 140 to 154,389 mg of prednisone or its equivalent for 7 to 8,717 days before the eye examination (Table 1). All patients followed a similar corticosteroid regimen. At the time of examination, 18 patients had been weaned off prednisone for at least 6 months.

Table 1. Corticosteroid treatment information for the population of 50 treated IBD patients. Range and mean ± standard deviation are given for each variable.

Variable	Range (mean±S.D.)
Total dose	140 to 154,389 (29,123±37,260) mg
Duration of treatment	7 to 8,717 (1,615±1,710) days
Average daily dose	5 to 38.89 (17.57±7.5) mg/day
Average daily dose 30 days prior to examination	0 to 40 (7.32±10.46) mg/day
Number of days on ≥ 25 mg	0 to 3,287 (438.5±640.73) days
Percent alternate day treatment	0 to 81 (10.86±16.88) %

PSC (Figures 1 and 2) were detected in 25 of the 50 steroid-treated patients (50%); 15 were Grade 1, 8 were Grade 2, and 2 were Grade 3. Of these 25 patients, who ranged in age from 21 to 68 years, 11 were male, 14 were female; 15 had Crohn's disease and 10 had ulcerative colitis. Twenty of the 25 patients (80%) had bilateral PSC. We found no significant correlation between the age, sex, or subtype of disease and the development of lens opacities (P>0.05). T-test comparisons between the patients with and without PSC demonstrated that duration of treatment (P=0.05) (Figure 3), total dose of prednisone (P=0.05) (Figure 4) and days on high dose therapy (P=0.03) (Figure 5) were significantly greater in the group with PSC than in those patients without lens opacities.

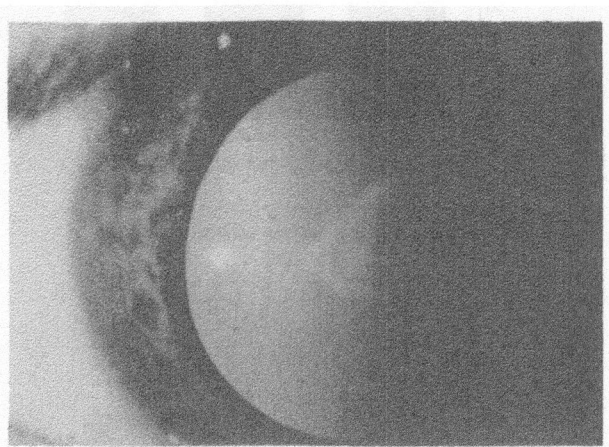

Figure 1. Photograph of lens with posterior subcapsular cataract.

The mean IOP in the corticosteroid-treated population was 13.62 ± 3.29 mm Hg. Four of the 50 patients (8%) had raised IOP (i.e., ≥ 21 mm Hg in either eye, or a difference in IOP of ≥ 6 mm Hg between the two eyes). Seven patients with IOP in the normal range had an asymmetric cup/disc ratio ≥ 0.2. Of those, only one patient had a family history of glaucoma. We found no positive correlation between the age, sex, or subtype of disease and IOP (P>0.05). No significant differences existed in the measured indices between the patients with or without raised IOP.

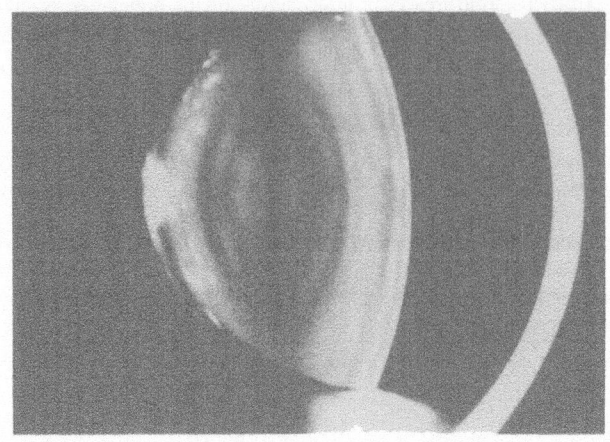

Figure 2. Biomicroscopic appearance of posterior subcapsular cataract.

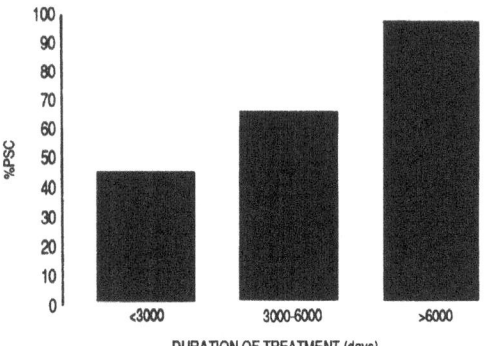

Figure 3. Bar graph showing relationship between the occurrence of PSC and the duration of steroid treatment.

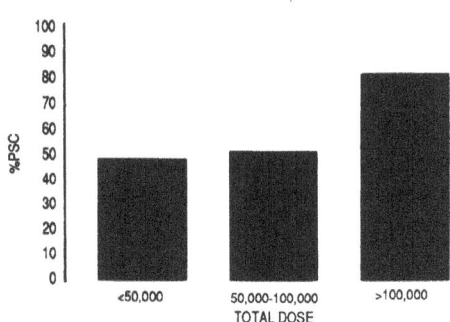

Figure 4. Bar graph showing the relationship between the occurrence of PSC and the total dose of steroids received during the period of treatment.

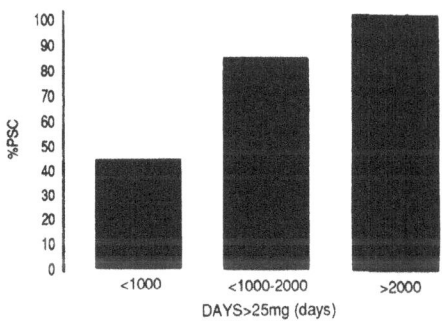

Figure 5. Bar graph showing the relationship between the occurrence of PSC and the number of days on daily dose of ≥ 25 mg.

Twenty-five patients (50%) were diagnosed with IBD prior to age 21. Of these, 10 (40%) had PSC, while 1 (4%) had raised IOP. Of the 25 patients who were diagnosed with IBD as adults (i.e., >21 years), 15 (60%) had PSC and 3 (12%) had raised IOP.

One patient with Grade 3 PSC experienced glare sensation during night driving. No other patients with PSC complained of functional visual disturbances. Four patients with Grades 1-3 PSCs but no other ocular pathology had significantly decreased visual acuity on Snellen chart examination (ranging from 20/40 to 20/100). None of the four patients with raised IOP had visual disturbances, decreased visual acuity or visual field loss. Only one patient (2%) displayed both raised IOP and PSC. Thus, 28 of the 50 corticosteroid-treated patients (56%) exhibited either steroid-induced PSC, raised IOP or both.

DISCUSSION

The incidence of PSC in the general adult population ranges from 0.2% to 6.0%[6-9] and that of raised IOP in subjects of 40 years old is approximately 1.5%.[10] The high incidence of PSC and raised IOP (50% and 8%, respectively) in our population of adult patients with IBD at a mean age of 38.5 years, implicates corticosteroids as the causative factor for the development of these ocular abnormalities. Association of IBD with certain inflammatory eye lesions such as uveitis, episcleritis, and keratoconjunctivitis has been reported.[11-16] However, cataracts (PSC) and raised IOP, have not been ascribed as direct ocular side effects of IBD. Likewise, the supplementary medications which the IBD patients received have not been incriminated in inducing PSC or raised IOP.[3,4]

The incidence of PSC in adult IBD patients treated with corticosteroids (50%) is much higher than those in pediatric patients (21%). This may be attributable to the fact that adult IBD patients, on average, were treated with 3 times the total amount of prednisone and for twice as long as the pediatric group.[3,4] The predominantly nonlabile nature of PSC may be an additional explanation for this observation. The lower incidence of raised IOP in the adults as compared to the pediatric patient population (8% vs. 36% respectively) is most probably related to discontinuation of prednisone in the adults for months prior to our ocular examination.

A statistical treatment of the data revealed that total dose of prednisone, duration of treatment and number of days on high doses (≥25 mg) of prednisone correlates significantly, though not strongly, with the development of PSC. Previous studies of steroid-induced PSC, in both children and adults, have produced contradictory results.[2,5,17-30] In our study of pediatric patients with IBD, we found a significant correlation between days on high doses of prednisone and PSC ($P=0.04$).[3] Therefore, an increased number of days on high doses of prednisone (i.e. $\geq$ 25 mg) in both adults and children appears to be a significant risk factor for the development of PSC. Tapering the high doses of corticosteroids as quickly as possible would seem beneficial in reducing this risk.

The onset of IBD, whether before or after the age of 21, does not correlate significantly with the incidence of PSC (40% vs. 60%) and raised IOP (4% vs. 12%) in our population. One might expect that patients who were diagnosed with IBD at a young age would have a high incidence of PSC because of a nonlabile nature of the lesion in most patients. However, factors such as average daily dose and total dose would seem to be important for this counter intuitive observation.

Although none of the patients with PSC have undergone cataract extraction, four patients had decreased visual acuity by Snellen chart examination and one patient with a grade 3 PSC complained of glare during night driving. Of note, two of the patients with decreased acuity had Grade 1 opacities and three of them showed decreased acuity in one eye only. The location of PSC and visual requirements of the patients may explain these phenomena. In those patients with unilateral defects, the opacity in the fellow eye may not be situated in the central visual axis, thus not obstructing vision; likewise, even a small opacity located directly in the visual axis can cause visual impairment. With continued corticosteroid treatment for IBD and as these patients age, these opacities are likely to cause more severe impairment warranting a cataract extraction.

It is possible that our incidence of 8% patients with raised IOP is erroneously low. However, seven patients who had IOPs within normal limits at the time of examination had asymmetric cup/disc ratios. Only one of these patients had a family history of glaucoma. This asymmetry could represent previously raised IOP causing damage to the disc. Because a signficant number of our patients were weaned off steroids prior to ocular examination, those who may have had raised IOP probably had reverted to a normal pressure at the time of examination. If we include six of the seven patients with asymmetric cup/disc as having had raised IOP, then our incidence of raised IOP in this population becomes 20% (10/50).

In our study of pediatric IBD patients, 11 of the 12 patients with PSC had Grade 1 opacities and one patient had a Grade 2 opacity. None of the pediatric patients had functional visual disturbances and none of them showed decreased visual acuity.[3] Thus, we predict that as the children with IBD continue to be treated with prednisone, even at low doses and with occasional breaks in treatment, more patients will develop PSC and the opacities will be of higher grade. Additionally, fewer patients may have raised IOP even with prolonged therapy, provided that the dose of steroids is kept low, preferably below 10 mg per day.[3]

Our protocol did not included patients treated with non-steroid medication or baseline patients because of the tertiary nature of our clinic. Therefore, the study estimates the prevalence of PSC and raised IOP in the majority of IBD patients who are treated with steroids. The correlations of ocular disease with steroid dose and exposure serve as internal controls. Subsequent studies would consider such controls to verify the likely associations.

The pathology of steroid-induced PSC involves a progression of biologic events. Under pathologic conditions, lens epithelial cells proliferate and migrate posteriorly, reaching the posterior pole of the lens. Proliferation proceeds until the entire posterior lens capsule is lined by a continuous layer of large cells, the so-called bladder cells of Wedl. The two major mechanisms for corticosteroid damage to the lens epithelial cells have been proposed: (1) inhibition of the $Na^+/K^+/ATPase$ pump, and (2) reaction of steroids with the amino group of lysine in the lens crystallins which causes a conformational change in the proteins, increased disulfide cross-linkages, and production of insoluble complexes that refract light. The relationship between the pathologic changes and the action of steroids on lens cells is yet to be verified. However, it is well established that the administration of glucocorticoids induces endoreplication of the DNA in trabecular cells, with an average increase of 36% in genomic activity, and synthesis of aberrant proteins in the aqueous outflow pathway.[31,32]

Our study reveals that adult patients with IBD who are treated with corticosteroids have a high incidence (56%) of PSC, raised IOP, or both. These patients, therefore, are at risk for continued opacification of their lenses and the development of steroid-induced glaucoma. Upon lowering the dose of steroids, raised IOP is reversible in the majority of patients and PSC, in its early stages, is reversible in some. To avoid ocular and other systemic complications of therapy, acute and chronic doses of steroids should be minimized. Because of individual susceptibility for glaucoma and cataract and their time- and dose-dependent nature, each patient receiving corticosteroids for IBD or any other condition must be carefully followed by an experienced ophthalmologist.

Acknowledgements: This study was supported by a grant from Research to Prevent Blindness, Inc., New York and the Vision Research Foundation.

Address correspondence to: Professor Ramesh C. Tripathi, M.D.,Ph.D.,F.A.C.S., Department of Ophthalmology, The University of South Carolina School of Medicine, South Carolina Eye Institute, 4, Richland Medical Park, Suite 100, Columbia, SC 29203

REFERENCES

1. S.B. Hanauer, Inflammatory bowel disease, in: "Cecil Textbook of Medicine," 19th ed., W.B. Saunders Company, Philadelphia (1992).
2. J. Williamson, R.W.W. Paterson, D.D.M. McGavin, M.K. Jasani, J.A. Boyle, and W.M. Doig, Posterior subcapsular cataracts and glaucoma associated with long-term corticosteroid therapy, Br J Ophthalmol. 53:361(1969).
3. R.C. Tripathi, B.S. Kirschner, M. Kipp, B.J. Tripathi, D. Slotwiner, N.S.C. Borisuth, T. Karrison, and J.T. Ernest, Corticosteroid treatment for inflammatory bowel disease in pediatric patients increases intraocular pressure, Gastroenter. 102:1957(1992).
4. R.C. Tripathi, M. Kipp, B.J. Tripathi, B.S. Kirschner, N.S.C. Borisuth, and J.T. Ernest, Ocular toxicity of prednisone in pediatric patients with inflammatory bowel disease, Lens and Eye Toxicity Res. 9:469(1992).
5. S.J. Crews, Posterior subcapsular lens opacities in patients on long-term corticosteroid therapy, Br Med J. 5346:1644(1963).
6. I. Adamsons, B. Munoz, C. Enger, and H.R. Taylor, Prevalence of lens opacities in surgical and general populations, Arch Ophthalmol. 109:993(1991).
7. R. Hiller, R.D. Sperduto, and F. Ederer, Epidemiologic associations with nuclear, cortical, and posterior subcapsular cataracts, Am J Epidemiol. 124:916(1986).
8. B.E.K. Klein, R. Klein, and K.L.P. Linton, Prevalence of age-related lens opacities in a population. The Beaver Dam eye study, Ophthalmol. 99:546(1992).
9. R.D. Sperduto and R. Hiller, The prevalence of nuclear, cortical and posterior subcapsular lens opacities in a general population sample, Ophthalmol. 91:815(1984).
10. M.F. Armaly, On the distribution of applanation pressure, Arch Ophthalmol. 73:11(1965).
11. E.A. Petrelli, M. McKinley, and F.J. Troncale, Ocular manifestations of inflammatory bowel disease, Ann Ophthalmol. 14:356(1982).
12. B.I. Korelitz and R.S. Coles, Uveitis (iritis) associated with ulcerative and granulomatous colitis. Gastroenter. 52:78(1967).
13. D.J. Hopkins, E. Horan, I.L. Burton, S.E. Clamp, F.T. DeDombal, and J.C. Galigher, Ocular disorders in a series of 332 patients with Crohn's disease, Br J Ophthalmol. 58:732(1974).

14. D.L. Knox, R.C. Snip, and W.J. Stark, The keratopathy of Crohn's disease, *Am J Ophthalmol.* 90:862(1980).

15. D.L. Knox, A.P. Schachat, and E. Mustonen, Primary, secondary, and coincidental ocular complications of Crohn's disease, *Ophthalmol.* 91:163(1984).

16. J.F. Salmon, J.P. Wright, and A.D. Murray, Ocular inflammation in Crohn's disease, *Ophthalmol.* 98:180(1991).

17. A. Loredo, R.S. Rodriguez, and L. Murillo, Cataracts after short-term corticosteroid treatment, *New Engl J Med.* 286:160(1972).

18. Y. Kobayashi, K. Akaishi, T. Nishio, Y. Kobayashi, Y. Kimura, and M. Nagata, Posterior subcapsular cataract in nephrotic children receiving steroid therapy, *Am J Dis Child.* 128:671(1974).

19. M. Bihari and B.J. Grossman, Posterior subcapsular cataracts, *Am J Dis Child.* 116:604(1968).

20. R.G. Bhagat and H. Chai, Development of posterior subcapsular cataract in asthmatic children, *Ped.* 73:626(1984).

21. D.C. Havre, Cataracts in children on long-term corticosteroid therapy, *Arch Ophthalmol.* 73: 818(1965).

22. H.J. Bachmann, P. Schildberg, I. Olbing, D. Kramer, and T. Waubke, Cortisone cataract in children with nephrotic syndrome, *Eur J Ped.* 124:277(1977).

23. R.N. Fine, G. Offner, W.A. Wilson, M.R. Mickey, A.J. Pennisi, and M.H. Malekzadeh, Posterior subcapsular cataracts: posttransplantation in children, *Ann Surg.* 182:585(1975).

24. S.K. Dikshit and P.N. Avasthi, Posterior subcapsular cataracts in children on long-term corticosteroid thearapy, *Indian J Ped.* 32:93(1965).

25. H. Shiono, M. Oonishi, M. Yamaguchi, F. Sakamoto, A. Umetsu, J. Kadowaki, M. Ooguchi, and S. Oono, Posterior subcapsular cataracts associated with long-term corticosteroid therapy, *Clin Ped.* 16:726(1977).

26. R.L. Black, R.B. Oglesby, L. von Sallmann, and J.J. Bunim, Posterior subcapsular cataracts induced by corticosteroids in patients with rheumatoid arthritis, *J Amer Med Assoc.* 174: 166(1960).

27. C.L. Giles, G.L. Mason, I.F. Duff, and J.A. McLean, The association of cataract formation and systemic corticosteroid therapy, *J Amer Med Assoc.* 182:719(1962).

28. R.W. Spencer and S.Y. Andelman, Steroid cataracts, *Arch Ophthalmol.* 74:38(1975).

29. R.B. Oglesby, R.L. Black, L. von Sallmann L, and J.J. Bunim, Cataracts in rheumatoid arthritis patients treated with corticosteroids, *Arch Ophthalmol.* 66:519(1961).

30. D.A. Braver, R.D. Richards, and T.A. Good, Posterior subcapsular cataracts in corticosteroid-treated children, *J Ped.* 69:735(1966).

31. B.J. Tripathi, R.C. Tripathi, and H.H. Swift, Hydrocortisone-induced DNA endoreplication in human trabecular cells in vitro, *Exp Eye Res.* 49:159(1989).

32. B.J. Tripathi, C.B. Millard, and R.C. Tripathi, Corticosteroids induce a sialated glycoprotein (Cort-GP) in trabecular cells in vitro, *Exp Eye Res.* 51:735(1990).

IN VITRO METHODS IN OCULAR TOXICOLOGY: INTRODUCTORY REMARKS

Martine Cottin

Advanced Research Center
L'OREAL
1, avenue Eugène Schueller
F93600, Aulnay sous Bois

IN VITRO METHODS TO REPLACE ANIMAL TESTING

Toxicologists should be aware of the rapid development of *in vitro* methods over the 10 last years, as they will have a major impact on this field (Frazier, 1993). The two main driving forces behind this development are a better understanding of cell biology, which has led to improvements in the use of cell culture models, and ethical pressures from animal rights movements (Balls, 1991; Goldberg and Frazier, 1989).

It is clearly impossible to replace animal testing in all areas of ocular toxicology, but major progress has been made in eye irritancy testing *in vitro* (Wilcox and Bruner, 1990). Indeed, *in vitro* methods are now commonly used by many companies as screening tools for new chemicals, and this has already led to a significant reduction in animal experimentation (Figure 1). In practice, companies use either a single method with multiple endpoints important for ocular irritation, e.g. the BCOP-test (Gautheron et al., 1992), or several methods for the assessment of a set of toxicological parameters (Bruner et al., 1991; Rougier et al., 1992; Cottin et al, 1994). These *in vitro* methods were chosen after a selection process known as "in house validation", based on results with well-characterized test substances.

It must, however, be stressed that no *in vitro* methods have yet been recognized by the authorities to replace the Draize eye test (Draize et al., 1944), considered as the only method suitable for evaluating eye irritation in a licensing dossier. For regulatory acceptance, an *in vitro* method must fulfil certain conditions (Balls et al., 1990). First, it must be reliable; this means that it must be reproducible both in a given laboratory and between different laboratories. This can only be validated by drawing up and applying well-defined protocols. The second condition for *in vitro* methods is relevance to *in vivo* events: each *in vitro* method must investigate one well-characterized event known to occur in vivo.

Before an *in vitro* method can be accepted as a replacement for animal testing, it must undergo a validation process. The European Center for the Validation of Alternative Methods (ECVAM) was created to coordinate and initiate validation exercises (Balls, 1994).

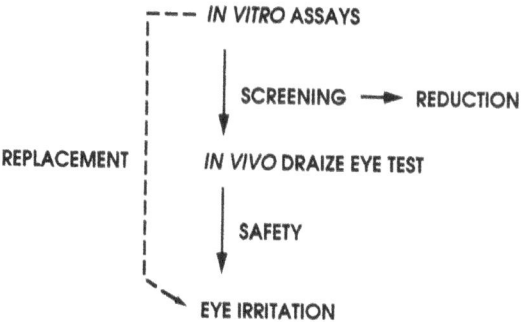

Figure 1. Use of *in vitro* methods in eye irritation assessment.

EYE IRRITATION

When a substance comes into contact with the eyes, its bioavailability (Figure 2), which is highly dependent on its chemicophysical properties (Saettone, 1993), will largely determine its effects. Clearly, a chemical that does not reach the corneal or conjunctival epithelium in amounts sufficient to affect cell biology will produce no irritation at all. Unfortunately, bioavailability is impossible to reproduce *in vitro*. Most *in vitro* tests simply consist of exposing the target system to the test substance for a certain period, with no regard to bioavailability (which is often unknown). This will clearly lead to an overestimation of toxicity when the exposure time is longer than *in vivo*, and to an underestimation with products which remains on the ocular surface.

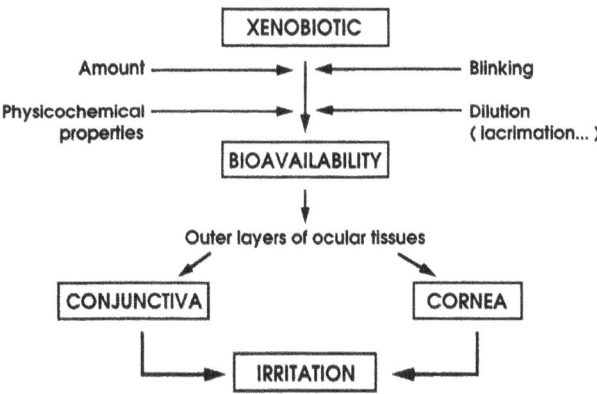

Figure 2. Early events in ocular irritation.

The main events occurring early in eye irritation involve the cornea and conjunctiva. In the case of the conjunctiva (Figure 3), inflammation is reflected by the onset of redness and chemosis. Microscopic examination shows the usual features of this inflammatory process, including cellular infiltration (monocytes and neutrophils), vasodilation and oedema of the connective tissue. It can also reveal fine alterations of cellular morphology with no clinical expression, such as oedema, necrosis or desquamation of epithelial cells, which clearly point to adverse cellular effects of the test chemical.

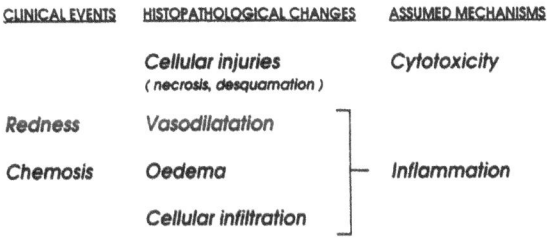

Figure 3. Main conjunctival events in ocular irritation.

As regards the cornea (Figure 4), fluoresceine staining directly reflects microscopic damage to the epithelium. Opacity can be due to direct effects on stromal microfibril organization, but is more commonly caused by functional impairment of the epithelium or endothelium. This again shows the pivotal role of altered cell physiology in ocular irritation.

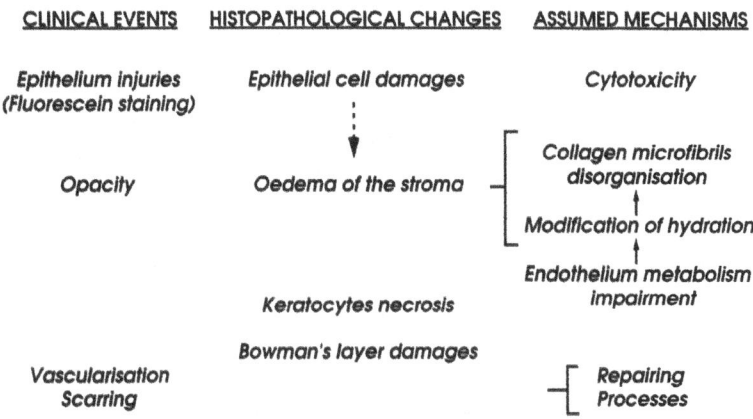

Figure 4. Main acute corneal events in ocular irritation

About 100 *in vitro* methods have been proposed as alternatives to the Draize eye test, most involving cell culture systems. This reflects the fact that no single *in vitro* method will be able to cover the whole range of events occurring in vivo: it is now accepted that various complementary *in vitro* methods will be necessary to replace the Draize eye test. Moreover, few methods have so far been designed to study the mechanisms of ocular irritation. The usual methods are rather linked to events described *in vivo* (see figures 3 and 4). This is due in particular to a lack of knowledge regarding certain mechanisms involved in the onset of eye irritation.

CELL CULTURE METHODS: PROMISING TOOLS TO STUDY THE MECHANISMS OF EYE IRRITATION

Cell cultures have been extensively investigated for the prediction of eye irritancy and have been shown to provide interesting information on the mechanisms of xenobiotic injury (Figure 5).

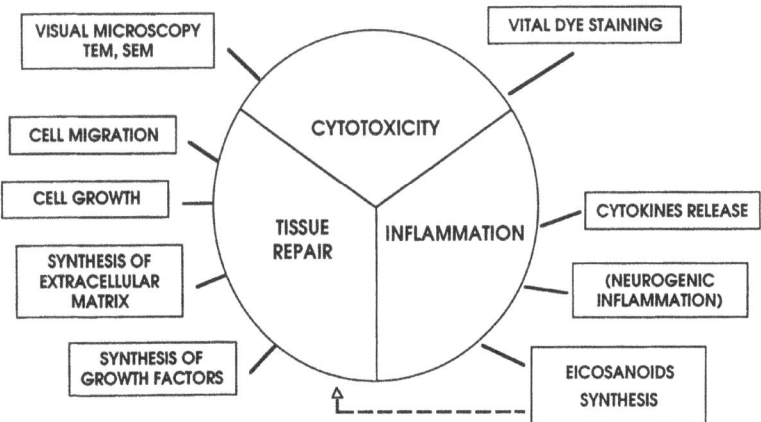

Figure 5. Endpoints in cell culture methods and their relationship to eye irritation.

Basic effects such as those on cell morphology can be evaluated by using optical and electron microscopy. In this way one can detect, for example, detrimental effects on cell-cell junctions which could have a major impact on paracellular penetration of chemicals through the corneal epithelium and subsequent damage to underlying structures (Anderberg and Artursson, 1993). Most teams evaluate cell viability by using UV-absorbant or fluorescent dyes which specifically colour living or dead cells (Borenfreund and Puerner, 1985).

Tissue repair is a very important process in eye irritation, particularly corneal lesions, but has rarely been studied. Epithelial migration and proliferation are the primary events occurring after epithelial injury. It has been shown that fibronectin stimulates epithelial cell migration, whereas hyaluronic acid is more active on proliferation (Salonen et al., 1991; Inoue and Katakami, 1993). Growth factors (EGF, FGF, etc.) have also been shown to play a role in corneal epithelial and endothelial wound healing (Dabin and Courtois, 1991; Raphael et al. 1993; Hoppenreijs et al., 1994). The effects of chemicals on the synthesis of these components by corneal cells could be extremely important in the modulation of repair processes.

Inflammation is another essential aspect of eye irritation which is poorly reflected by the usual "alternative" methods. In addition to the release of cytokines by epithelial and stromal cells (Cubitt et al., 1993), the synthesis of eicosanoids such as prostaglandins, leukotrienes and hydroxyeicosatetraenoic acids is also important in ocular inflammation (Edelhauser et al., 1993; Phillips et al., 1993). Eicosanoids can be divided into three categories according to the enzymes involved in their synthesis (Figure 6).

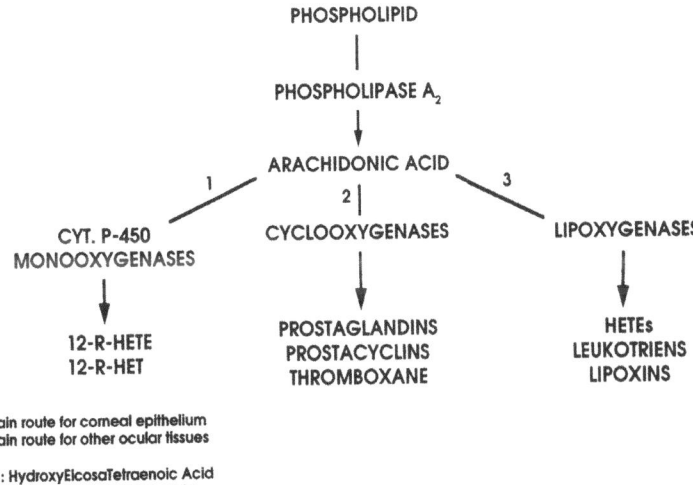

PHOSPHOLIPID

PHOSPHOLIPASE A$_2$

ARACHIDONIC ACID

1

2

3

CYT. P-450
MONOOXYGENASES

CYCLOOXYGENASES

LIPOXYGENASES

12-R-HETE
12-R-HET

PROSTAGLANDINS
PROSTACYCLINS
THROMBOXANE

HETEs
LEUKOTRIENS
LIPOXINS

1) main route for corneal epithelium
2) main route for other ocular tissues

HETE : HydroxyEicosaTetraenoic Acid
HET : HydroxyEicosaTrienoic Acid

Figure 6. Pathways of eicosanoid synthesis

The first step in the synthesis of these mediators is the <u>release</u> of <u>arachidonic acid</u> from membrane phospholipids. This step is common to the three pathways of eicosanoid synthesis and could thus prove useful as an early marker of the inflammatory process (Klöcking et al., 1994).

CONCLUSION

In vitro methods will continue to mature and, little by little, replace animal tests. However, a great deal of work first remains to be done on *in vivo* toxicological mechanisms. Therefore *in vitro* methods are already being used both to reduce animal testing (screening) and to study the mechanisms involved in ocular toxicity (research).

REFERENCES

Anderberg, E.K. and Artusson, P., 1993, Epithelial transport of drugs in cell culture, *J. Pharm. Sc.* 82:392.

Balls, M., 1991, The replacement of animal testing: ethical issues and practical realities, *Int. J. of Cosmet. Sci* 13:23.

Balls, M., Blaauboer, B., Brusick, D., Frazier, J., Lamb, D., Pemberton, M., Reinhardt, C., Roberfroid, M., Rosenkranz, H., Schmid, B., Spielmann, H., Stammati, A.L. and Walum, E., 1990, Report and recommendations of the CAAT/ERGATT workshop on the validation of toxicity test procedures, *ATLA* 18:313.

Balls, M., 1994, Replacement of animal procedures: Alternatives in research, education and testing, *Laboratory Animals* 28:193.

Borenfreund, E. and Puerner, J.A., 1985, Toxicity determined *in vitro* by morphological alterations and neutral red absorption, *Toxicol. Letts.* 24:119.

Bruner, L.H., Kain, D.J., Roberts, D.A., Parker, R.D., O'brien, K.A.F., Uttley, M. and Walker A.P., 1991, An evaluation of five potential alternatives *in vitro* to the rabbit eye irritation test *in vivo*, *Fundam. Appl. Toxicol.* 17:136.

Cottin, M., Dossou, K.G., De Silva, O., Tolle, M., Roguet, R., C. Cohen, Catroux, P., Delabarre, I., Sicard, C. and Rougier A., 1994, Relevance and reliability of *in vitro* methods in ocular safety assessment, *In vitro toxicol.* 7:3.

Cubitt, C.L., Tang, Q., Monteiro C.A., Lausch, R.N. and Oakes J.E., 1993, IL-8 gene expression in cultures of human corneal epithelial cells and keratocytes, *Invest. Ophthalmol. & Vis. Sci.* 34:11.

Dabin, I. and Courtois, Y., 1991, Acidic fibroblast growth factor overexpression in corneal epithelial wound healing, *Growth Factors*, 5:129.

Draize J.H., Woodard G. and Calvery H.O., 1944, Methods for the study of irritation and toxicity of substances applied topically to the skin and mucous membranes. *J. Pharmacol. Exp. Ther.* 82:377

Edelhauser, H.F., Geroski, D.H., Woods, W.D., Holley, G.P. and Laniado-Schwartzman, M., 1993, Swelling in the isolated perfused cornea induced by 12(R) hydroxyeicosatetraenoic acid, *Invest. Ophthalmol. & Vis. Sci.* 34:10.

Frazier, J.M., 1993, *In vitro* models for toxicological research and testing, *Toxicol. Letts* 68:73.

Gautheron, P., Dukic, M., Alix, D. and Sina, J.F., 1992, Bovine corneal opacity and permeability test: an *in vitro* assay of ocular irritancy, *Fundam. Appl. Toxicol.* 18:442.

Goldberg, M. and Frazier, M., 1989, Alternatives to animals in toxicity testing, *Scientific American* 261:2.

Hoppenreijs, V.P., Pels, E., Vrensen, G.F., Treffers, W.F., 1994, Basic fibroblast growth factor stimulates corneal endothelial cell growth and endothelial wound healing of human corneas, *Invest. Ophthalmol. Vis. Sci.* 35:931.

Inoue, M., and Katakami, C., 1993, The effect of hyaluronic acid on corneal epithelial cell proliferation, *Invest. Ophthalmol. & Vis. Sci.* 34:7.

Klöcking, H.P., Schlegelmilch, U. and Klöcking, R., 1994, Assessment of membrane toxicity using arachidonic acid release in U937 cells, *Toxic. In Vitro* 8:775.

Phillips, A.F., Szerenyi, K., Campos, M., Krueger, R., McDonnell, P.J. 1993, Arachidonic acid metabolites after excimer laser corneal surgery, *Arch Ophthalmol.* 111:1273.

Raphael, B., Kerr, N.C., Shimizu, R.W., Lass, J. H., Crouthamel, K.C., Glaser, S.R., Stern, G.A., McLaughlin, B.J., Musch, D.C., Duzman, E., Conway, J. and Schultz G.S., 1993, Enhanced healing of cat corneal endothelial wounds by epidermal growth factor, *Invest. Ophthalmol. & Vis. Sci.* 34:7.

Rougier, A., Cottin, M., De Silva, O., Roguet, R., Catroux, P., Toufic, A. and Dossou, K.G., 1992, *In vitro* methods: Their relevance and complementarity in ocular safety assessment. *Lens Eye Toxic. Res.* 9:229.

Salonen, E.-M., Vaheri, A., Tervo, T, Beuerman, R., 1991, Toxicity of ingredients in artificial tears and ophthalmic drugs in a cell attachment and spreading test, *J. Toxicol.-Cut. & Ocular Toxicol.* 10:157.

[3H]-ARACHIDONIC ACID RELEASE AS AN ALTERNATIVE TO THE EYE IRRITATION TEST

Hans-Peter Klöcking[1], Ulf Schlegelmilch[1], and Renate Klöcking[2]

Friedrich-Schiller-University, Faculty of Medicine, [1]Center for Vascular Biology and Medicine and [2]Institute of Antiviral Chemotherapy, Nordhäuser Str. 78, 99089 Erfurt,Germany

ABSTRACT

Eye irritation as monitored by the Draize test is primarily caused by the membrane-toxic effect of chemical substances. Arachidonic acid (AA) is an integral part of the cell membrane phospholipids and a substrate for inflammatory mediators formed in response to membrane-toxic events. It is rapidly released as a result of membrane disintegration or of enzymatic cleavage of phospholipids. In order to replace the Draize test by alternative methods, we examined the [3H]-AA release of U937 cells using the following substances: dimethylsulphoxide (DMSO), formamide, chloramine, dimethoate, 2,4-dichlorophenoxyacetic acid (2,4-D), sodium dodecyl sulphate (SDS), and lysolecithin. As revealed by the determination of maximum tolerated concentrations (MTC) and by calculation of both the linear correlation coefficient (r^*) and the rank correlation coefficient according to Spearman (r_s), a positive correlation ($r^* = 0.92$; $r_s = 0.98$; $\alpha = 5\%$) between the [3H]-AA release and the results of the Draize test was seen. It was attributed to the fact that the release of AA represents a key reaction of the inflammation process. The sensitivity of the *in vitro* method surpassed the Draize test by 1-2 orders of magnitude demonstrating the [3H]-AA release test to be a potentially suitable alternative to the eye irritation test.

INTRODUCTION

Half a century after the eye irritation test (EIT) in the rabbit had been standardized by Draize, Woodard and Calvery (1944), there are worldwide attempts to replace EIT and other animal tests by *in vitro* methods. The success of such attempts essentially depends on finding the closest relation between *in vitro* tests and the *in vivo* pathogenetic mechanisms.

Our studies are based on the assumption that the *in vitro* cell membrane-damaging effect of skin-toxic chemicals (Marks and Kingston, 1985) is a crucial event for eye irritation in rabbits, too.

This prompted us to study the [3H]-arachidonic acid release test ([3H]-AART) (Klöcking et al., 1994b) which is highly sensitive to membrane-toxic agents for its suitability to replace the EIT according to Draize.

Ocular Toxicology, Edited by I. Weisse *et al.*
Plenum Press, New York, 1995

MATERIALS AND METHODS

Chemicals

[³H]-Arachidonic acid (sp. act. 23.8 GBq/mg) was obtained from Amersham Buchler GmbH & Co. KG (Braunschweig, Germany); chloramine was a product of Fahlberg-List Pharma GmbH (Magdeburg, Germany); 2,4-dichlorophenoxyacetic acid (2,4-D) was obtained from Aldrich Chemie (Steinheim, Germany); dimethyl-sulphoxide (DMSO) was purchased from Merck-Schuchardt (Hohenbrunn, near Munich, Germany); and dimethoate as Bi58EC from Chemie AG Bitterfeld-Wolfen (Bitterfeld, Germany). Other chemicals were obtained from the following sources: formamide from Merck, Darmstadt, Germany, lysolecithin from Calbiochem-Novabiochem GmbH, Bad Soden/Ts., Germany, and sodium dodecyl sulphate (SDS) from Ferak, Berlin, Germany.

Cells

The promonocytic human cell line U937-ATCC (CRL1593) or ECACC (No. 87010802) was used.

Test Procedure

Prelabelling of U937 cells. For AA release studies, cells were grown in 10% FCS-containing RPMI 1640 for 2-3 days, washed twice with serum-free RPMI by centrifugation (200 x g, 5 min) and resuspended in RPMI at a density of about 10^6 cells/ml. After incubation at 37°C and 5% CO_2 for 1 h, FCS to a final concentration of 10 % and 0.1 µCi/ml [³H]-AA were added and cells were further incubated for 20 (16-24) hours. Then, the labelling medium was removed by washing twice with serum-free RPMI. Cells were resuspended in cold (4°C) serum-free RPMI and kept at that temperature until use.

In all experiments, 24-hours uptake of [³H]-AA was about 80% of the radioactivity added to the labelling medium.

Determination of [³H]-AA release. Aliquots (1 ml) of [³H]-AA-prelabelled U937 cells were placed in sterile 8 ml polystyrene tubes (Falcon) and test substances dissolved in cold serum-free RPMI were added at graduated concentrations. Control cells received an appropriate volume of RPMI without test substances. Cell cultures were kept for 1 hr at 4°C, after which the temperature was raised to 37°C. The cells were further incubated for 1 hr (dose-response relationship). After incubation, [³H]-AA was determined in the 200 g supernatants of cultures by liquid scintillation counting (liquid scintillation counter, Wallac 1410, Wallac Oy, Turku, Finland). Three experiments were carried out in every given series. All assays were performed in triplicate.

Calculation of the maximum tolerable concentration (MTC). MTC is the highest substance concentration which has no significant effect on the release of arachidonic acid under the described experimental conditions. To determine the MTC of the test substance, a confidence interval was calculated by means of variance analysis for both the RPMI cell control and the dose-response curve up to the 10-fold [³H]-AA release compared to the cell control. The first concentration at which a significant difference was found between the AA release of the test substance and that of the cell control was determined. The next lower concentration of the test substance was taken as maximum tolerable concentration (MTC).

Eye Irritation Test (EIT). Test substances were dissolved in saline. If necessary, pH was adjusted to 7.4 using 0.1 mol/l HCl and 0.1 mol/l NaOH, respectively. Five different concentrations of each substance were studied in four rabbits each. To this end, 0.1ml test solution was given into the conjunctival sac and the degree of irritation was evaluated 1, 24, 48 and 72h post expositionem (p.e.). The untreated eye served as control. The symptoms observed at the cornea, iris, and conjunctiva were graded according to the score given by Draize et al. (1944). MTC was taken 1 h p.e. as the highest substance concentration causing a mean score ≤ 2.

Statistical evaluation. The maximum tolerated concentrations (MTC) obtained by the *in vivo* test procedure served as a basis to rank the test substances. The following statistical tests were performed: Calculation of the rank correlation coefficient according to Spearman (r_s) for distribution-free dependence, calculation of the linear regression and the linear correlation coefficient (r^*). In all tests the level of significance was $\alpha = 5\%$.

RESULTS

Figure 1 illustrates the [^{3}H]-AA release of U937 cells under the influence of lysolecithin, SDS, dimethoate, chloramine, 2,4-D, formamide, and DMSO.

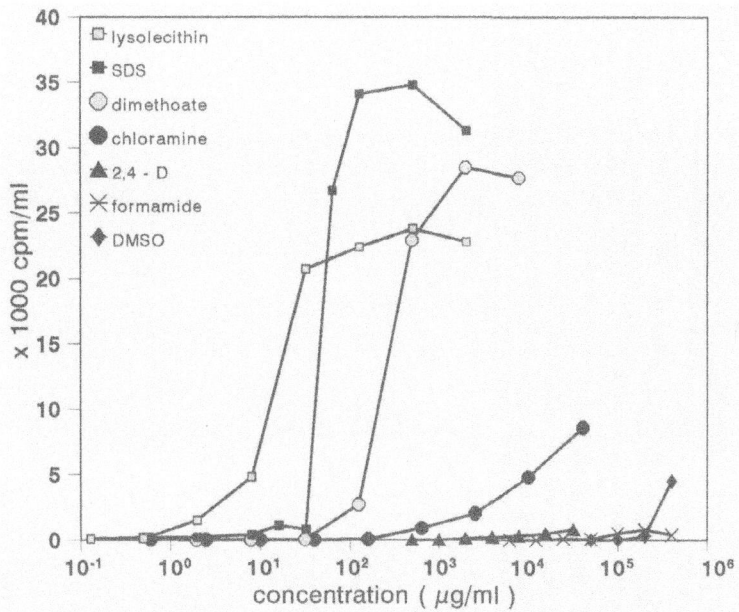

Figure 1. Release of [^{3}H]-AA in U937 cells by different chemicals after at 37°C 1 h p.e.

The dose-response curves clearly demonstrate that the cells respond to all the substances with a concentration-dependent increase in [^{3}H]-AA release. However, the effective ranges of substance concentrations differed by some orders of magnitude. Correspondingly, this was also true for the maximum tolerable concentrations (MTC values, Table 1). For lysolecithin and SDS, the MTC values amounted to 0.5 and 2.0 µg/ml, respectively, for formamide and DMSO 50 and 100 mg/ml, respectively. The MTC values of the remaining substances - dimethoate, chloramine and 2,4-D - (31, 160 and 1000 µg/ml) demonstrated their position between the extremely toxic and the well tolerable substances.

Table 1. Maximum tolerated concentrations (MTC) of seven test substances determined from the Draize eye irritation test (EIT), and the [^{3}H]-AA release test ([^{3}H]-AART)

Test substances	MTC (µg/ml)	
	EIT*	[^{3}H]-AART**
DMSO	500 000	100 000
Formamide	250 000	50 000
2,4-D	> 50 000	1 000
Dimethoate	> 50 000	31.3
Chloramine	10 000	160
SDS	3 125	2.0
Lysolecithin	481	0.5

* 1h after exposition; ** 1h at 37°C

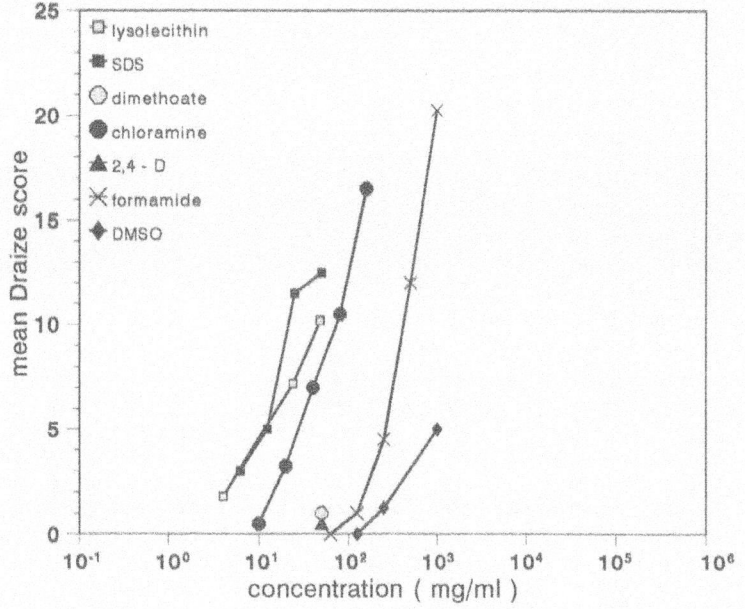

Figure 2. Mean Draize scores obtained for seven test substances at different concentrations 1 h after dosing.

The EIT results are given in Figure 2. First, all the substances were tested to find out the irritation concentrations which caused the lowest possible discomfort to the animals. Lysolecithin caused a slight irritation already at low substance concentra-tions (2.5 mg/ml). Comparable effects were only caused by undiluted DMSO. The following substances ranked between them with increasing MTC values: SDS < chloramine < dimethoate < 2,4-D, < formamide (see also Table 1).

Up to a concentration of 50 mg/ml the two plant-protective agents 2,4-D, and dimethoate did not irritate the rabbit eye. Higher concentrations could not be tested because of the limited solubility of the substances.

As shown in Figure 3, the MTC values obtained from EIT correlate with those obtained from [^{3}H]-AART (r^*= 0.92, r_s = 0.98 for [^{3}H]-AART/EIT).

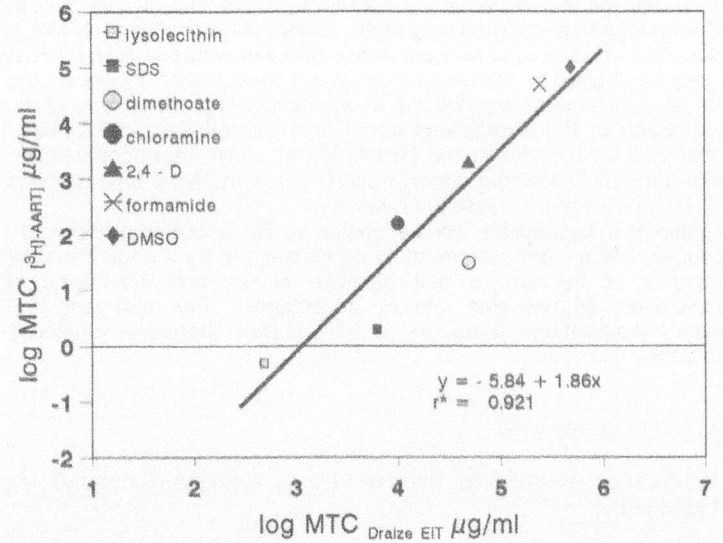

Figure 3. MTC values of Draize eye irritation test (EIT) plotted versus MTC values of [^{3}H]-AART. The linear regression line, the corresponding equation, and the correlation coefficient (r^*) are shown in the figure.

DISCUSSION

All the official recommended methods for determining the ocular irritation potential of a chemical derive from the Draize rabbit eye test (Draize et al., 1944). Despite of its historical impact, to day most scientists as well as the general public are disapproved of the Draize test for ethical and scientific reasons (Sharpe, 1985; Swanston, 1985). A number of *in vitro* test systems were described, e.g. the isolated eyes (Price and Anders, 1985), the embryonated hen's egg-choriallantoic membrane (HET-CAM) test (Luepke, 1985), the neutral red/kenacid blue method (Borenfreund and Puermer, 1985; Knox et al., 1986; Riddell et al., 1986), or the EYTEX[R] method (Martin, 1993; Regnier, 1994).

However, all tests are not directly linked with membrane alterations. A more causative pathogenetic event of eye irritation is the release of arachidonic acid.

Arachidonic acid is a particularly suitable marker for early membrane changes because it is an integral part of cell membrane phospholipids and rapidly released into the cell culture medium indicating changes in the cell environment. Furthermore, arachidonic acid represents the substrate for inflammatory mediators - leucotrienes and prostaglandins - which are formed enzymatically in response to the membrane-toxic events according to various metabolic routes.

It has previously been shown that various cell lines in culture, similar to their in vivo counterparts, respond to certain chemical irritants such as the phorbol ester tumor promoter 12-0-tetra-decanoylphorbol-13 acetate or the carcinogen benzo(a)pyrene. The cells respond by deacylation of cellular lipids in a process which results in the increased release of arachidonic acid and prostaglandins into the medium (Hassid and Levine, 1977; Levine and Chuchi, 1978; Mufson et al.,

1979; Fürstenberger et al., 1981). These studies prompted investigators to explore the likelihood of an *in vitro* release of arachidonic acid by cells in response to expo-sure to a series of irritants. It was shown that the release of arachidonic acid from [^{3}H]-AA-prelabelled hepatoma cells (Stark et al., 1983) and from [^{14}C]-prelabelled human keratinocytes correlates with the irritant potential of chemicals. These findings have been confirmed and extended by using [^{3}H]-AA-prelabelled U937 cells to study the membrane toxicity of chemicals (Klöcking et al., 1994b).

Dependent on the incubation temperature, membrane toxicity may be caused by different mechanisms (Klöcking et al., 1994b). An enhanced [^{3}H]-AA release at 4°C speaks in favour of a non-enzymatic process whereas a [^{3}H]-AA release at 37°C may be caused by activation of enzymes, in particular, by phospholipase A$_2$.

For all substances, we noticed a remarkably high sensitivity of the *in-vitro* method. Each of the substances found to be irritating by the Draize test was characterized as harmful in the [^{3}H]-AART at much lower concentrations. This leads to the conclusion that concentrations below the MTC values found by [^{3}H]-AART, will probably not irritate the rabbit eye.

In case this hypothesis will be confirmed for a larger number of chemical compounds, this *in-vitro* system could be considered as a good candidate for the replacement of the Draize test because of its high sensitivity, objectivity, automatization degree and ethical acceptance. This test only reflect the inflammatory alterations of the Draize EIT and must therefore completed by other *in vivo* tests.

ACKNOWLEDGEMENTS

The technical support of Fritz-Thyssen-Stiftung, Cologne (Germany), is gratefully acknowledged.

REFERENCES

Draize, J.H., Woodward, G., and Calvery, H.O., 1944, Methods for the study of irritation and toxicity of substances applied topically to the skin and mucous membranes. *J. Pharmacol. Exp. Ther.* 82: 377 - 390.

Borenfreund, E., and Puerner, J.A., 1985, Toxicity determined in vitro by morphological alterations and neutral red absorption. *Toxicology Letters* 24: 119 - 124.

Klöcking, H.-P., Eigenwillig, K., and Klöcking, R., 1994a, Studies on the temperature dependency and the reversibility of xenobiotic-induced membrane lesions. *Naunyn-Schmiedeberg's Arch. Pharmacol.* 349 (Suppl): R 112.

Klöcking, H.-P., Schlegelmilch, U., and Klöcking, R., 1994b, Assessment of membrane toxicity using [^{3}H]-AA release in U937 cells. *Toxic. in Vitro* 8: 775-777.

Knox, P., Uphill, P.F., Fry, J.R., Beuford, J., and Balls, M., 1986, The FRAME multicentre project on in vitro cytotoxicology. *Fd. Chem. Toxic.* 24: 457-463.

Levine, L., and Chuchi, K., 1978, Retinoids as well as tumor promotors enhance deacylation of cellular lipids and prostaglandin production in MDCK cells. *Nature* 276: 274 - 275.

Luepke, N.P., 1985, Hen's egg chorioallantoic membrane test for irritation potential. *Fd. Chem. Toxic.* 23: 287 - 291.

Marks, R., and Kingston, T., 1985, Acute skin toxicity reactions in man - tests and mechanism. *Fd. Chem. Toxic.* 23: 155 - 163.

Martin, Cl.G., 1993, Qualification of EYTEX^{R} data: user's guide. *ATLA* 21: 239 - 259.

Müller-Decker, K., Fürstenberger, G., and Marks, F., 1992, Development of an in vitro alternative assay to the Draize skin irritancy test using human keratinocyte-derived proinflammatory key mediators and cell viability as test parameters. *In Vitro Toxic.* 5: 191 - 209.

Price, J.B., and Anders, I.J., 1985, The in vitro assessment of eye irritancy using isolated eyes. *Fd. Chem. Toxic.* 23: 1313 - 1315.

Regnier, J.-F., Imbert, Ch., and Boutonnet, J.-Ch., 1994, Evaluation of the EYTEX[R] system as a screening method for the ocular irritancy of chemical products. *ATLA* 22: 32 - 50.

Riddell, R.J., Clothier, R.H., and Balls, M., 1986, An evaluation of three in vitro cytotoxicity assays. *Fd. Chem. Toxic.* 24: 469 - 471.

Sharpe, R., 1985, The Draize test: motivations forchange. *Fd. Chem. Toxic.* 23: 139-143.

Stark, D. M., Shopsis, C., Borenfreund, E., and Walberg, I., 1983, Alternative approaches to the Draize assay: Chemotaxis cytology, differentiation, and membrane transport studies. *in:* Alternative Methods in Toxicology Vol.1: Product Safety Evaluation, A. M. Goldberg, ed., Mary Ann Liebert, New York, pp. 179 - 203.

Swanston, D.W., 1985, Assessment of the validity of animal techniques in eye-irritation testing. *Fd. Chem. Toxic.* 23: 169 - 173.

CYTOTOXIC EFFECTS OF ANTIFUNGAL DRUGS
ON CULTURED HUMAN CONJUNCTIVAL CELLS

Nobuo Takahashi[1,2], Teiichiroh Murayama[2], Minoru Miyakoshi[1], and
Takayuki Kurihara[1]

Medical Research Institute[1], Department of Ophthalmology[2],
Kanazawa Medical University, 1-1, Daigaku, Uchinada, Kahoku
Ishikawa, Japan

ABSTRACT

We evaluated the cytotoxicity of 3 antifungal drugs using cultured human conjunctival cells. Cell growth curve, electron microscopic appearance and analysis of DNA histograms were studied after 2 to 4 min exposures to the test solution. Amphotericin B inhibited cell growth dose-dependently. Amphotericin B from 50 µg/ml to 100 µg/ml revealed loss of microvilli and a remarkable decrease in cell population. Miconazole (10 mg/ml) destroyed the cells completely. Fluconazole, at a concentration usually used (1 mg/ml), did not cause inhibition of cell growth or damage to the cell surface. None of the drugs studied resulted in abnormal pattern on DNA histograms.

INTRODUCTION

A fungal infection on the ocular surface is hard to cure and the term of the disease is likely to be prolonged. Since the long-term instillation of antifungal drugs may cause cytotoxic effects on the ocular surface, we do not have any basic *in vitro* data on the cellular toxicity of the drug. In this study, we selected 3 drugs which are usually administered systemically and are sometimes prepared for ophthalmic solutions from parenteral preparations in order to elucidate some effects on cell physiology. The cell surface was examined by a scanning electron microscope and the cell cycle was evaluated by DNA histograms which were drawn by flow cytometry. The agent used in these experiments include amphotericin B, miconazole and fluconazole. Amphotericin B is a polyene antibiotic produced by streptomyces nodusus[1]. The antibiotic binds rapidly to susceptible sterols in fungal and mammalian membranes. It causes increased permeability of the cellular membranes and results in leakage of essential intracellular constituents[2]. It binds more avidly to ergosterol in the fungal membrane than in mammalian membranes.

Miconazole is a derivative of the imidazole compounds which interfere with the synthesis of ergosterol needed for the fungal membrane. It causes an accumulating surplus of

α-methylsterol and alters cell membrane permeabitity[3]. Since the fluidity of fungal cell membrane is maintained by ergosterol, ergosterol deficient membrane makes it difficult to keep cell function and structure.

Fluconazole is a synthetic antifungal agent of the triazole group[4,5] which inhibits demethylation of 24-methylene dihydroxylanosterol, a precursor of ergosterol in fungal membrane. This study was performed to find out if the agents produce the same effects on cultured human cells as on fungal cells.

MATERIALS AND METHODS

Chang's human conjunctival cells[6] with a population of 10^5/ml were cultured in Eagle's minimum essential medium supplemented with 10% fetal calf serum for 48hrs in 5% CO_2 in a 37°C incubator. Cell sheets were exposed to various concentrations of amphotericin B (Bristol-Myers Squibb Co., purity 100%), miconazole (Janssen Pharmaceutica Co., purity 100%), and fluconazole (Pfizer Pharmaceuticals Inc. Co., purity 100%) for 2 or 4 min. Test drug concentrations were adjusted to clinical use. Cells were prepared, immediately after exposure to the test solutions, for scanning electron microscopy and flow cytometry or cultured for a further 24 hrs to examine cell growth.

To prepare scanning electron microscopic specimens, the cells were fixed in 2.5% glutaraldehyde for 30 min and in 1% osmium tetraoxide for 30 min. After dehydration with serial ethanol, the cells were treated with the carbon dioxide critical point drying technique followed by a gold-platinum coating in vacuum evaporation[7,8] and examined by a scanning electron microscope (Japan Electric Co., Model TSM 840).

To get DNA histograms, after separating by tripsinization, cells were fixed with 20% ethanol. They were treated with 0.25% ribonuclease for 1 hr followed by the staining of intranuclear DNA with 0.005% propidium iodide. DNA histograms were drawn by flow cytometry (Cytofluorograf 50H, Ortho Co.) followed by cell cycle analysis[9].

RESULTS

Amphotericin B

Cell growth was inhibited dose-dependently after exposure to the test solutions with concentrations from 10 µg/ml to 100 µg/ml (Fig. 1). Fig. 2 shows a normal cell surface as a control. Four min exposure to 50 µg/ml of the drug caused a decrease in cell population of 20% and a partial loss of microvilli (Fig. 3). Flow cytometry did not reveal any abnormal DNA histograms (Fig. 4).

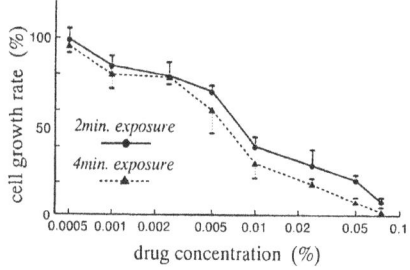

Fig. 1.Cell growth curve of amphotericin B.

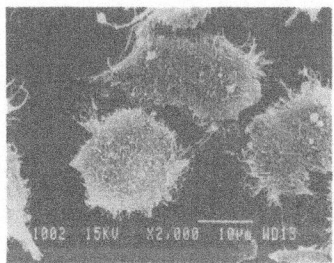

Fig. 2. Normal microscopic appearance of cells (control).

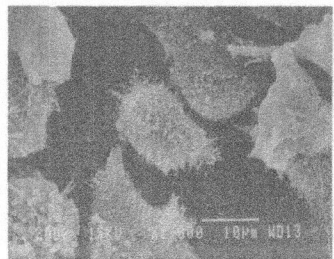

Fig. 3. Scanning electron microscopic finding after exposure for 4 min to 50 μg/ml of amphotericin B.

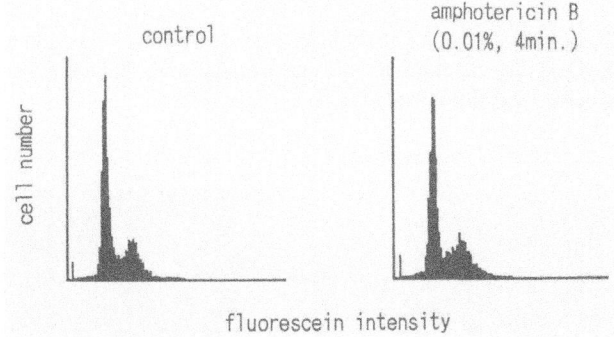

Fig. 4. DNA histogram after exposure for 4 min to 100 μg/ml of amphotericin B. No abnormal pattern.

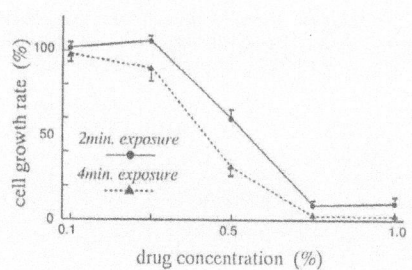

Fig. 5. Cell growth curve, miconazole.

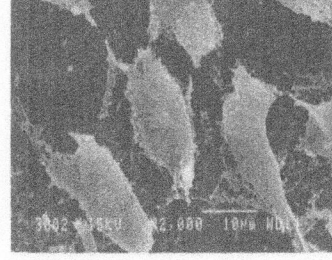

Fig. 6. Scanning electron microscopic finding. Miconazole (10 mg/ml) caused loss of microvilli and filopodia and a lot of small holes formation.

Miconazole

Cell growth was suppressed dose-dependently by 4-min exposure to the drug solutions (Fig. 5). The cells were completely destroyed, lost almost all microvilli and filopodia

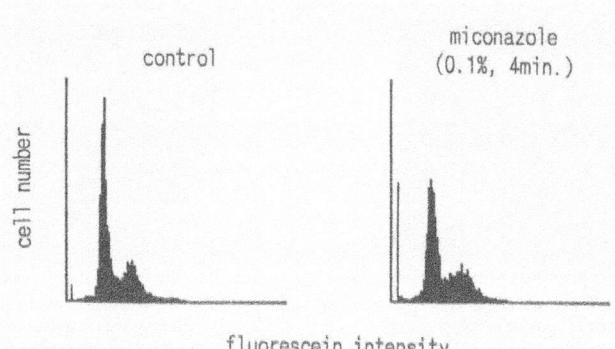

Fig. 7. DNA histogram after exposure to miconazole (1 mg/ml). No abnormal pattern.

and numerous small holes formed on the cell surface after 4-min exposure to a 10 mg/ml drug solution (Fig. 6). The exposure of cells to a 1 mg/ml drug solution did not result in any abnormality in the DNA histograms (Fig. 7).

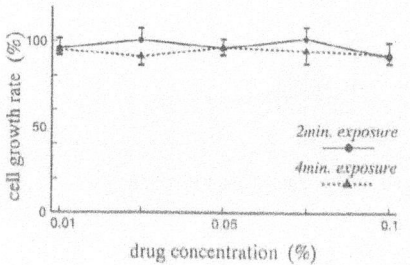

Fig. 8. Cell growth curve, fluconazole (1 mg/ml).

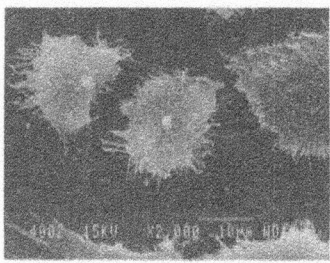

Fig. 9. Scanning electron microscopic finding. No abnormal appearance is seen after exposure for 4 min to fluconazole (1 mg/ml).

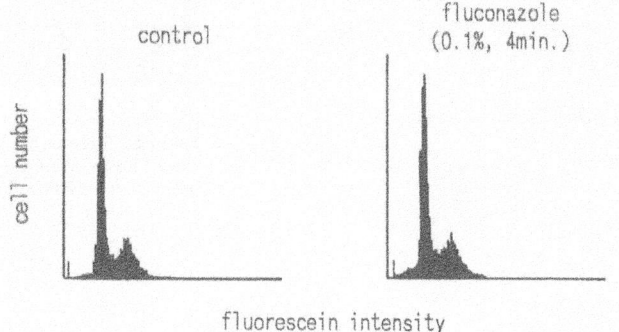

Fig. 10. DNA histogram after exposure for 4 min to fluconazole (1 mg/ml).

Fluconazole

Four-min exposure with the highest concentration (1 mg/ml) did not inhibit cell growth (Fig. 8), damage the cell surface (Fig. 9) or cause any abnormal pattern in the DNA histogram (Fig. 10).

DISCUSSION

It has been reported that continuous topical appliation of 10 mg/ml amphotericin B causes a progressive worsening of corneal epithelial defects and stromal opacities[2]. In this study, it is clear that even 4-min exposure to 100 μg/ml amphotericin B severely damages cell growth and the cell surface. Since 0.05 to 0.15% amphotericin B is topically used[10], there is a high possibility that drug side effects will occur in human eyes. The topical application of miconazole (10 mg/ml) has been reported to be relatively well tolerated by the conjunctiva and the cornea[10]. However, in this study, miconazole (10 mg/ml) completely destroyed the cells. Less than 1 mg/ml of miconazole is recommended when topically applied. The exposure to fluconazole (1 mg/ml) did not result in the inhibition of cell growth or damage to the cell surface and did not delay cell cycle progression. Toxic effects of many kinds of topical agents have been revealed after they had been clinically used. The fact demonstrates low sensitivity of *in vivo* experiments. Because cell culture assay has higher sensitivity compared to tissues, it may predict drug cytotoxicity. In this study, we got precise toxic parameters for antifungal drugs which have not been elucidated in *in vivo* experiments. These experimental procedures should be applied as a matter of course to evaluate the cytotoxicity of topical agents.

References

1. American Medical Association: Amphotericin B *in* : Drug Evaluations, 6th. ed., W.B. SAUNDERS CO., Philadelphia (1986)
2. Havener, W.H.: Antibiotics *in* : Ocular pharmacology, 5th. ed., The C.V. Mosby CO., St Louis (1983)
3. American Medical Association : Miconazole *in* : Drug Evaluations, 6th. ed., W.B. SAUNDERS CO. Philadelphia (1986)
4. Richardson, K., Brammer, K.W., Marriott, M.S., Troke, P.F.: Activity of UK-49858, a bis-triazole derivative, against experimental infections with Candida albicans and Trichophyton metagrophytes. *Antimicr. Agent & Chemother.* 27: 832-835 (1982)
5. Odds, F.C., Chessman, S.L., Abbott, A.B.: Antifungal effects of fluconazole (UK-49858), a new triazole antifungal, in vitro. *J. Antimicr. Chemother.* 18: 473-478 (1986)
6. Chang, R.S.: Continuous subcultivation of epithelial-like cells from normal human tissue. *Proc. Soc. exp. Biol. Med.* 87: 440-443 (1954)
7. Takahashi, N., Mukai, Y., Nakaizumi, H., Sasaki, K.: An Evaluation of the cytotoxicity of ophthalmic solutions in cell culture: aminoglycosides and dexamethasone sodium phosphate *in* : Concepts Toxicol. 4, Drug-Induced Ocular Side Effects and Ocular Toxicology, Karger, Basel (1987)
8. Anderson, T.E.: Techniques for preparation of 3-dimentional structure in preparing specimens for electron microscopy. *Trans. N.Y. Acad. Sci.* 13: 130-134 (1951)
9. Takahashi, N., Fujikawa, K., Miyakoshi, M., Teraoka, K., Taniuchi, K.: Flow cytometric study of effects of benzalkonium chloride on the cell cycle. *J. Jpn. ophthalmol. Soc.* 96: 823-827 (1992)
10. Liesegang, T.J.: Bacterial and fungal keratitis *in* : The Cornea, edited by Kaufman, H.E. McDonald, M.B., Barron, B.A., Waltman, S.R., Churchill Livingstone, New York (1988)

CHARACTERIZATION OF SIALOMUCINS EXPRESSED BY HUMAN CONJUNCTIVAL GOBLET CELLS

W. Naib-Majani[1], W. Breipohl[1], U. Sterzinsky[1], and M. Takeda[2]

[1]Department of Experimental Ophthalmology, University of Bonn,
D-53105 Bonn, Germany
[2]Department of Oral Anatomy II, School of Dentistry
Higashi Nippon-Gakuen-University
Hokkaido 061, Japan

INTRODUCTION

Tear sialomucins are of prime importance for the wettening of the cornea. So far their production almost unanimously has been allocated by other authors to the conjunctival goblet cells. However, two major bodies of findings led us to question the prime importance of conjunctival goblet cells for an appropriate tear attachment to the corneal surface[1]. First, and according to other authors, Dry Eye syndromes are not always associated with a marked reduction of conjunctival goblet cells[2]. Second, own previous lectin-histochemical investigations on the main and accessory lacrimal glands have documented considerable glycoprotein expression, amongst them different types of sialomucins, also in these organs[3-5]. In addition, electrophoretic analyses revealed different sialomucins in human tears[6,7].

Thus the question to be addressed in this study was, whether a lectin histochemical study on human conjunctival goblet cells could help to explain the discrepancy regarding the assumed key importance of goblet cells for tear sialomucins and the lack of numerical goblet cell reduction in some Dry Eye patients.

MATERIALS AND METHODS

Remains of cadaveric human conjunctiva (maximum 36 hours after death) were fixed in formalin and Bouin's solutions respectively. The paraffin embedded material was cut serially and systematically screened for the presence of mucosa and goblet cells by counterstaining with hematoxylin and eosin. Parallel sections were treated with a panel of six FITC labeled lectins (30 μg/ml over night) identifying and discriminating glycoproteins with regard to their terminal bound neuraminic acid (Table 1). Lectins applied included *Triticum vulgare* (wheat germ agglutin) (**WGA**), *succinylated Triticum vulgare* (**sWGA**), *Limax flavus* (**LFA**), *Limulus polyphemus* (**LPA**), *Maackia amurensis* (**MAA**), and *Sambucus nigra* (**SNA**).

Table 1. Survey on applied lectins, including their origin and the specific carbohydrate moieties identified by them.

GROUP	LECTIN	ORGIN	SUGAR SPECIFITIY
	WGA	Tritium vulgare	(GlcNac-β1,4)$_3$ > (GlcNac-β1,4)$_2$ = GlcNac > NeuNAc
II			
	sWGA	Succinyl.-Tritium vulgare	(GlcNac-β1,4)$_3$ > (GlcNac-β1,4)$_2$ = GlcNac
	LFA	Limax flavus	Neu5Ac > Neu5Gc
	LPA	Limulus polyphemus	Neu5Gc-α2,3 GalNAc > Neu5Ac-α2,6 GalNAc > Neu5Ac = Neu5Gc
V			
	MAA	Maackia amurensis	NeuNAc-α2,3 Gal
	SNA	Sambucus nigra	NeuNAc-α2,6 Gal = NeuNAc-α2,6 GalNAc

Table 2. Affinity of human conjunctival goblet cells to selected group II and V lectins.

LECTIN	CONJUNCTIVAL GOBLET CELLS
WGA	+++
sWGA	-/+
LFA	++
LPA	-
MAA	++/+++
SNA	-

Legend: -, +, ++, +++ = no, moderate (week), strong, and very strong affinity.

Controls included: i) section pretreatment with *Vibrio cholerae* neuraminidase for the specificity of LFA reactivity (indicating strong general sialomucin expression), ii) section pretreatment with *Newcastle disease virus* to check for the specificity of MAA binding (indicating sialomucins characterized by 2,3 bound sialic acid), iii) lectin pretreatment with

Fetuin (a bovine embryonic glycoprotein especially rich in terminal sialic acid) to check for the specifity of sialic acid receptor reactions of LFA and MAA lectins.

RESULTS

The obtained results are specific for glycoproteins, as glycolipids were washed out during the histological treatment and thus have not to be considered here any further. The overall results on lectin affinity to the human conjunctival goblet cells are summarized in Table 2. As documented there, lectin staining was observed with all but LPA and SNA.

A more sophisticated differentiation on the lectin affinity of human conjunctival cells reveals the following. Reactions with group II lectins were highly different. With **WGA** the strongest staining results could be obtained for the goblet cells. These did not stain evenly, but the diameter of the goblet cells seen in the actual plane of the section had no influence on the staining intensity. In other words, goblet cells with the largest diameters did not necessarily stain most intensively. Affinity of WGA with the other epithelial cells was faint though more pronounced than with the subepithelial mucosal components (Figure 1a). In contrast to WGA, affinity with **sWGA** was moderate to absent for the conjunctival goblet and the other epithelial cells, but strongly for the subepithelial conjunctival cells (Figure 1b). Experiments with group V lectins allowed for a further differentiation of sialomucin expression in human conjunctival cells. **LFA** affinity was strong and almost even for all goblet cells, regardless of their diameters. Only rarely some weeker or stronger zones of fluorescence could be seen within the mucous compartment of a given goblet cell. Weak to absent reactivity was seen for the other epithelial and subepithelial cells (Figure 1c).

LPA affinity was not observed for the conjunctival goblet cells. Conjunctival basal cells revealed some reactivity in their perinuclear (presumably nuclear membrane) region (Figure 1d). **MAA** affinity to human conjunctival goblet cells was strong to very strong (Figure 2a). Non-goblet epithelial cells had no or only a week affinity, while the sub-epithelial cells reacted moderate to strong. No affinity of human conjunctival goblet cells could be observed for **SNA** (Figure 2b). The other epithelial cells showed no or only a week affinity to SNA. Occasionally, a week reactivity was restricted to the perinuclear (presumably nuclear membrane) region of the non-goblet epithelial cells. Subepithelial conjunctival cells showed an overall moderate to strong affinity to SNA (Figure 2b).

Neuraminidase (from *Vibrio cholerae)* pretreatment of the sections prior to LFA incubation prevented lectin binding (Figure 3a). Pretreatment of LFA with Fetuin almost abolished the lectin binding to the goblet cells (Figure 3b). Neuraminidase (from *Newcastle disease virus*) pretreatment of the sections prior to MAA incubation almost prevented MAA binding to the goblet cells (Figure 3c). The same results occurred after preincubation of MAA with Fetuin (Figure 3d).

DISCUSSIONS

This study, the first in a series of investigations on goblet cells in different locations, has revealed overall differences in glycoprotein expression of human conjunctival goblet cells and especially sophisticated differences in their sialomucin expression. The obtained data are in accordance with statements in the literature that tear mucins are preferentially produced by the conjunctival goblet cells[8]. However, the above data appear to contradict reports in the literature which assume a sole production of tear sialomucins by the conjunctival goblet cells.

While none of the applied lectins showed a strong affinity to non-goblet conjunctival epithelial cells, the experiments with WGA (affinity to glycoproteins with terminal gluco-

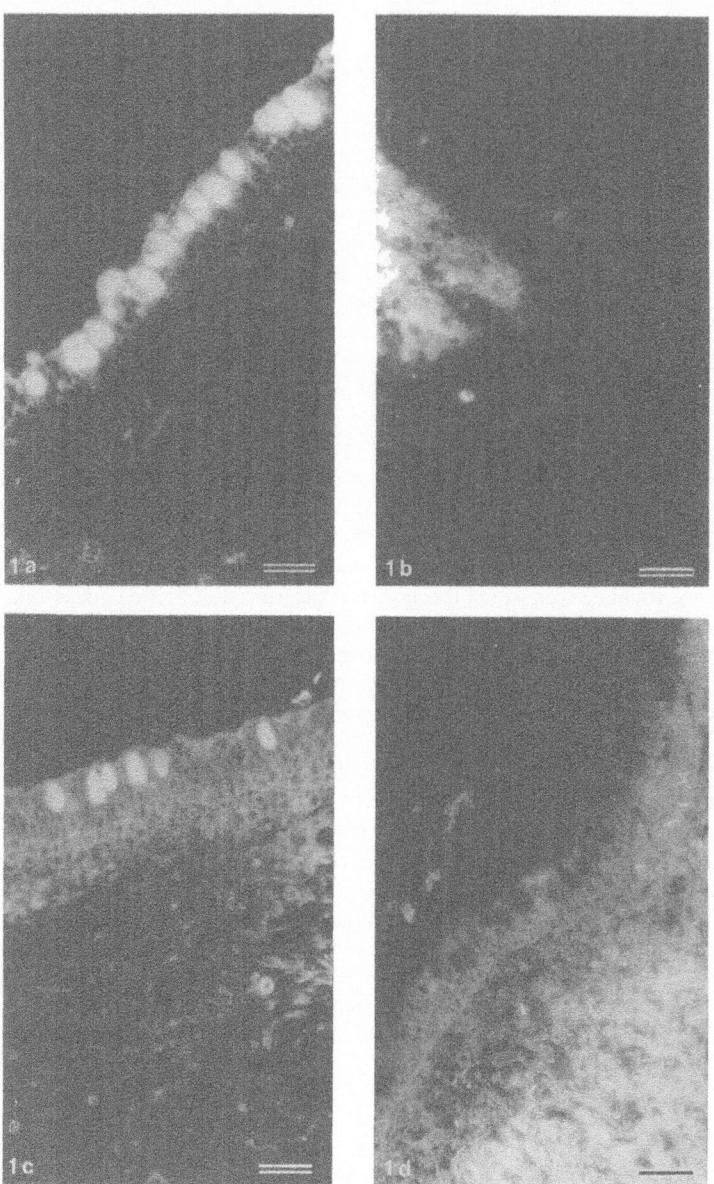

Figure 1. Human conjunctival mucosa following reaction with FITC labeled lectins. 1a) Reaction with WGA. Strong to very strong affinity to goblet cells. Weak reaction with other epithelial cells. Almost no reaction with subepithelial cells. 1b) Reaction with sWGA. Moderate to absent affinity to goblet and other epithelial cells, while the subepithelial cells often stain strongly. 1c) Reaction with LFA. Strong affinity to goblet cells. Weak to absent reaction with other epithelial and subepithelial cells. 1d) Reaction with LPA. No affinity to goblet cells. As for LFA, basal epithelial cells revealed some reactivity in their perinuclear (presumably nuclear membrane) region. Subepithelial cells stained week to strong or very strong. Bar equals 50μm.

272

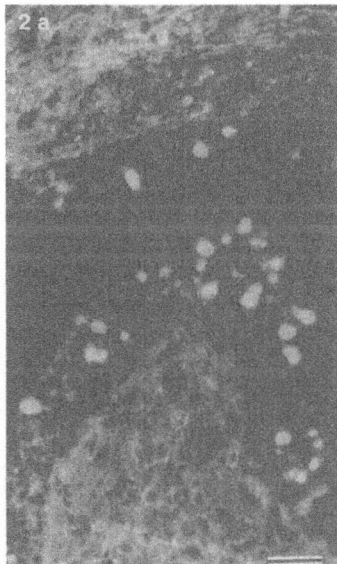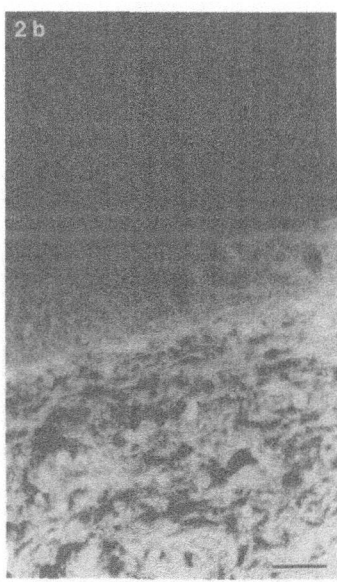

Figure 2. Human conjunctival mucosa following reaction with FITC labeled lectins. 2a) Reaction with MAA. Strong to very strong affinity to goblet cells. No or moderate reaction with other epithelial and subepithelial cells. 2b) Reaction with SNA. No affinity to goblet cells. Only occasional moderate reaction with other epithelial but up to strong reaction with subepithelial cells. Bar equals $50 \mu m$.

samine and neuraminic acid) versus sWGA (affinity to glycoproteins with terminal glucosamine but not neuraminic acid residues), and the results with LFA and MAA revealed sialomucin production in the goblet cells. This is in agreement with the demonstration of sialic acid in human tear fluid and WGA positivity of tear proteins reported by others[7,9,10]. The strong reaction of conjunctival goblet cells with MAA is indicative of an abundance of 2,3 sialic acid residues, while 2,6 residues (lack of reaction with SNA) are apparently absent.

A few reports of others and ourselves are in support of sialomucins being produced not only in conjunctival goblet cells but also in the main and accessory lacrimal gland cells [4,5,11,12] and thus question further the unique importance of conjunctival goblet cell borne sialomucins with regard to proper corneal tear attachment[1].

Parallel to the above investigations we documented MAA and SNA positive sialomucins in the tears[6]. While the latter could corroborate with the presence of lacrimal gland cell produced lactoferrin[13], the former could reflect both, goblet cell produced sialomucins and the presence of tear IgA and its components[6,14,15]. MAA and SNA positivity of human tear glycoproteins could also result from specific proteins produced in the accessory lacrimal gland[4]. Additional but yet unpublished data of our group indicate that tears contain minimal amounts of LPA positive sialomucins, which according to the present study, are not expressed in the conjunctival goblet cells either. Alltogether then these data contradict the assumption of a sole responsibility of conjunctival goblet cells for tear sialomucin production.

The differences in human conjunctival goblet cell group V lectin affinity are of special interest. While LFA results do not differentiate between goblet cells of different activity discrimination appears possible on the basis of the WGA and MAA results. With WGA some goblet cells labeled especially strong. Differences in WGA affinity were never linked

273

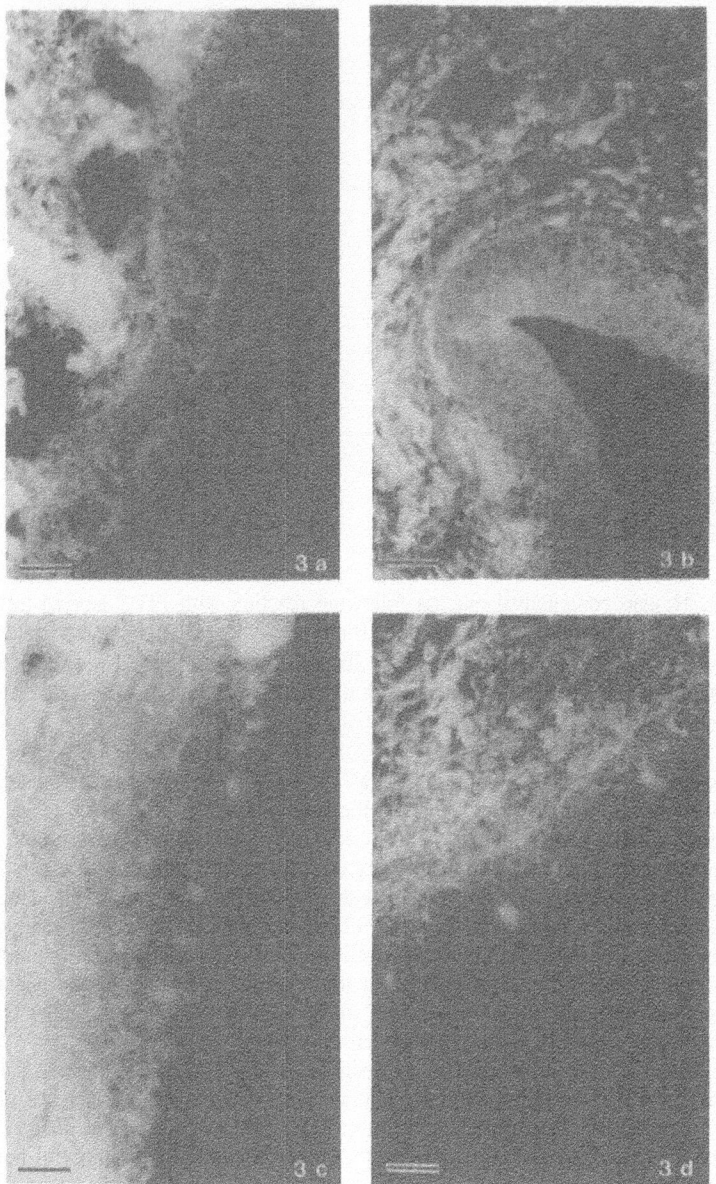

Figure 3. Human conjunctival mucosa following reaction with FITC labeled lectins. Controls. Pretreatment with neuraminidases of sections (3a *Vibrio cholerae* prior to LFA incubation, 3c *Newcastle disease virus* prior to MAA incubation) and preincubation of lectins with Fetuin[17] (3b with LFA, 3d with MAA) reduced or abolished the labeling results. Bar equals 50μm.

to the size of the goblet cell diameters in the plane of section. In contrast, MAA positivity appeared to be especially strong with those goblet cells which were largest in the plane of section. Thus MAA positivity might reflect the mass of mucous preserved in the plane of section, while WGA, in contrast, might differentiate between different goblet cells according to the quality (maturity) of mucous. This hypothesis, however, needs additional experimental clarification. The above date on neuraminidase reduction of lectin affinity are in accordance with investigations demonstrating a very strong though incomplete abolishment of lectin binding[16].

CONCLUSIONS

Taken together, the obtained data suggest expression of some but not all tear sialomucins by the human conjunctival goblet cells. The MAA data together with WGA versus sWGA and LFA suggest preferential expression of sialomucins with 2,3 terminal bound sialic acid in human conjunctival goblet cells. Comparing the obtained results with own previous reports one can assume differences in the type of sialomucins produced in human conjunctival goblet, main and accessory lacrimal gland cells. The findings further suggest variation between goblet cells regarding their sialomucin producing activity.

The conflicting results on goblet cell reduction and Dry Eye symptoms[2] could mean, that reduction of goblet cell numbers could eventually be overcome by a stimulation of the sialomucin production in the remaining cells. Together with previous reports, suggesting a tear sialomucin production also in other sources than conjunctival goblet cells, this study supports the hypothesis of a variety of Dry Eye syndromes, caused by impairments in the specific spectrum of sialomucin production. Thus different Dry Eye syndromes could re-sult from a different involvement of conjunctival goblet, main and accessory lacrimal gland cells, and one day might be classified by a sophisticated lectin diagnostic of tears. It might even become possible in the future to compose and prescribe patient related or Dry eye type specific articifial tears.

Definitely the data is requesting the extention of tear analyses of different groups of patients by additional neuraminic acid specific lectins in conjunction with specific neuraminidase controls. The above described investigations and efforts must also be complemented in future by studies on the respective corneal sialomucin type receptors. It is postulated that this way a fingerprint like typization of Dry Eye patients in individuals could be achieved.

ACKNOWLEDGEMENTS

This study, the first in a series of light and electron microscopic histochemical investigations on goblet cells in different species and locations, was in part supported by a Japanese Society for the Promotion of Science, fellowship granted to W.B.

REFERENCES

1. F.J. Holly and M.A. Lemp, Wettability and wetting of corneal epithelium, Exp. Eye Res. 11:239-250 (1971).
2. S.K. Kinoshita, T.C. Kiorpes, and J. Friend, R.A. Thoft, Goblet cell density in ocular surface disease, Arch. Ophthal. (Chicago) 101:1284-1287 (1983).
3. W. Breipohl, M. Spitznas, F. Sinowatz, O. Leip, W. Naib-Majani, and A. Cusumano, Galactose-binding sites in the acinar cells of the human accessory lacrimal gland, In: Lacrimal gland, tear film and dry eye syndromes, D. Sullivan, ed., Plenum, New York - London, pp 45 - 48 (1994).
4. W. Breipohl, W. Naib-Majani, F. Sinowatz, T. Naguro, and A. Wegener, Sialomucin expression in the human accessory lacrimal gland, In: Sjögrens Syndrome. State of the Art, M. Homma M. et al., eds, Kugler, Amsterdam - New York, pp 553 - 557 (1994).
5. W. Breipohl, W. Naib-Majani, and U. Sterzinsky, Classification of glycoprotein expression in human conjunctival, main and accessory tear gland cells, Invest. Ophthalmol. Vis. Sc. 35:1795 (1994).

6. W. Breipohl, C. Reitz, M.H.J. Ahrend, F.H. Grus, and J. Bours, Characterization of human tear glycoproteins by Phast electrophoresis, western blotting and lectin binding, This Volume.

7. A. Kuizenga, N.J. van Haeringen, and A. Kijlstra, Identification of lectin binding proteins in human tears, Invest. Ophthalmol. Vis. Sci. 32:3277-3284 (1991).

8. L. Hazlett, D. Dudzik, and B. Harries, Development of ocular mucin: scanning EM analysis, Ophthalmic Res. 18:28-33 (1986).

9. K. Bjerrum, P. Halken, and J.U. Prause, The normal tear glycoprotein profile detected with lectin probes, Exp. Eye Res. 53:431-435 (1991).

10. A. Kuizenga, E.J. van Agtmaal, N.J. van Haeringen, and A. Kijlstra, Sialic acid in human tear fluid, Exp. Eye Res. 50:45-50 (1990).

11. O.A. Jensen, I. Falbe-Hansen, T. Jacobsen, and A. Michelsen, Mucosubstances of the acini of the human lacrimal gland (orbital part). I. Histochemical identification, Acta Ophthalmol. 47:605-619 (1969).

12. I. Falbe-Hansen, O.A. Jensen, and D.J. Karossa, Mucosubstances of the acini of the human lacrimal gland (orbital part). II. Biochemical identification, Acta Ophthalmol. 47:620-627 (1969).

13. G. Spik, G. Strecker, B. Fournet, and S.B. Montreuil, Primary structure of the glycans from human lactotransferrin, Europ. J. Biochem. 121:413-419 (1982).

14. A.T. Sapse, B. Bonavida, W. Stone jr., and E.E. Sercarz, Proteins in human tears, Arch. Ophthal. 81:815-819 (1969).

15. A. Kuizenga, Identification and characterization of proteins in human tear fluid, Academisch Proefschrift, Amsterdam, (1992).

16. A. Kluge, G. Reuter, H. Lee, B. Ruch-Heeger, and R. Schauer, Interaction of rat peritoneal macrophages with homologous sialidase-treated thrombocytes in vitro: biochemical and morphological studies. Detection of N-(O-acetyl)glycoloylneuraminic acid, Europ. J. Cell Biol. 59:12-20 (1992).

17. R.L. Miller, A sialic acid-specific lectin from the slug *Limax flavus*, J. Invertebrate Path. 39:210-214 (1982).

CRITICAL EVALUATION OF THE EVIDENCE FOR AN ASSOCIATION BETWEEN OCULAR DISEASE AND EXPOSURE TO ORGANOPHOSPHORUS COMPOUNDS

Michael D. Stonard,[1] Peter H. Berry,[2] Sandra J. Kennedy,[3] George J. Krinke,[4] Derek A. Stringer,[5] and Ingo Weisse[6]

[1]Zeneca Central Toxicology Laboratory, Alderley Park, Nr. Macclesfield, Cheshire, SK10 4TJ, England
[2]Smith, Kline and Beecham, The Frythe, Welwyn, Herts, AL6 9AR, England
[3]Unilever Research, Sharnbrook, Bedford, MK44 ALQ, England
[4]Ciba Geigy AG, CH-4002, Basel, Switzerland
[5]European Centre for Ecotoxicology and Toxicology of Chemicals, B-1160 Brussels, Belgium
[6]Boehringer Ingelheim KG, D-552A8, Ingelheim/Rh., Germany

INTRODUCTION

The ECETOC Task Force carried out a critical evaluation of the evidence for an association between ocular disease and exposure to organophosphorus compounds (OPs).

Acute Syndrome

Organophosphorus compounds have been used safely for many years as crop protection chemicals, primarily because of their effectiveness against a wide range of insects. However, examples of toxicity, including to the eye, have been described. In humans, the appearance of ocular signs and symptoms eg. blurred vision, miosis, palpebral tremor and ciliary muscle spasm immediately after systemic absorption of many OPs is well documented (Murphy, 1986). For the most part, the biological effects of the acute exposure to OPs in humans can be induced in a range of animal species and these effects are considered attributable to inhibition of acetylcholinesterase (AChE), at cholinergic receptor sites within the eye.

Intermediate Syndrome

Subsequent to the acute cholinergic manifestations of OP toxicity in humans, and approximately 24-96 hours after exposure, the onset of an "intermediate syndrome" which includes ocular effects has been recognised more recently for some OPs (Senanayake and Karalliedde, 1987; Karademir *et al.*, 1990). The associated clinical signs, which are characteristically different from those seen in OP-induced delayed polyneuropathy, are paralysis and weakness of proximal limbs, respiratory, neck and cranial muscles, including those innervated by the oculomotor nerve. The occurrence of myopathy in rats exposed to diisopropylfluorophosphate, paraoxon or soman (Wecker *et al.*, 1978; Vanneste and Lison, 1993) resembled the features of the "intermediate syndrome". The severity and duration of the myopathy in rats appeared directly related to the degree of inhibition of AChE.

Long Term Effects

Prolonged exposure to OPs has been suspected to have a causal relationship to the entity known as "Saku Disease" in Japan (Ishikawa, 1973; Ishikawa and Miyata, 1980; Dementi, 1994). The major ocular signs of this disease entity are reduced vision, a narrowing of the peripheral visual field and/or central scotoma and abnormal refraction or myopic tendency with or without vertical corneal astigmatism. The epidemiological feature of the disease is characterised by its restriction to a fraction of the Japanese population and to certain geographical regions only. The difficulty in defining "Saku Disease" led the Japanese Ministry of Public Welfare to list the diagnostic criteria for which at least five out of the eight must be present to be considered compatible with diagnosing the disease (Plestina and Piukovic-Plestina, 1978). The major OPs used in Japan up to the early 1970s included malathion, 0-ethyl-0-P nitrophenyl benzenphosphorothioate (EPN), ethyl parathion and methylparathion. These were replaced by fenthion, dipterex, fenitrothion and diazinon as the latter group was considered to be less toxic to humans. All of these OPs have been implicated with the development of "Saku Disease" (Ishikawa and Miyata, 1980).

The findings of visual impairment in humans allegedly attributable to chronic exposure to OPs have prompted the development of animal models for studying the ocular effects of OPs and elucidating the mechanism of action. Repeat dose studies in dogs with either fenitrothion or disulfoton have shown that degeneration of ciliary muscle was obviously related to myopia (Tokoro *et al.*, 1973; Suzuki and Ishikawa, 1974; Ishikawa and Miyata, 1980). Also, a reduction in AChE activity and the occurrence of degeneration in extraocular muscle of dogs treated with disulfoton resembled findings in humans (Mukuno and Imai, 1973). Retinal pigment degeneration reported in humans was also paralleled by similar retinal findings in dogs or rats treated with disulfoton, fenthion or parathion (Uga *et al.*, 1976; Imai, 1977; Miyata *et al.*, 1979; Uga *et al.*, 1979). Likewise, the electroretinographic defects reported in humans have been reproduced in some but not all strains of rats (Miyata *et al.*, 1979; Uga *et al.*, 1979; Imai *et al.*, 1983). Recently, in two year rat carcinogenicity bioassays with fenthion and tribufos (DEF), chronic ocular effects have been observed. Dietary exposure to these compounds was associated with retinal changes and with an increased incidence of corneal dystrophy and cataract with uveitis in one or both sexes (Stuart, 1992).

EVALUATION

Although the pathogenesis of "Saku Disease" has not been delineated in detail, there is no reason to presume that mechanisms other than AChE inhibition are involved as appears to occur following acute exposure and in the "intermediate syndrome". It has been suggested, however, that chronic AChE inhibition alone does not explain all of the ocular changes and that other mechanisms may be involved (Boyes *et al.*, 1994). If the development of "Saku Disease" occurs by a mechanism not involving direct inhibition of AChE, then it is not via OP-induced delayed polyneuropathy as there is only limited overlap between the two groups of chemicals (Lotti, 1992). Reports of electroretinographic changes at levels of OP exposure below those which inhibit brain and retinal AChE must be corroborated, as the findings could reflect a low sensitivity of the AChE assay, or alternatively, erroneous findings arising from the variability inherent in the technique of electroretinography. Obviously, more fundamental research is needed before any conclusive statements on other possible mechanisms for ocular effects of OPs can be made.

Changes observed in chronic rat studies may reflect for the most part species-specific senile changes which are not relevant to the human situation or they may reflect possible chronic dysfunction of ocular structures which are innervated through cholinergic pathways, eg. changes in the secretory activity of the Harderian and lacrimal glands. The adnexa have a secretory function, a failure of which may facilitate the development of secondary lesions in the eye. An interference with, or exacerbation of spontaneous, age-related changes in chronic rodent studies may confound the interpretation of treatment-related effects and therefore the rat is considered not to be a suitable model for chronic human exposure. In the absence of information on the structure-activity relationships or mechanism of action for the ocular toxicity arising from exposure to OPs, it is not possible to determine whether the dog or rat is the more relevant species.

CONCLUSION

The publication of a proposed regulatory protocol, targetted at the determination of the potential ocular effects of OPs, appears unduly premature (Hamernik, 1994). This is well illustrated by the findings from a recent study using a protocol similar to that proposed by the US-EPA in which repeat oral dosing of dogs with ethyl parathion produced no functional or histopathological changes indicative of ocular toxicity (Atkinson *et al.*, 1994). A practical testing strategy is required which has the potential to identify and characterise ocular toxicity produced by all chemicals in appropriate test systems. This is the subject of the next paper in this publication (Kennedy *et al.*, 1994).

REFERENCES

Atkinson, J.E., Bolte, L.F., Rubin, L.F. and Sonawane, M., 1994, Assessment of ocular toxicity in dogs during 6 months exposure to a potent organophosphate. *J. Appl. Toxicol.* 14:145.

Boyes, W.K., Tandon, P., Barone, S. and Padilla, S., 1994, Effects of organophosphates on the visual system of rats. *J. Appl. Toxicol.* 14:135.

Dementi, B., 1994, Ocular effects of organophosphates : a historical perspective of Saku disease. *J. Appl. Toxicol.* 14:119.

Hamernik, K.L., 1994, Proposed protocols for the determination of potential ocular effects of organophosphorus pesticides. *J. Appl. Toxicol.* 14:131.

Imai, I., 1977, Experimental retinal degeneration due to organophosphorus agents. *Acta Soc. Ophthal. Jap.* 81:925.

Imai, H., Miyata, M., Uga, S. and Ishikawa, S., 1983, Retinal degeneration in rats exposed to an organophosphate pesticide (fenthion). *Env. Res.* 30:453.

Ishikawa, S., 1973. Chronic optico-neuropathy due to environmental exposure of organophosphate pesticides (Saku disease) - clinical and experimental study. *Nippon Ganka Gakkai Sasshi.* 77:1835.

Ishikawa, S. and Miyata, M., 1980, Development of myopia following chronic organophosphate pesticide intoxication: an epidemiological and experimental study, in: "Neurotoxicity of the Visual System," W. Merigan and B. Weiss, eds., Raven Press, New York.

Karademir, M., Erturk, F. and Kocak, R., 1990, Two cases of organophosphate poisoning with development of intermediate syndrome. *Human Exper. Toxicol.* 9:187.

Kennedy, S., Berry, P., Krinke, G.J., Stonard, M.D., Stringer, D.A. and Weisse, J., 1995, A practical testing strategy for the evaluation of the oculotoxic potential of chemicals, in: Proceedings of the 4th Congress of the International Society of Ocular Toxicology, I. Weisse, O. Hockwin, K. Green, R.C. Tripathi, eds., Plenum Publishing Corporation, New York.

Lotti, M., 1992, The pathogenesis of organophosphate polyneuropathy. *Crit. Rev. Toxicol.* 21:466.

Miyata, M., Imai, H. and Ishikawa, S., 1979, Experimental retinal pigmentary degeneration by organophosphorus pesticides in rats. *Excerpta Med. Int. Cong. Ser. 450. 1. Ophthalmology* :901

Mukuno, K. and Imai, H., 1973, Histological research on dogs given long term administration of organophosphorus pesticides - especially the changes in the extraocular muscles. *Nippon Ganka Gakkai Sasshi* 77:1246.

Murphy, S.D., 1986, Toxic effects of pesticides, in: "Toxicology. The Basic Science of Poisons." 3rd Edition, C.D. Klaassen, M.O. Amdur and J. Doull, eds, Macmillan, England.

Plestina, R. and Piukovic-Plestina, M., 1978, Effect of acetylcholinesterase pesticides on the eye and on vision. *Crit. Rev. Toxicol.* 6:1.

Senanayake, N. and Karalliedde, L., 1987, Neurotoxic effects of organophosphorus insecticides. *New Eng. J. Med.* 316:761.

Stuart, B.P., 1992, Experiences with retinopathy in the F344 rat, in "A Histopathology Seminar on the Eye and Ear of Laboratory Animals," San Diego, California.

Suzuki, H. and Ishikawa, S., 1974, Ultrastructure of the ciliary muscle treated by organophosphate pesticide in beagle dogs. *Brit. J. Ophthal.* 59:931.

Tokoro, T., Suzuki, S., Nakano, H. and Otsuka, J., 1973, Experimental studies of organic phosphorus pesticide on beagle dog : long-term observations on the refraction and the intraocular pressure. *Acta Soc. Opthal. Jap.* 77:1237.

Uga, S., Ishikawa, S. and Mukuno, K., 1976, Microscopic changes in the retina of dogs administered organophosphorus pesticides for prolonged periods. *Jap. Rev. Clin. Ophthal.* 70:282.

Uga, S., Imai, H., Miyata, M. and Ishikawa, S., 1979, Retinal degeneration in Long-Evans rats induced by fenthion intoxication : an electron microscopic study. *Excerpta Med. Int. Cong. Ser. 450. I. Ophthalmology* :915.

Vanneste, Y. and Lison, D., 1993, Biochemical changes associated with muscle fibre necrosis after experimental organophosphate poisoning. *Human Exper. Toxicol.* 12:365.

Wecker, L., Laskowski, M.B. and Dettbarn, W.D., 1978, Neuromuscular dysfunction induced by acetylcholinesterase inhibition. *Fed. Proc.* 37:2818.

A PRACTICAL TESTING STRATEGY FOR THE EVALUATION OF THE OCULOTOXIC POTENTIAL OF CHEMICALS

Sandra J. Kennedy,[1] Peter H. Berry,[2] Georg J. Krinke,[3] Michael D. Stonard,[4] Derek A. Stringer,[5] and Ingo Weisse[6]

[1]Environmental Safety Laboratory, Unilever Research, Colworth House, Sharnbrook, Bedford, MK44 1LQ, England
[2]SmithKline Beecham Pharmaceuticals, The Frythe, Welwyn, Herts. AL6 9AR, England
[3]Ciba-Geigy AG, CH-4002 Basel, Switzerland
[4]Zeneca, Alderley Park, Nr. Macclesfield, Cheshire, SK10 4TJ, England
[5]European Centre for Ecotoxicology and Toxicology of Chemicals, B-1160 Brussels, Belgium
[6]Boehringer Ingelheim KG, D-55218 Ingelheim/Rh., Germany

INTRODUCTION

The ECETOC Task Force carried out a critical evaluation of the evidence for an association between ocular disease and exposure to organophosphorus compounds (OPs). This has been reported in the previous paper in this publication (Stonard et al., 1994). As a result of these deliberations a practical testing strategy was devised for the identification and characterisation of oculotoxicity in animal studies. The details of this strategy will now be described.

STRATEGY FOR TESTING FOR OCULOTOXICITY

The following testing strategy should apply equally to the testing of agrochemicals, food additives, industrial chemicals and pharmaceuticals, although testing of ophthalmic medicaments requires a specific approach. It involves the extension of existing guidelines to allow for the conduct of studies in such a way as to identify potential oculotoxicity. The probability of detecting ocular toxicity is enhanced when both rodent and non-rodent species are used.

The testing for oculotoxicity should be performed in a stepwise manner starting with routine toxicity studies (Figure 1). It is recommended, in addition to requirements specified in some regulatory guidelines, that histopathology of the eye should be incorporated into those studies where the design includes histopathological examination of the nervous system, as a means of assessing the neurotoxic potential of a chemical.

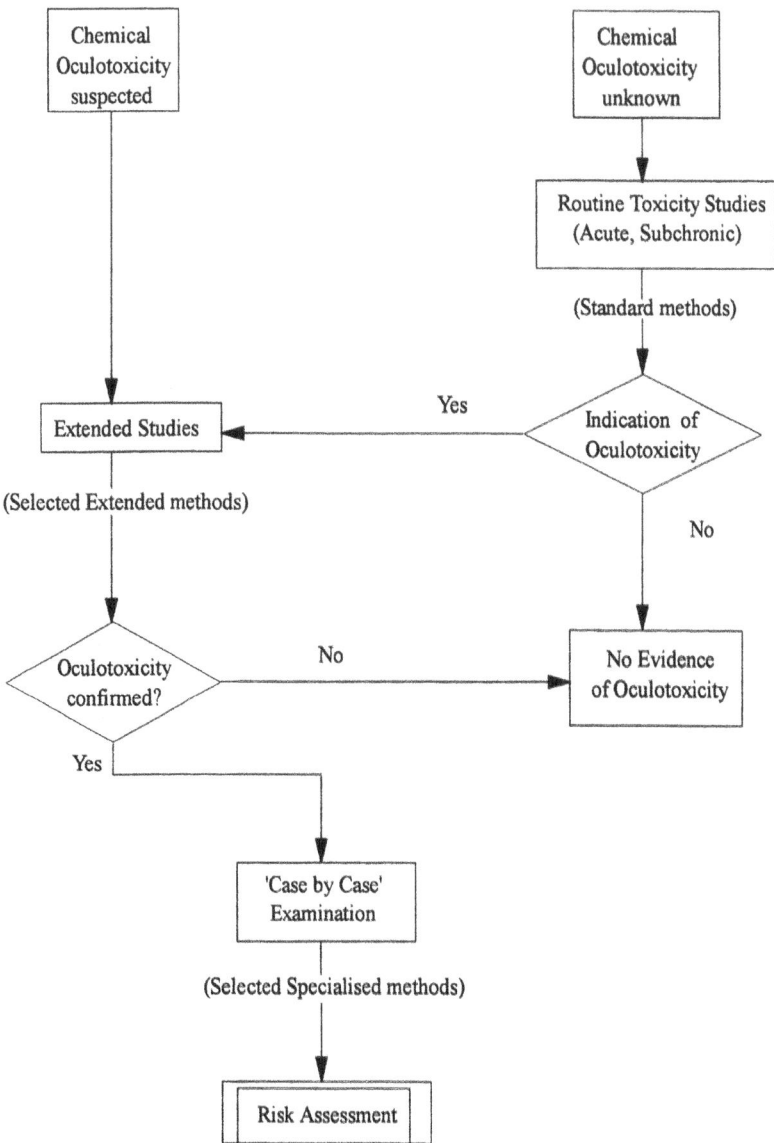

Figure 1. Order of activities for testing oculotoxicity

282

Furthermore, in routine studies where ophthalmology and histological examination are the main procedures used, the ocular adnexa such as the lacrimal and Harderian glands should be preserved for histopathological examination in case of findings in the eye and the optic nerve, since the changes observed in the ocular adnexa may contribute to their interpretation.

When the potential for oculotoxicity has been identified with a compound, it may be necessary to extend the existing techniques of ophthalmology and histology by performing additional relevant measurements and by using more extended or specialised techniques. Examples are provided in Table 1.

Table 1. Clinical and post mortem methods of eye examination in toxicity studies.

	STANDARD	EXTENDED	SPECIALISED
Clinical methods:			
Anterior eye segment			
dog monkey rabbit (pig)	- examination with focal illumination - direct/indirect ophthalmoscopy	- slit lamp biomicroscopy - slit lamp photography - external ophthalmic stains - Schrimer tear test - esthesiometry - pupillometry - tonometry	- pachymetry - examination of the refraction
rat mouse	- slit lamp biomicroscopy - direct/indirect ophthalmoscopy	- slit lamp photography	- Scheimpflug photography/biometry
Ocular fundus			
dog monkey rabbit (pig)	- direct/indirect ophthalmoscopy	- fundus photography - fluorescein angiography	- Electro-retinography (ERG)
rat mouse	- indirect ophthalmoscopy	- fundus photography - fluorescein angiography	- Electro-retinography (ERG) - visual evoked cortical potential (VECP)
Microscopical methods:	- light microscopy	- transmission electron microscopy (TEM) - scanning electron microscopy (SEM)	- perfusion fixation - transmission electron microscopy (TEM) - scanning electron microscopy (SEM)

Extended or specialised methods, when considered necessary, should be tailored to characterise the suspected oculotoxicity of particular chemical agents. "Case by case" decisions about selection of additional procedures and "custom made" design of special studies, including the desirability to demonstrate the reversibility of any observed changes are recommended.

There is insufficient scientific database for defining detailed testing rules for specific chemical or biological classes of chemicals. This is evident from the recent proposed protocols for the determination of potential ocular effects of OP pesticides (Hamernik, 1994), where a variety of examinations is suggested, but simultaneously identified as "optional" (cholinesterase assay in various tissues) or "open for discussion" (ERG, VECP). However, the various animal models developed for studying chronic human effects have yielded vast quantities of data demonstrating a spectrum of functional, biochemical and morphological effects of OPs on the animal ocular system. If animal studies performed to study alleged human effects of OPs are reviewed, it is revealed that most changes are detected in routine studies using ophthalmology and histopathology. It is only rarely that other more specialised techniques are needed to provide further clarification. For example, astigmatism can be detected by ophthalmometry, or measurement of corneal curvature and measurement of corneal thickness by pachymetry can be used, electroretinography for testing retinal abnormalities and visual evoked potentials for testing visual pathways. The main advantages of electrophysiological techniques are that they provide an assessment of functional integrity and can be used in the in-life phase of studies. However, non-invasive techniques are not essential in toxicity studies where ophthalmology and histology provide a sensitive and reliable assessment of the oculotoxicity.

For selected compounds, it may be necessary to define the toxicokinetics and mechanism of toxic action in order to place the observations into context for human exposure and to provide a basis for a risk assessment to be made. Moreover, the predictive value of animal findings for man must not be exaggerated, since the human visual system is able to perform functions which are developed differently to those of animals and therefore practical testing is inappropriate.

Ocular toxicity in man following long term exposure to chemical substances is a matter of particular concern. In general, there is poor correlation between the ocular toxicity observed from routine animal studies and eye lesions observed in man. Changes observed in chronic rodent studies reflect for the most part species-specific senile changes which are considered not to be predictive of long term effects to the human ocular system. Furthermore, the interpretation of ocular findings can be confounded by physiological changes. For instance, when OPs are tested, there is a sustained excitation of cholinergic systems which can result in secondary effects such as failure of lacrimation. Thus, carefully designed studies of shorter duration appear more appropriate for studying the possible effects in man.

CONCLUSION

Therefore the ECETOC Task Force is recommending a practical strategy for the identification and characterisation of oculotoxicity in animal studies. The basic principle is to perform the testing in a stepwise manner starting with the more routine screening studies, which can then be supplemented by additional technical procedures when oculotoxicity is expected to occur. Most chemically-induced changes are detected using a combination of ophthalmology and histopathology; other more specialised techniques are rarely needed. The existing regulatory guidelines largely cover the necessary testing requirements, but their harmonisation by the various agencies would be of benefit to both industry and the toxicology community. It is recommended, that in addition to the requirements of repeat dose toxicity studies, histopathology of the eye should be incorporated in those studies where the design includes histopathological examination of the nervous system, as a means of assessing the neurotoxic potential of a chemical. Also, microscopic examination of the ocular adnexa such as the lacrimal and Harderian glands may be essential to facilitate the interpretation of eye lesions.

In summary, a practical testing strategy for oculotoxicity which utilises the framework of existing guidelines but which equally retains the flexibility to extend the range of technical procedures to address specific oculotoxic effects is considered to offer the best approach to hazard identification in man.

REFERENCES

Hamernik, K.L., 1994, Proposed protocols for the determination of potential ocular effects of organophosphorous pesticides, J.Appl.Toxicol. 14:131-134.

Stonard, M.D., Berry, P., Kennedy, S.J., Krinke, G.J., Stringer, D.A. and Weisse, I. 1995, Critical evaluation of the evidence for an association between ocular disease and exposure to organophosphorus compounds, in: Proceedings of the 4th Congress of the International Society of Ocular Toxicology, I. Weisse, O. Hockwin, K. Green, R.C. Tripathi; eds. Plenum Publishing Corporation, New York.

AESTHESIOMETRY– AZELASTINE EYE DROPS REDUCE CORNEAL SENSITIVITY IN RABBITS, BUT NOT IN DOGS AND HUMANS

Klaus Krauser,[1] Edith Schneider,[2] Robert Hermann,[2] and Wolfgang Jahn[1]

ASTA Medica AG
[1]Institute of Toxicology
D-33790 Halle/Westfalen, Germany
[2]Clinical Pharmacology Unit
D-60314 Frankfurt am Main, Germany

INTRODUCTION

The active principle of Azelastine Eye Drops is Azelastine.HCl. Azelastine is a phthalazinone derivative which was synthetized and developed by ASTA Medica AG as an antiasthmatic and antiallergic compound. It is marketed as tablets and/or nasal spray in several countries as U.K., France, Spain, Germany, Japan, and others. A NDA is submitted in the United States.

The preclinical development of ophthalmic solutions of Azelastine was performed according to the Note for Guidance on Non-Clinical Local Tolerance Testing of Medicinal Products issued by the Committee for Proprietary Medicinal Products (CPMP) of the Commission of the European Communities. According to this guideline the evaluation of ocular tolerance for medicinal products intended for administration to the human eye requires: a) An ocular tolerance test by a single administration, usually conducted in rabbits; tests for the detection of anesthetizing properties of the administered compound should be included; and b) A repeat dose ocular tolerance test, usually conducted in rabbits, with daily administration for 4 weeks. In the following it is reported on tests for the detection of anesthetizing properties.

Several methods are available to measure corneal sensitivity[1-3]: The Cochet-Bonnet aesthesiometer with a filament producing mechanical stimuli, warming the cornea with a jet of warm saline, chemical stimulation of the cornea with e.g. capsaicin, thermal stimulation of the cornea with a carbon dioxide laser, air-impulse aesthesiometry, and stimulation with a low electric current. In most experimental animal and human studies the Cochet-Bonnet aesthesiometer was used[4-11].

Therefore, in the present studies measurement of the corneal sensitivity was performed with the Cochet-Bonnet aesthesiometer in experimental animals as well as in humans. The aim was to detect anesthetizing properties of Azelastine Eye Drop solutions and to evaluate the relevance for the treatment in man.

MATERIALS AND METHODS

The measurements of the corneal sensitivity were performed with a Cochet-Bonnet aesthesiometer[12] supplied by Luneau Ophthalmologie, F-28001 Chartres, France. This instrument consists of a calibrated nylon filament, 0.12 mm in diameter, who´s length may be continuously controlled from a gradation of 0-6, the higher number indicating the greater length. The longer the filament the less pressure it can exert on the cornea and vice versa. Each numerical grade on the aesthesiometer corresponds to an actual pressure which is given in a conversion table of measurements (table 1).

Table 1. Conversion table of aesthesiometer measurements into pressure applied to the cornea (filament diameter: 0.12 mm)

	Filament length, cm											
	6.0	5.5	5.0	4.5	4.0	3.5	3.0	2.5	2.0	1.5	1.0	0.5
Mean values of pressures, g/mm^2	0.96	1.08	1.16	1.40	1.84	2.40	3.20	4.60	6.64	8.84	12.84	17.68

For the measurement of the corneal sensitivity in experimental animals the tip of the nylon filament was slowly applied perpendicularly to the central cornea until the filament bent slightly. The examination was started at the longest filament length of 60 mm. Then the filament length was shortened in 5 mm increments until a blink response occurred on at least 3 of 5 trials. The longest filament length sufficient to elicit a blink response consistently was recorded as corneal sensitivity. If even at a filament length of only 5 mm no blink reflex could be induced, a complete loss of sensitivity respectively an anesthesia of the cornea was assumed.

As in experimental animals also in human volunteers the Cochet-Bonnet aesthesiometer was used. The sensation was measured in the inferior cornea at the 6 o´clock position. The quantification of the corneal sensitivity was achieved by determination of the length of the fibre, which was necessary to provoke a notification from the subject. The corresponding pressure in g/mm^2 was recorded.

The following studies were performed:

1. In a preliminary study the anesthetic effect of proxymetacaine hydrochloride (5 mg/ml) was tested in 5 male and 5 female albino rabbits (White Himalayan). One drop of the anesthetic was instilled in one eye per animal. The contralateral eye was treated with physiological saline solution as control. Measurements were performed before treatment as well as 1, 30, and 60 minutes after treatment.

2. Azelastine ophthalmic solutions were tested in 3 albino rabbits (White Himalayan) each per concentration. The concentrations used were 0.01%, 0.05%, 0.1%, and 0.5%. A single application of one drop into the conjunctival sac of one eye per animal was given.

The contralateral eye remained untreated as control. Measurements of the corneal sensitivity were performed before treatment as well as 1, 5, 10, 15, 20, 25, 30, 40, 50, 60, 70, and 80 minutes after the treatment. Additionally Azelastine ophthalmic solutions with concentrations of 0.05% or 0.1% were tested after single application in pigmented Fauve de Bourgogne rabbits.

3. During a 4-week study with 4 daily administrations of Azelastine ophthalmic solutions on the eye of pigmented rabbits (Fauve de Bourgogne) measurement of the corneal sensitivity was performed in satellite animals before start of the study as well as before the second administration each on days 7, 13, 22, and 27. During this study Azelastine concentrations of 0.05% and 0.1% were used. Four animals each received 50 µl at each application into the right conjunctival sac. The left eye remained untreated. An additional group of animals received physiological saline solution as controls.

4. An 0.1% Azelastine solution was applied 5 times per day for 14 days in 5 female Beagle dogs. Each animal received 100 µl per application into one eye. The contralateral eye remained untreated as control. Aesthesiometry was performed prior to the first administration, on days 2 and 9 during the first 10 minutes after the second administration on the respective day, and after the treatment period on day 16.

5. In 6 male and 6 female healthy human volunteers the local tolerability and effect on corneal sensitivity of an 0.1% Azelastine ophthalmic solution, following a single dose instillation, were investigated. The trial was performed according to a 3-period crossover design with both placebo and verum control. Vehicle solution was used as placebo; proxymetacaine hydrochloride (0.55%) was used as verum. Wash-out intervals were 7 days between each test drug application. The ophthalmic target parameter "corneal sensitivity" was measured before the administration, as well as 5, 10, 15, 30, 45, 60, 90, and 120 minutes after administration.

6. During a partially double-blind, placebo-controlled, randomised, parallel-group study the ocular tolerability and safety of 0.05% and 0.1% Azelastine ophthalmic solutions and 2% disodium chromoglycate (DSCG) were investigated in 36 healthy human volunteers. The test drugs were administered 3 times daily into the right eyes for 7 days. The left eyes were treated with vehicle solution. The corneal sensitivity measurement was performed using a Cochet-Bonnet aesthesiometer before start of the study as well as twice each on study days 3, 5, and 7, respectively, always before administration as well as 15 minutes after administration.

RESULTS

During measurement of the corneal sensitivity with the Cochet-Bonnet aesthesiometer in both albino and pigmented rabbits the pressure base values for untreated, physiological saline solution treated, or vehicle solution treated animals was approximately 5 g/mm^2. In Beagle dogs the mean pressure to elicit a blink reflex was higher than in rabbits and reached approximately 9 g/mm^2. In human volunteers, where the subjective notification of the touch of the filament tip on the cornea was taken as criterion, pressure base values were much lower than in experimental animals, i.e. approximately 1 g/mm^2.

During the different experimental studies the following results were compiled:

1. (see figure 1) Proxymetacaine hydrochloride proved to induce a complete anesthesia of the cornea with no sensitivity measurable (mean pressure >20 g/mm^2) within less than one minute after application of one drop of the anesthetic. After 30 minutes in most animals a corneal sensitivity was present again (mean pressure ca. 10 g/mm^2), but still reduced. No differences were evident for males or females, respectively. Physiological saline solution, which was used as control, had no effect on the sensitivity of the cornea in the albino rabbits.

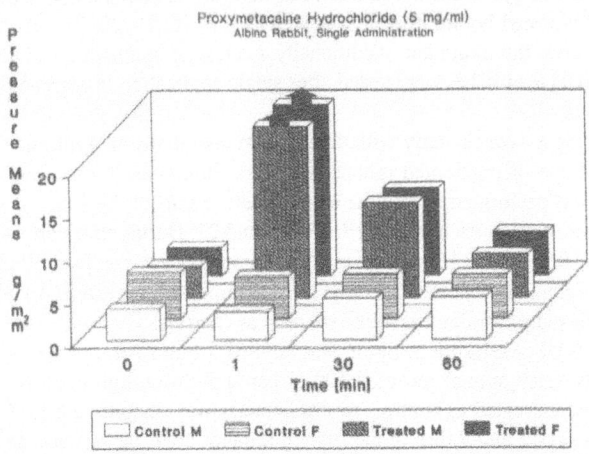

Figure 1

2. (see figure 2) Azelastine had an anesthetic effect on the cornea of the albino rabbit when applied as an 0.5%, 0.1%, or 0.05% solution, respectively. At a concentration of 0.5% of Azelastine no corneal sensitivity was measurable for up to 60 minutes after administration. At 0.1% and 0.05% the corneal sensitivity was reduced (mean pressure for induction of a blink response up to ca. 15 g/mm^2) but still measurable with the Cochet-Bonnet aesthesiometer. No obvious differences existed between these two concentrations. No clear surface anesthetic effect on the cornea was evident at 0.01%. The slightly increased pressure means at the 10 and 15 minutes time points are considered to be incidental.

An acute anesthetic effect was also confirmed in pigmented Fauve de Bourgogne rabbits, when 0.1% or 0.05% Azelastine ophthalmic solutions were applied.

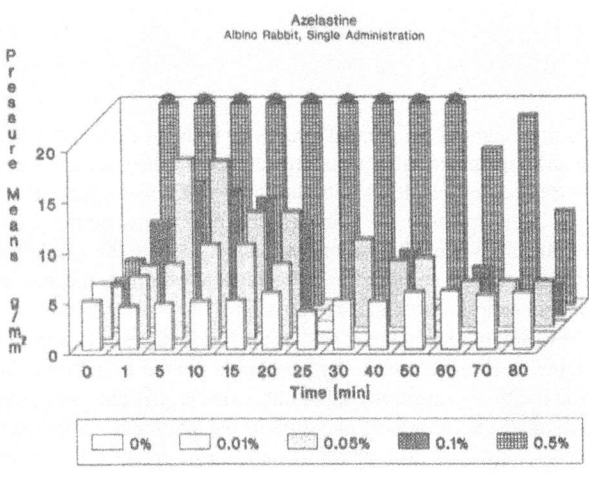

Figure 2

3. (see figure 3) No Azelastine related changes in general corneal sensitivity were revealed in pigmented rabbits over the 4-week treatment period, compared with untreated eyes or with control eyes treated with physiological saline solution. During this study no measurements of acute effects on the cornea were performed.

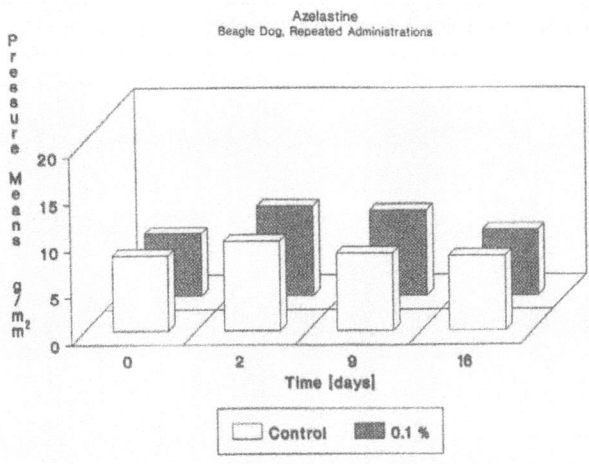

Figure 3

4. (see figure 4) When aesthesiometry using the Cochet-Bonnet aesthesiometer was performed in Beagle dogs after repeated application of an 0.1% Azelastine ophthalmic solution, there were no differences between the pressure mean values before, during, and after the treatment period, as well as between control and test substance treated eyes. Neither an acute nor a general reduction of the corneal sensitivity were noted.

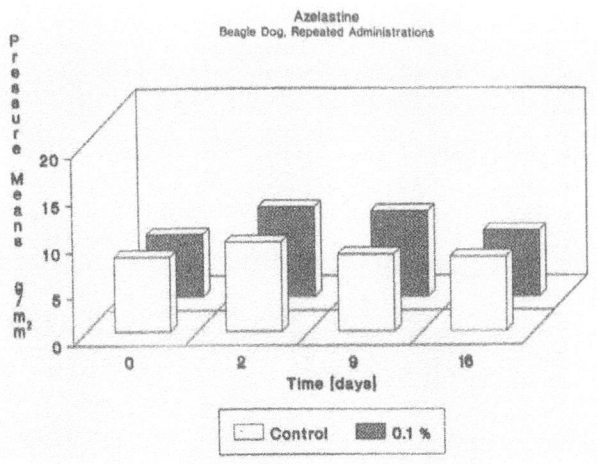

Figure 4

5. (see figure 5) In human volunteers it was apparent that proxymetacaine hydrochloride was able to induce a distinct and measurable local anesthesia respectively reduction of the sensitivity of the cornea (mean pressure up to ca. 15 g/mm^2) with a fast onset of action and a duration of more than 15 minutes. In contrast to proxymetacaine hydrochloride neither the Azelastine ophthalmic solution nor the vehicle solution showed any significant changes from pressure base values. In particular there was no difference between 0.1% Azelastine ophthalmic solution and vehicle solution at all during the aesthesiometrical investigations with the Cochet-Bonnet aesthesiometer.

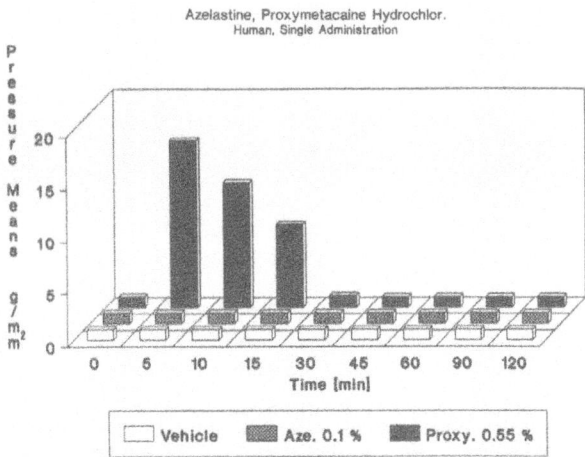

Figure 5

6. (see figure 6) When 0.1% and 0.05% Azelastine ophthalmic solutions and 2% disodium chromoglycate ophthalmic solution were tested in human volunteers after repeated administrations during 7 days, the aesthesiometrical investigations with the Cochet-Bonnet aesthesiometer did not reveal any decrease in corneal sensitivity.

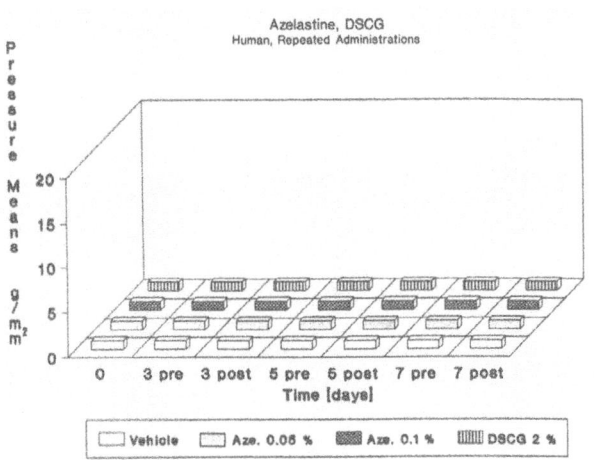

Figure 6

DISCUSSION

During the experimental studies reported pressure base values were approximately 5 g/mm^2 in rabbits and 9 g/mm^2 in Beagle dogs, when corneal sensitivity was measured with the Cochet-Bonnet aesthesiometer. Harris et al.[4] and Trevithick et al.[10] reported base values of 2-3 g/mm^2 for rabbits; approximately 7 g/mm^2 are the mean pressure base value given by MacRae et al.[6] for dogs of mixed breeds. In contrast to the relatively high pressure base values in experimental animals in man the values were approximately 1 g/mm^2 during the presented studies in human volunteers as well as reported in the literature[4,5,9,11]. All measurements were performed with a Cochet-Bonnet aesthesiometer containing a filament of 0.12 mm in diameter. The clear differences in pressure base values between experimental animals and humans are considered to be due to the different endpoints measured. While in experimental animals the blink reflex must be taken as criterion for the determination of the corneal sensitivity, in man the subjective notification is taken, which is a much more sensitive parameter. Therefore, it seems likely that slight reductions of corneal sensitivity after application of ophthalmic solutions cannot be detected under experimental conditions, but carefully performed clinical studies are necessary.

When eye drop formulations of the antiallergic Azelastine were tested in both albino and pigmented rabbits a clear hypoesthetic or even anesthetic effect was noted at concentrations of 0.05% or higher. The reduction of the corneal sensitivity was a concentration-dependent, acute, transient effect. However, when Azelastine eye drops were administered repeatedly no changes in the general corneal sensitivity were revealed. Even after a 4-week treatment period with 4 daily applications in pigmented rabbits no relevant differences in the pressure base values were noted.

To prove the relevance of the acute, transient corneal hypoesthesia or even anesthesia found in rabbits after topical administration of Azelastine ophthalmic solutions, testing was additionally performed in Beagle dogs. In contrast to rabbits no indication of any acute or general reduction of the corneal sensitivity was noted in the Beagle dogs.

Concerning the effects on corneal sensitivity different results were obtained from experimental studies in rabbits and dogs. From the literature it is known, that studies on corneal anesthesia in rabbits should not be directly extrapolated to the human eye because there may be a lack of correlation. Harris et al.[4] reported on investigations on soaps and surfactants, which induced prolonged and profound corneal anesthesia in rabbits but not in humans. They discussed the absence of Bowman´s membrane in the rabbit cornea, differences in corneal innervation, and other unknown factors as possible reason for this marked difference between the rabbit and human cornea. As evident from the presented results such a difference exists also between the rabbit and dog cornea. Other factors possibly responsible for the discrepancies between rabbits and humans concerning corneal sensitivity are more loosely arranged stomal lamellae in rabbits, a lower number of epithelial layers of the cornea of rabbits than in humans, differences in the enzyme pattern of the corneal epithelium, and differences in tear composition and turnover rate as well as in the blinking frequency which is much lower in rabbits compared to humans[13, 14].

According to the results of the experimental studies and to the findings of Harris et al.[4] the acute, transient reduction of the corneal sensitivity only in rabbits was considered not to be prohibitive for the further development of Azelastine ophthalmic solutions. Clinical phase I studies were performed, where special consideration was given to the measurement of the corneal sensitivity. As in rabbits also in man the positive reference test drug proxymetacaine hydrochloride was able to induce a distinct and measurable local anesthesia with a fast onset of action and a duration of approximately 15-30 minutes. Azelastine ophthalmic solutions at concentrations of 0.05% and/or 0.1%, however, did not produce any changes of the corneal sensitivity after both single or repeated applications. Concerning these results it must especially be noted, that in human volunteers the more sensitive parameter of subjective notification of the touch of the filament tip on the cornea was used, in contrast to experimental animals, where the blink reflex was taken as criterion for determination of the corneal sensitivity. Azelastine ophthalmic solutions at concentrations of up to 0.1% do not possess any hypoesthetic potential on the human cornea, even under the more sensitive condition of measurement compared to experimental animals.

CONCLUSIONS

Aesthesiometry using the Cochet-Bonnet aesthesiometer is a reliable method for measuring the corneal sensitivity during preclinical studies with medicinal products for topical application to the eye.

In the rabbit, which is the predominantly used species in preclinical safety studies with ophthalmics, the susceptibility of the cornea against substances with a hypoesthetic potential is obviously much more higher than in other species, e.g. in dogs or even in man, so that there could be a lack of correlation.

A reduction of the corneal sensitivity in rabbits should, therefore, not be considered prohibitive for the further development of ophthalmic drugs for topical use in man, but induce special consideration to this parameter during clinical trials.

Azelastine ophthalmic solutions, which show good antiallergic efficacy in a concentration of 0.025%, do not reduce the corneal sensitivity in man in the tested concentrations of up to 0.1%.

REFERENCES

1. N.A. Brennan and A.S. Bruce, Esthesiometry as an indicator of corneal health, Optom Vis Sci 68(9):699 (1991).
2. V. Rasch and D. Schulze, Zur klinischen Anwendung der Luftimpulsaesthesiometrie, Folia Ophthalmol 11:131 (1986).
3. H. Biermann, G. Grabner, I. Baumgartner, and M. Reim, Zur Hornhautsensibilität nach Epikeratophakie, Klin Mbl Augenheilk 201:18 (1992).
4. L.S. Harris, Y. Kahanowicz, and M. Shimmyo, Corneal anesthesia induced by soaps and surfactants, lack of correlation in rabbits and humans, Ophthal Basel 170:320 (1975).
5. J.Y. Hung, Corneal sensation in retinal detachment surgery, Ann Ophthalmol 19:313 (1987).
6. S.M. MacRae, R.L. Engerman, D.L. Hatchell, and R.A. Hyndiuk, Corneal sensitivity and control of diabetes, Cornea 1:223 (1982).
7. W.D. Mathers, J.V. Jester, and M.A. Lemp, Return of human corneal sensitivity after penetrating keratoplasty, Arch Ophthalmol 106: 210 (1988).
8. M. Millodot and H. Owens, The influence of age on the fragility of the cornea, Acta Ophthalmol 62:819 (1984).
9. B.C.K. Patel and A.B. Tullo, Corneal sensation in acute angle closure glaucoma, Acta Ophthalmol 66:44 (1988).
10. J.R. Trevithick, T. Dzialoszynski, M. Hirst, and A.P. Cullen, Esthesiometric evaluations of corneal anesthesia and prolonged analgesia in rabbits, Lens and Eye Tox Res 6(1&2):387 (1989).
11. R. Vogel, C.M. Clineschmidt, H. Hoeh, St.F. Kulaga, and R.W. Tipping, The effect of timolol, betaxolol, and placebo on corneal sensitivity in healthy volunteers, J Ocular Pharmacol 6(2): 85 (1990).

12. P. Cochet and R. Bonnet, L´Esthésie Cornéenne, Extrait de "La Clinique Ophthalmolo-
    gique", No. 4, Paris (1960).
13. E.J. Calabrese. "Principles of Animal Extrapolation", John Wiley and Sons, New York
    (1984).
14. V.H.L. Lee and J.R. Robinson, Review: topical ocular drug delivery: recent develop-
    ments and future challenges, J Ocular Pharmacol 2(1):67 (1986).

INFLUENCE OF CHRONIC ALCOHOLIC INTOXICATION ON HEALING OF CORNEAL EPITHELIAL DEFECTS. EFFECTIVITY OF TREATMENT BY PROTEASE INHIBITOR CONTRYCAL (APROTININ) AND AUTOLOGOUS FIBRONECTIN

I.A. Makarov, A.N. Ovchinnikov, and G.S. Polunin

Research Institute of Eye Diseases
Russian Academy of Medical Sciences
Moscow, Russia

ABSTRACT

Clinical observations of 23 patients (23 eyes) with persistent corneal defects after traumatic injury of eye were discussed. 8 patients were treated in special narcological hospital and had not alcohol drinks. 5 patients had small and strong alcohol drinks systematically. We studied activity of plasmin-like enzymes of tear and influence of protease inhibitor contrycal (aprotinin) and autologous fibronectin on healing of corneal defects. At the first day of observation the activity of lacrimal plasmin-like enzymes was 234.5 ± 19.0 arbitrary units (AU) for control group, 249.0 ± 21.5 AU for patients from narcology hospital and 352.6 ± 24.2 AU for patients who had alcohol drinks (50.72 ± 7.73 AU for normal persons). Combined use of contrycal and autologous fibronectin accelerated regeneration process of corneal defect: 6.60 ± 1.28 days for control group, 5.75 ± 1.25 days for patients from the narcology hospital and 19.4 ± 4.48 days for patients who had small and strong drinks during long time before and at the moment of the present study.

INTRODUCTION

Inflammation processes of cornea may cause persistent corneal defects and ulcers. In spite of different modern methods of treatment, these processes may result in development of cornea destruction with the following rough opacities in the cornea (Krasnov M.M., 1988). Healing of corneal epithelial defects depends on both appropriate effective treatment and common state of patient. One of a state of patient, which may result in different eye diseases (especially to traumatic wounds), is alcohol intoxication. This factor may explain the well-known fact that the most part of complications with traumatic eye wounds are observed for ambulatory patients (in comparison with hospital ones). The aim of our work is a study of influence of alcohol intoxication on corneal epithelial defects healing after eye trauma and effectiveness of protease inhibitor contrycal (aprotinin) and autologous fibronectin for treatment of such defects.

MATERIALS AND METHODS

We observed 23 patients (23 eyes) with persistent corneal epithelial defects after previously endured eye traumatic injuries. These injuries were caused by metal shaving or chemical reagents and were obtained during production and everyday activity of the patients. Treatment was carried out by traditional medicaments and ways (local use of antibacterial and antiviral ophthalmic solutions, solcoseril) but was not effective during 3-4 weeks.

All patients were subdivided into 3 groups. The first group included 8 patients from a special narcological hospital who were on the second stage of chronic alcoholism and did not take alcoholic drinks during 1-4 months before our study. The second group included 5 patients who systematically took alcohol drinks and were not observed by narcologist during the time of the present study. Using anamnesis and talks with relatives of patients we found that 4 patients from this group were previously treated at special narcological hospital in connection with chronic alcoholism. All patients of the second group used small and strong alcohol drinks (more than 100 - 150 grams of 100% alcohol every day) during the time of this study. The third (control) group included 10 practically healthy patients who did not use alcohol drinks at all or periodically used small amount of alcohol. All patients from the control and experimental groups had not any diseases of liver and intestinal-gastric tract.

Complex of clinic-biochemical investigations (included cytological and bacteriological analysis of conjunctiva) was performed for all patients.

The patients of experimental and control groups were treated by instillations of protease inhibitor contrycal (Germany) (six times per day), instillations of autologous fibronectin (five times per day), and instillations of antibacterial medicament (Ophthalmic solution of Furacillin 0.02%) (four times per day).

Every day control for effectiveness of treatment was performed by biomicroscopy at slit lamp 75 SL (Opton Feintechnik GmbH) with photoregistration, vital paint of cornea by solution of 1% fluorescein, and determination of area of corneal defects by millimeter net in ocular of slit lamp.

About 25 μl of tear from every patient was collected by automatic micropipette for study of plasmin-like activity of tear proteases.

Study of Activity of Plasmin-Like Enzymes in Tear

Activity of plasmin-like enzymes was measured with synthetic peptide substrate - Tos-Gly-Pro-Lys-p-nitroanilide ("Serva", Germany). Tear samples (5-25 μl) were placed into microliter plate wells. 150 μl of 0.05 M K-phosphate (pH 7.9) and 40 μl of substrate (2.4 mg/ml) were added in plate well for reaction initiation. Microtiter plate was thermostated at 250 °C. Optical density changes were measured using Microrider (Uniscan 11, Labsystems, Finland) at 405 nm. Measurements were made for 3-4 times during 5 hours. Plasmin-like activity of tear was calculated as tangent of slop of line in coordinates: optical density via time. For accurate calculation we used a special software - Enzfitter (version 1.05 - EGA). We determined arbitrary unit of plasmin-like activity of tear as change of 1.0 unit of optical density per minutes per 1 ml of tear.

Fibronectin Separation and Purification

50 ml of venous blood of patients with epithelium defects of cornea were placed in sterile centrifuge tube containing 5 ml of 0.1 M K-phosphate buffer (pH 7.2) with Na-citrate f or prevention of blood clotting. The blood sample was centrifuged immediately at Beckman J2-21/E centrifuge at 1700 g and 4° for blood cell separation. Blood plasma was a start material for fibronectin purification.

We used affinity chromatography on gelatin-sepharose (Pharmacia Fine Chemicals, Sweden) for one stage fibronectin purification. Column I x 10 cm with about 6-8 ml of gelatin-sepharose was equilibrated by 100 ml of isotonic solution containing 0.015 M K-phosphate (pH 7.2). After blood plasma loading (about 20 ml), the column was washed by initial buffer. Elution was performed using isotonic solution with pH 2.1 (HCl), and fibronectin was eluted in sharp peak (4-6 ml).

Fibronectin sample was dialyzed against 1 L of 0.1 M ammonium carbonate solution and then against 1 L of isotonic solution with 0.015 M K-phosphate (pH 7.2). 0.25 mg/ml of levomicitin was added as microbial inhibitor.

The fibronectin solution was filtered using Millex-GV filters (0.22 mm, "Millipore", USA) and then divided in 1 ml portions for storage. Samples of pure fibronectin were stored at -20°C. Fibronectin concentration in the samples varied from 0.5 to 1 mg/ml. Fibronectin concentration in the samples was determined spectrophotometrically taking into account that 1.0% fibronectin solution absorbs 12.8 optical units at 280 nm.

Electrophoresis in PAAG in the presence of Na-dodecylsulfate showed absence of any additional components. Similar data were obtained using HPLC technique (HP 1090 M chromatograph, "Hewlett-Packard").

RESULTS AND DISCUSSIONS

Activity of plasmin-like enzymes of tear of healthy patients with intact cornea was 50.72 ± 7.73 AU. At the first day of observation the activity of lacrimal plasmin-like enzymes of patients with corneal epithelial defects in the control group increased more than 4 times and was 234.5 ± 19.0 AU. These data did not significantly differed from the data obtained for the patients from the first experimental group (249.0 ± 21.5 AU) (table 1). On the contrary, the activity of lacrimal plasmin-like enzymes in patients who had small and strong drinks during the time of the present study (second group) increased almost 1.5 time and was 352.6 ± 24.2 AU ($p < 0.01$).

Table 1. Activity of plasmin-like enzymes of the tear of patients with corneal epithelial defects.

Group of patients	The activity of plasmin-like enzymes of the tear (AU).		
	1st day	p	2nd day
lst study	249.0 ± 21.5		153.7 ± 19.6
		< 0.01	
2nd study	352.6 ± 24.2		294.2 ± 18.0
		< 0.01	
Control	234.5 ± 19.0		168.5 ± 18.6

At the second day of observation use of the protease inhibitor contrycal allowed to reduce activity of plasmin-like enzymes to 168.5 ± 18.6 AU in the control group and to 153.7 ± 19.6 AU in the first experimental group. This activity was also reduced to 294.2 ± 18.0 AU in the second experimental group, but the decrease of activity was not so significant as in the other groups.

At the same time a clinic status of patients was characterized by beginning of epithelization which expressed in active migration of epithelial cells in a region of the corneal defect place, decrease of square of this defect, relaxation of eye inflammation and pain syndrome. The improvement was better pronounced at the control and the first experimental group than at the second group.

From the second day of observation all patients were also treated by instillations of autologous fibronectin (five times a day).

The most considerable therapeutic effect from the combined use of contrycal and autologous fibronectin was observed among the patients with chronic alcoholism who treated at the special narcology hospital (the first experimental group). Complete healing of corneal epithelial defects occurred during 5.75 ± 1.25 days in this group. These patients received treatment of various vitamins, medicaments, which stimulated metabolic processes, tranquillizers. This fact allowed us to suppose that the treatment created Protection power of constitution" in the patients from this group and therefore the healing of their corneal epithelial defects was more effective than in patients from the control group (6.60 ± 1.28) after use of identical therapy by protease inhibitor contrycal and autologous fibronectin (table 2).

On the contrary, the patients, who had small and strong drinks during long time before and during the present study (the second experimental group), had considerably more prolonged course of corneal epithelial defects after use of contrycal and autologous fibronectin and finished healing was at 11-28 days (19.4 ± 4.48).

Increase of activity of plasmin of tear was found in patients with traumatic corneal damage (Tervo T. et al., 1988). A significant increasing of tissue plasmin activator, urokinase-type plasminogen activators and plasminogen/plasmin were found for patients with corneal ulcers and thermal or chemical burns relative to the pattern observed in the control subjects (Barlati S. et al., 1990).

Table 2. Date of corneal epithelial defects healing with used protease inhibitor contrycal and autologous fibronectin.

Group of patients	Date of corneal defects healing (days)	p
1st study	4-8 (5.75 ± 1.25)	< 0.001
2nd study	11-28 (19.4 ± 4.48)	< 0.001
Control	3-10 (6.60 ± 1.28)	

Unregulated content of plasminogen activators leads to plasmin accumulation in the field of contact between cell border of epithelium and subepithelial basal membrane. Plasmin cleaves fibronectin molecular with separation of the cell-binding and matrix-binding domains. The nonfunctional fragments of fibronectin compete with intact fibronectin for binding on the cell surface and for heparin-sulfate of basal membrane. This process blocks a normal cell binding and migrating. Excess of plasmin leads to destroying other adhesive proteins - laminin and integrin and to activating of type VI collagenase which destroys type IV collagen in subepithelial basal membrane. (Berman M.B., 1989; Hynes R.O., 1990). Kininogens and splitting compliment C-3 by plasmin to result in migration keratocytes and polymorphonuclear leukocytes to corneal defect place from limb blood vassals. They free latent collagenases which are activated by plasmin in active collagenases to degrade corneal stroma (Pickij V.I. et al., 1991; Berman M. et al., 1988). Aprotinin is applied topically to inhibit plasmin (for patients with persistent cornea defects) on the corneal surface when endogenous or topically administered fibronectin is degraded inappropriately (Salonen at al., 1987; Tervo T. et al., 1991).

The results of our study confirm that all patients with corneal epithelial defects have increased activity of plasmin-like enzymes of tear, which was almost 1.5 times higher in the second group than in the control one.

REFERENCES

Barlati S., Marchina E., Quaranta C.A. et al., 1990, Analysis of fibronectin, plasminogen activators and plasminogen in tear fluid as markers of corneal damage and repair, *Exp Eye Res.* 51:1.

Berman M.B., 1989, The pathogenesis of corneal epithelial defects, *Acta Ophthalmol (Copenh.)(Suppl).* 192, 67:55.

Berman M., Kenyon K., Hayashi K. et al., 1988, The Pathogenesis of Epithelial Defect Formation and Stromal Ulceration, *in*: The Cornea: Trans World Congr. Cornea III, D. Cavanagh (ed.), NY. Raven Press.

Hynes R.O., 1985-1986, Fibronectins: a family of complex and versatile adhesive glycoproteins derived from a single gene, *Harvey Lect.*, 81:133.

Hynes R.O., 1990, Fibronectins, Springer-Verla, NY.

Krasnov M.M., 1988, Contemporary Ophthalmology and Perspectives of its Development, **in**: Big Medical Encyclopaedia, Vol.29., Medicine, Moscow.

Mosesson M.W. and Umfleet RA., 1970, The cold-insoluble globulin of human plasma. Purification, primary characterization and relationship to fibrinogen and other cold-insoluble fraction components, *J BioL Chem.*, 7-4 245:11:5728.

Pickij V.I. Allergic Diseases, 1991, Medicine, Moscow.

Salonen E.M., Tervo T., Torma E. et al., 1987, Plasmin in tear fluid of patients with corneal ulcers: basis for new therapy, *Acta. Ophthalmol (Copenh)*, 65:13.

Tervo T., van Setten G., Joutsimo L. and Tarkkanen A., 1991, The fibrinolytic system and use of aprotinin for the eye, *Klin Monatsbl Augenheilkd*, 198:1:66.

Tervo T., Salonen E.M., Vahen A. et al., 1988, Elevation of tear fluid plasmin in corneal disease, *Acta Ophthalmol (Kbh)*, 66:4:393.

THE USE OF CYCLOSPORINE A IN VETERINARY OPHTHALMOLOGY

Willy Neumann and Andrea L. Schulte-Neumann

Veterinary Surgical Clinic
University of Giessen, Germany
35392 Giessen, Germany

INTRODUCTION

A clinical field trial and a controlled study were carried out in France, Germany and the United Kingdom between 1992 and 1993 with the help of Schering Plough, USA in order to assess the efficacy of Cyclosporine A ointment in the treatment of „Kerato-conjunctivitis sicca" (KCS) and a breed specific ocular disease, „Keratitis Überreiter" in the German Shepherd Dog.

I. KERATOCONJUNCTIVITIS SICCA (KCS)

Keratoconjunctivitis sicca (KCS) in dogs is a common prevalent ophthalmological disorder, leading to chronic irritation of one or both eyes and in its advanced stages. KCS is associated with mucopurulent conjunctivitis, superficial keratitis with vascularisation and pigmentation of the cornea and corneal ulceration. KCS is in most cases a vision threatening condition in affected dogs.

The absolute incidence of KCS in the general population of dogs is unknown, but a review of the incidence of this disease over the past 25 years in the USA reveals a continuing progressive increase in the rate of reporting of canine KCS. In 1988 more than 50% of all canine cases of conjunctivitis were attributed to KCS (Kaswan and Salisbury, 1990).

Although KCS in many cases represents a condition of unknown origin, many theories of possible causes have been discussed:

Distemper, congenital alacrimia, neurologic xerosis, Vitamin A deficiency, mechanic obstruction of lacrimal ductules etc. In most cases individual causes could not be determined and predominant opinion now is based on histopathologic and serological findings, suggesting an immune-mediated destruction of the lacrimal glands revealing immunological similarities between canine KCS and human "dry-eye" disorders or "Sjögren's Syndrome" (Kaswan and Salisbury, 1990; Olivero, 1994).

The disease is often misdiagnosed by veterinarians as "bacterial, or non-specific chronic conjunctivitis". Therefore, in the past dogs were often treated with topical antibiotics and steroids, which obviously cannot give more than transient relief. Cases of correctly diagnosed KCS were treated in addition with artificial tears and cholinergic tear stimulants as a more symptomatic treatment without marked improvement on long term basis.

The treatment of KCS by artificial tears in most cases is unsatisfactory in dogs, since to be effective, artificial tears must be applied very frequently (10-15 times/day) which makes this kind of treatment very inconvenient, if not impossible, for many owners. Until today there are no approved products for the treatment of KCS in dogs and desire for various cocktails of different ingredients (tear stimulants, antibiotics, corticosteroids, acetylcystein) have led veterinarians to custom compounding of ophthalmic products with questionable quality control.

Since medical management of KCS often fails completely, surgical treatment (parotid duct transposition) is performed frequently, causing additional problems later on like excessive flow, facial dermatitis, precipitates, superficial keratopathy or total failure to salivate.

As a result of mismanagement by veterinarians on one hand and due to the often unknown aetiology of the particular disease on the other hand, many dogs develop progressive corneal opacities and blindness associated with pain and discomfort as a result of corneal ulceration and massive exsudation formation.

For the future the topical use of Cyclosporine A, a noncytotoxic immunosuppressant, offers a new possibility in treatment of KCS in dogs and a major advance in the management of this chronic eye disease.

INCLUSION CRITERIA

Eighty seven dogs (45 females and 42 males; age ranging from 0.9 to 14 years) from a total of eighty eight dogs enrolled were statistically evaluated in this study, designed to confirm the efficacy of 0.2% Cyclosporine A (CsA) ophthalmic ointment for the treatment of chronic idiopathic keratoconjunctivitis sicca (KCS) in dogs. 31 different breeds were represented with the West Highland White Terrier and Yorkshire Terrier accounting for 41% of all dogs.

The study was conducted as an open clinical field trial. All dogs included in the studies were taken from the general dog population (representing more than 40 different breeds), thus representing a realistic cross section of the KCS population.

The cases selected met stringent requirements, which included having the characteristic symptoms associated with long-standing idiopathic xerophthalmia, one or both eyes affected with KCS, presence of conjunctivitis with or without keratitis with a Schirmer Tear Test (STT) value of 10 mm/min or less, and having no prior exposure to Cyclosporine A in any form.

Fifty five dogs qualified in both eyes (bilateral cases) while 32 qualified in only one eye (22 left eyes, OS; 10 right eyes, OD). These cases were contributed by 4 veterinary ophthalmologists under field conditions in four geographic regions of Europe (Newmarket, UK; Gießen, Germany; Paris and Lyon, France).

An initial diagnostic evaluation including the dog's medical history and a pre-treatment, physical and ophthalmic examination was performed on Day 0. Tubes containing 0.2% Cyclosporine A in a corn oil/petrolatum/lanolin based ophthalmic ointment, identical to Optimmune® (Schering Plough, USA) but with 0.5% of preservative, were dispensed to the client, who was instructed to apply a 2/3 cm ribbon of ointment to each qualifying eye every 12 hours. The client was allowed to remove excessive mucus prior to treatment by gentle flushing of the eye with an eye wash or physiologic saline solution. Concurrent therapy was not allowed and the treatment continued for six consecutive weeks.

The response to therapy with the test article was assessed by ophthalmic examinations (Days 7, 21, and 42 post-treatment initiation) at which time the clinical appearance of the conjunctiva, cornea, and internal ocular structures were scored, and STT values were determined. The results for incidence of eyes showing improvement in Schirmer Tear Test were defined as follows: „Marked improvement" (STT increase ≥4 mm/min)"im-proved" (STT increase ≥3 mm/min and ≤4mm/min), or "not improved" (STT increase <2mm/min). Presence of epiphora, discomfort, vision, lid-related conditions, and optionally, intraocular pressure was also assessed at these examinations. Client assessment of the dogs immediate and delayed reactions after ointment application on Days 7, 21 and 42 were made.

STATISTICS

Statistical analyses were performed by use of SAS software version 6.07 (SAS Institute, Cary NC), and StatXact version 2.04 (Cytel Software Corporation, Cambridge, MA). The a priori level of statistical significance was defined as alpha<0.05. Preliminary statistical significance was defined as 0.05<alpha<0.10. All analyses used a 1-sided alternative hypothesis of improvement with Cyclosporine A therapy as compared to pre-treatment levels. Analyses were separately performed for OS and OD.

Schirmer Tear Test results were analysed for change from pre-treatment levels (for individual dogs) by paired T-tests, for each post-treatment observation day. In addition to the separate evaluations of OS and OD, bilateral cases were analysed for mean STT change. STT scores were further evaluated after dividing the cases into two subgroups: an initial (Day 0) STT of 0 or 1, or an initial (Day 0) STT of≥2. Ordered categorical variabies and binomial variables were evaluated by the Marginal Homogeneity Test (K x K)/McNemars Test (2 x 2). Each ordered categorical or binomial variable was evaluated for change from Day 0 (pretreatment), for each post-treatment observation day.

RESULTS

The results of the study show that the increase in STT was associated with improvement in conjunctival and corneal parameters as well. In addition, increase in STT (mm/min) from Day 0 and overall investigator evaluation on Day 42 were recorded. The analysis of the immediate and delayed reactions of the dogs to the ointment application reported by the owner, showed a reduction in the frequency of these reactions throughout the study period. This apparent improvement in tolerance might be related to the improvement of the disease itself. A relatively high percentage of dogs was reported by the owners as having immediate or deferred reactions but most of those reactions (>63% depending on day of study and type of reaction) were considered to occur only occasionally.

Some adverse events were reported by the investigators. All of them were related either to reactions reported by the owner after application of the ointment or to the clinical progression of the disease. No unexpected drug-related adverse events were reported in any of the 87 dogs enrolled in this study.

The overall investigator assessment on Day 42 showed improvement (vast or some improvement) in 76% of OS and 87% of OD.

The results of this study demonstrate that 0.2% Cyclosporine A ophthalmic ointment significantly improves tear production and clinical signs associated with chronic idiopathic KCS in dogs. Furthermore, there were no drug-related safety concerns recognised in any dog. A 2/3 cm ribbon of 0.2% Cyclosporine A ophthalmic ointment applied to the eye at 12 hour intervals is an effective treatment for chronic idiopathic KCS. The mean STT significantly increased throughout the study. The majority of the increase in STT was observed during the first week of therapy (Fig. 1).

The main criteria of efficacy, (STT, amount of conjunctival discharge, conjunctival hyperaemia/hypertrophy and corneal surface and corneal vascularisation) prove 0.2% Cyclosporine A ointment to be the recommended dose.

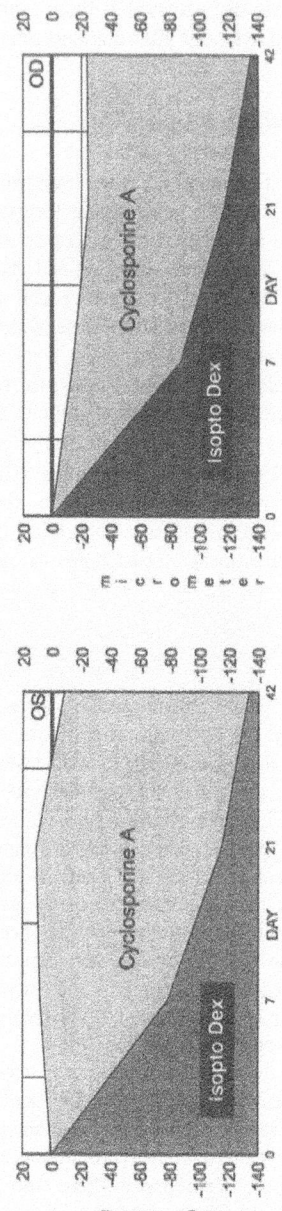

Figure 1. Pachymetry results

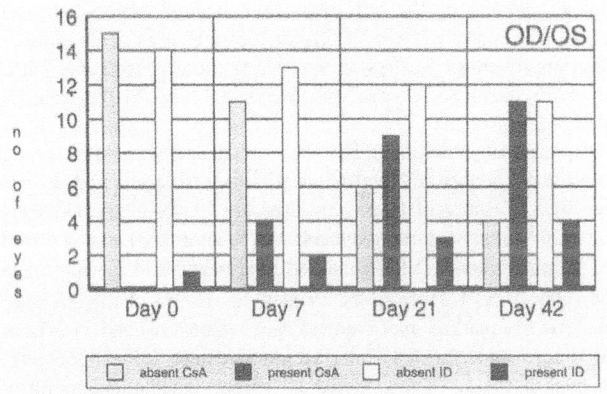

Figure 2. Results of STT readings (epiphora)

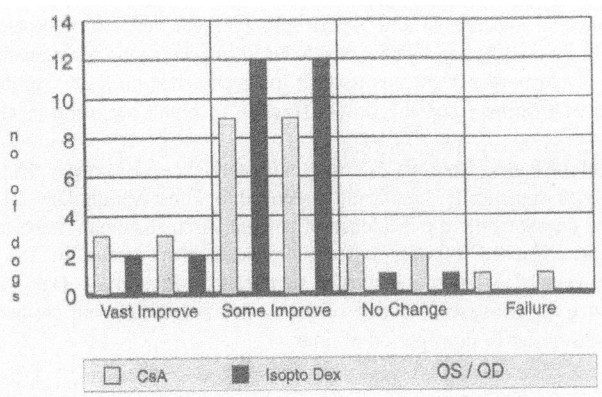

Figure 3. Investigator's overall assessment for initial phase

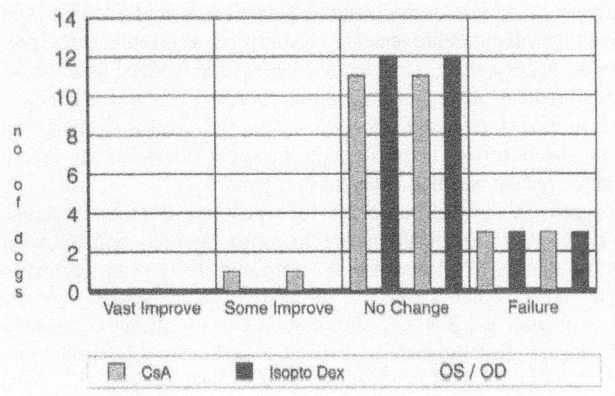

Figure 4. Investigator's overall assessment for withdrawl phase

By Day 42, 64.8% of the left eyes (OS) showed improvement (51.3% marked improvement, 13.5% improved) and 66.7% of the right eyes (OD) showed improvement (61.9% marked improvement, 4.8% improved). For the enrolled cases with bilateral KCS, improvement in the mean STT score was found in 71.7% of the cases (64.2% marked improvement, 7.5% improved).

As clinical response in Schirmer Tear Test was expected to differ for animals with very low STT scores, the incidence of "Improvement" was further subdivided. In those dogs with an initial (Day 0) STT score of 0 or 1 by Day 42, 50.0% of the left eyes (OS) showed "Improvement" (26.9% marked improvement, 23.1% improved) and 62.5% of the right eyes (OD) showed "Improvement" (58.3% marked improvement, 4.2% improved). Those dogs with an initial (Day 0) STT score of ≥2 by Day 42, 72.9% of the left eyes (OS) showed "Improvement" (64.6% marked improvement, 8.3% improved) and 71.1 % of the right eyes (OD) showed "Improvement" (65.8% marked improvement, 5.3% improved).

Conjunctival discharge (characterised as "absent, mucoid/mucopurulent or purulent") was listed for each observation day (Fig.2). Statistically significant reduction from Day 0 in the character of conjunctival discharge were found on all observation days post initiation of Cyclosporine A therapy for OS and OD (Fig.3). The amount of conjunctival discharge ("absent, mild or marked") also statistically significantly decreased on all days and in all eyes (OD+OS) post initiation of Cyclosporine A therapy.

Conjunctival hyperaemia and hypertrophy ("absent, mild to moderate and marked") was found to be statistically significantly reduced in severity on all examination days post initiation of Cyclosporine A therapy (except for hyperaemia on Day 7, probably due to the short period of treatment and the slower reaction of blood perfusion level in the specific tissue) (Fig.4).

Corneal thickness ("smooth, 1-2 times normal thickness or greater than 2 times normal thickness") was statistically significantly reduced on observation Day 21 and 42 (both OS+OD) and consequently the incidence of corneal vascularisation ("none or ghost vessels, superficial or collapsed vessels, superficial vessels that extend to the centre of the cornea/deep vessels") shows statistically significant reduction on Day 42. This can be explained since the neovascularisation of the cornea associated with chronic disease is not expected to disappear in short period of time.

CONCLUSION

Cyclosporine A appears to be effective and well tolerated. Two distinct therapeutic effects of Cyclosporine A ophthalmic ointment were observed, when used BID in dogs with KCS: Increased tear production in most cases and improved ocular surface lesions.

Improvement of the corneal and conjunctival lesions in dogs with KCS can be dramatic, with or without improvement in lacrimation, suggesting that Cyclosporine A has a direct antiinflammatory effect. Conjunctival hyperplasia, corneal granulation tissue (later on becoming scar tissue= "leukoplakia") and mucopurulent ocular discharge, improved in most of the Cyclosporine A-treated KCS dogs, within 2-3 weeks. Corneal vascularisation and pigmentation also resolved in most dogs, however, these lesions resolved much more gradually; improvement was first apparent by 3 months.

Cyclosporine A shows promise to be of benefit in a spectrum of chronic ocular surface inflammatory disorders as an alternative to topical steroids and NSAIDs. The apparent advantages of topical Cyclosporine A compared to topical corticosteroids are that Cyclosporine A does not appear to promote cataractogenesis, glaucoma or corneal collagenase activation which is very often associated with chronic complicated KCS. Current experience suggests that most dogs respond to ophthalmic Cyclosporine A administered twice daily. The frequency of application of ophthalmic Cyclosporine A might be reduced after several months under constant control of a veterinarian; rarely, however, can a dog be withdrawn completely without relapse. Necessary interruptions in treatment, f. e. due to trauma, secondary infection or development of deep corneal ulcers, precipitate relapses of KCS signs, but fortunately reintroduction quickly regains the maximal tearing effect.

Pigmentary keratitis has been recognised to be very slowly responsive to Cyclosporine A ophthalmic treatment. Therefore treatment with Cyclosporine A should not be considered unsuccessfull in regards to improving vision until a significant period of constant treatment has elapsed.

Cyclosporine A A 0,2% ointment represents a great improvement in the handling of KCS in dogs and clearly acts as a lacromimetic agent.

KERATITIS ÜBERREITER
(CHRONIC SUPERFICIAL KERATITIS=PANNUS)

INTRODUCTION

Ocular diseases in dogs mediated in part or in large part by the immune system are many and varied. They range from disorders initiated by well defined exogenous factors to those with putative autoimmune mechanisms. The proposed mechanisms for these disorders, however, need, in the main, to be more fully evaluated. In the past few years, improved clinical tools for the evaluation and new therapeutic concepts of these diseases as well as new therapeutic agents have provided us with greater information concerning these diseases. Results of clinical treatment and information gained from basic scientific work clearly indicate how naive we were in our attempts to explain immune phenomena in animals. Especially the use of Cyclosporine A (CsA), both in the basic research as well as the clinical sphere (e.g. KCS) has provided us with a valuable new tool from a therapeutic aspect and as a probe to the underlying mechanisms mediating these diseases.

Ocular inflammatory disorders for which CsA may or has been shown to be applicable in man and in animals can be loosely classified into three large categories: disorders of the ocular surface, transplantation, and intraocular inflammatory disease. Many of these disorders are thought to be T-cell mediated and except KCS, they have not been particularly amenable to more standard therapeutic approaches until today. A large number of disorders affect the ocular surface that are thought to be immune-mediated. Some of them are breed specific (Keratitis in Boxer or in the Long Haired German Dachshound, Corneal Dystrophy in the Sibirian Husky), others show a certain predisposition in particular breeds (KCS in the West Highland White Terrier).

Another corneal disease suspected to be of autoimmune origin frequently occurs in one of the most popular breeds in Germany: The German Shepherd Dog (GSD). The condition of this particular corneal disease which affects the cornea and can lead to corneal blindness if untreated, remained unnamed until the late 1950s, although first described by Coats, 1913. The Austrian ophthalmologist Überreiter (1956) was the first veterinarian, to perform basic scientific research on the cornea of affected dogs, therefore the disease, often called „Pannus" or „Keratitis superficialis vasculosa pannosa pigmentosa" became known as „Keratitis Überreiter" or „Überreiter's Syndrome". This use of more than one name arose because the aetiology of the disease was unknown, a position which still pertains to this day. The term „corneal pannus" has been adopted from Bedford, (1979) to describe the condition of the disease as the Latin word *pannus*, a cloth, aptly describes the appearance of the lesion, and the prefix „corneal" prevents confusion with similarly named conditions in orthopaedics.

The term pannus is used to refer to tissue changes characterised either by cellular infiltration and extensive vascularisation or by the replacement of normal tissue by granulation tissue. In man, the aetiology and histopathology of corneal pannus vary considerably, but in the dog common usage of the term is usually confined to a distinct disease entity which demonstrates a breed specificity for the German Shepherd Dog. Similar or identical canine ocular lesions have been described variously under the names of keratitis pannosa and pigmentosa, chronic superficial kerato-conjunctivitis, Überreiter's Disease or Syndrome and chronic superficial keratitis (Bedford, 1979). Since the pathological change is a chronical inflammation of the corneal epithelium and anterior corneal stroma, the term „chronic superficial keratitis" seems to be more appropriate. The aetiology of pannus in the dog remains obscure, but work in the USA and in Europe has demonstrated that environmental conditions are possibly of considerable importance in determining the origins of the disease and its response to therapy.

Treatment of Pannus within the last 40 years consisted of cautery, radiotherapy, plastic surgical techniques, tinted glass goggles, injections of blood and milk as well as corticosteroid injections, systemic and local application. The purpose of this paper is to describe the clinical features of pannus observed in GSD patients in Germany and to report the results of a clinical field trial comparing the efficacy of 0.2% Cyclosporine A (Optimmune® Schering Plough, USA) and dexamethasone ointments (Isopto Dex®, Alcon, USA) in the treatment of Pannus in GSD. The study was designed as a blind clinical field trial, based on a series of 30 GSD patients seen in our clinic over a period of four months (Sept.-Dec. 1993).

INCLUSION CRITERIA

30 German or Belgian shepherd dogs, ranging from 2-11 years of age, 17 female and 13 male, were enrolled in the study if they were diagnosed with Pannus at the pre-treatment examination on the basis of history, physical and ophthalmological examination.

They all fulfilled the following inclusion criteria: Chronic (> 5 days) bilateral cases, normal Schirmer Tear Test: STT (≥10 mm/min), presence in the cornea of superficial vessels and/or pigmented opacity and/or granulation tissue.

The following therapy was to be discontinued for specific periods of time before inclusion of the dog in the study: Topical or systemic use of Cyclosporine A for at least 14 days prior to inclusion. Topical ophthalmic or systemic use of a corticosteroid for at least 14 days prior to inclusion (In case of subconjunctival injection, this period was extended to 28 days for regular solutions and 90 days for long acting or unknown formulations). Use of systemic or topical atropine for at least 7 days prior to inclusion. Use of systemic or topical pilocarpine for at least 2 days prior to inclusion.

The following concurrent therapies were not permitted during the entire study period: Systemic use of Cyclosporine A, topical ophthalmic or systemic use of corticosteroid, use of systemic or topical atropine, use of systemic or topical pilocarpine, topical use of artificial tears.

After an initial diagnostic evaluation and review of the inclusion criteria, the dog's medical history was taken and pre-treatment physical and ophthalmic examinations performed (Day 0). A cortisol stimulation test was performed at that time as well. Blood was drawn and submitted to a referral laboratory for plasma cortisol level determination by radio-immunoassay prior to IM injection of 2 u ACTH/kg and 1-2 hr later on Days 0 and 42.

Once the ophthalmic examination was complete, the owner received a treatment box corresponding to the case number. The investigator instructed the owner as to the proper techniques of instilling the proper amount of ointment into each eye. The dosage of the investigational drugs was approximately 1 cm ribbon of ointment in each eye every 12 hours. If necessary, excessive discharge could be removed prior to treatment by gentle cleansing or flushing of the eye with an eye wash or physiologic saline solution, as instructed by the investigator.

Treatment continued for a full 6 weeks. Treatment was interrupted on Day 42. The ocular condition was reevaluated and the case terminated at the soonest of either significant worsening of the condition or Day 63 (3 weeks after cessation of treatment).

Ophthalmic examination was performed on Days 7, 21, 42 and 63. At each presentation the following ocular assessments were documented: Condition and disorders of visual function, lids, third eyelid, STT, conjunctiva, cornea (including pachymetry of corneal thickness) and the response to therapy was evaluated by both, the investigator and the client. In addition any adverse reaction or complicating medical factors were recorded individually.

RESULTS

Statistically significant differences between the two treatment groups were found for pachymetry, the incidence of eyes with „present" or „absent" epiphora and in the overall assessment of the investigator.

Pachymetry: A summary of the pachymetry results is found in Figure 5. This chart lists the mean pachymetry per treatment group, for each observation day. Each eye was measured three times, the minimum thickness was used as the pachymetry result for that eye. The statistical significant p-values for the comparison of Cyclosporine A treated eyes vs Isopto-Dex treated eyes (Analysis of covariance) are p=0.0060 on Day 7, p=0.0005 on Day 21 and p=0.0002 on Day 42 in the right eye and p=0.0021 on Day 7, p=0.0036 on Day 21 and p=0.0013 on Day 42 in the left eye. For the initial treatment phase (Day 7 to Day 42), the covariate was the Day 0 pachymetry value, per dog. For the treatment withdrawal phase (Day 63), the covariate was the Day 42 result. Figure 5 also lists the change in mean „minimum" pachymetry per treatment group for each observation day. Statistically significant differences were found between the treatment groups for mean "minimum" pachymetry on all observation days during the test drug therapy period. For each observation day, the positive control (Isopto-Dex) showed a statistically significantly greater decrease in pachymetry than Cyclosporine A ointment. When the within treatment group evaluations were reviewed, Isopto-Dex was found to statistically significantly reduce pachymetry on all observation days during the treatment phase. Cyclosporine A treated eyes did not show a statistically significant reduction in pachymetry on any observation day. After withdrawal of the test drug, the OS Cyclosporine A treated eyes showed a preliminary statistically significant increase in pachymetry; however, the OD did not show a change. For the Isopto-Dex treated eyes, both OS and OD showed a statistically significant increase in mean pachymetry after drug withdrawal.

Epiphora: A summary of the epiphora results is found in Figure 6. The chart lists the incidence of eyes with „present" or „absent" epiphora, per treatment group, for each observation day. The differences between the treatment groups for epiphora on Day 21 (p=0.060) and Day 42 (p=0.0027) for the right eye and on Day 21 (p=0.060), on Day 42 (p=0.066) and Day 63 (p=0.080) in the left eye indicate significant or preliminary significant differences between the two treatment groups.

Investigators overall assessment: Results for the investigator's overall assessment of the initial treatment phase (Day 0 up to Day 42) are found in Figure 7. The chart lists the incidence of dogs who were assessed as having "vast improvement", „some improvement", „no change", or „failure/worsening".

The statistical significance level for the analysis is p=0.8182 for both eyes. Cyclosporine A treated eyes showed a statistically significant higher percentage of „vastly improved" and „improved" than the Isopto-Dex group (OS and OD). The overall percentage of Cyclosporine A treated eyes with vastly improved or improved assessments were 81.4% (OS) and 81.3% (OD). This is contrasted to the Isopto-Dex group results of 46.2% (OS) and 47.6% (OD).

Results for the investigator's assessment of the withdrawal phase (Day 63) are found in Figure 8. The chart lists the incidence of dogs who were assessed as having "vast improvement", „some improvement", „no change", or „failure/worsening". The statistical significance level for the analysis is p=1.0000 for both eyes. All Cyclosporine A treated eyes (except one OD) and all Isopto-Dex vehicle treated eyes worsened without ocular therapy. No statistically significant differences were found between treatment groups.

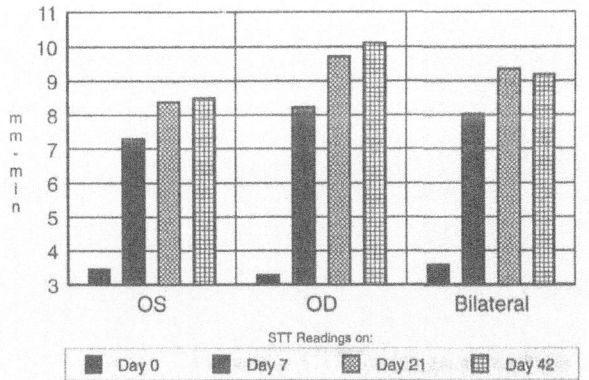

Figure 5. Mean STT increase

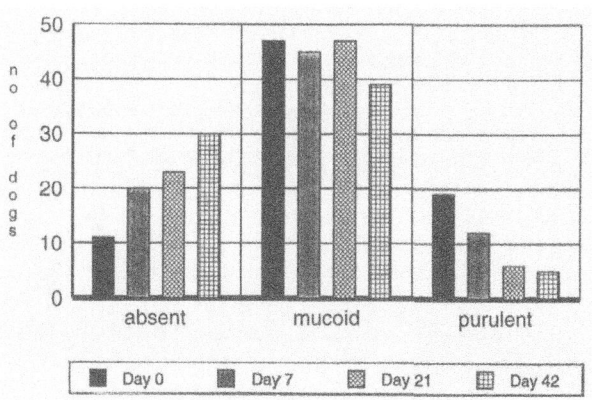

Figure 6. Presence and quality of conjunctival discharge

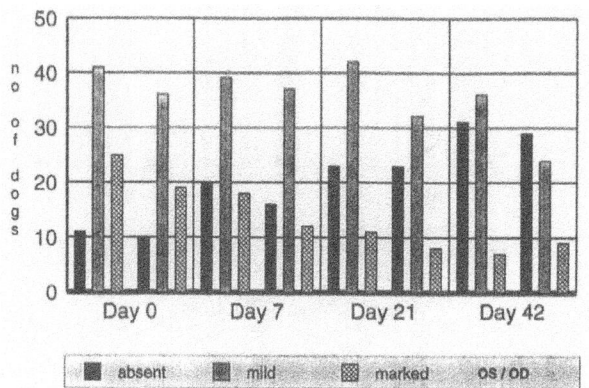

Figure 7. Volume of conjunctival discharge

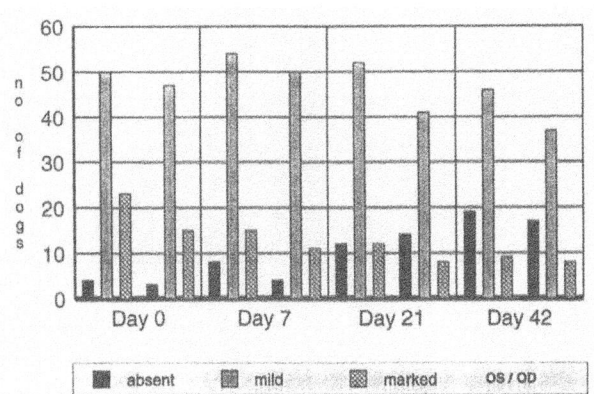

Figure 8. Conjunctival Hyperaemia

CONCLUSIONS

The present study supports the use of Cyclosporine A in the management of Pannus in the GSD. Although lesions associated with Pannus were not completely eliminated during therapy with Cyclosporine A within six weeks of treatment and corticosteroids show a better control of initial symptoms (corneal edema, decrease of pannus formation), improvement of ocular lesions was progressive and compared to Dexamethasone treatment the overall assessment of Cyclosporine A treated eyes was significantly better in the Cyclosporine A group.

Clinical experience over many years has demonstrated that continuous Dexamethasone treatment maintains a „silent" state of the disease with spontaneous relapse occurring. Dogs observed for longer treatment periods with Cyclosporine A show further continuous improvement (data obtained for five month after cessation of study) concerning amount of pigmentation and corneal clarity. Therefore continuous resolution of corneal lesions is likely to occur with continuous long-term treatment. Since Cyclosporine A is a selective immune modulator with reported absence of ophthalmic toxicity and other ocular complications (infectious diseases, corneal ulcer), which cannot be ruled out by using Dexamethasone on long term basis, especially when affected dogs are treated on a daily basis without routine reexamination, treatment with Cyclosporine A is an attractive, promising therapeutic agent for treatment of Pannus in the GSD. The combination of corticosteroid (subc.inj.+local application) in the acute phase and concurrent use of both, Cyclosporine A and corticosteroids, may provide increased efficacy in treating Pannus.

REFERENCES

Kaswan, R. L. and Salisbury, M. A. and Ward, D. A.., 1990, Spontaneous canine kerato-conjunctivitis sicca, A useful model for human keratoconjunctivitis treatment with cyclosporin eye drops, *Arch. Ophthalmol;* 107:1210.

Olivero, D. K., Davidson, M. G. and English, R. V., 1994, Clinical trial evaluating 1% topical cyclosporine A for canine keratoconjunctivitis sicca., *J. Am. Ve.t Med. Assoc., submitted for publication.*

Bedford, P. G. C. and Longstaffe, J. A., 1979, Corneal Pannus (chronic superficial keratitis) in the German Shepherd Dog, *J. Small Anim. Pract.,* 20: 41.

CHARACTERIZATION OF HUMAN TEAR GLYCOPROTEINS BY PHAST

SDS ELECTROPHORESIS, WESTERN BLOTTING AND LECTIN

BINDING

W. Breipohl[1], C. Reitz[1], M.H.J. Ahrend[1],
F.H. Grus[2], and J. Bours[1]

[1]Department of Experimental Ophthalmology,
[2]Department of Ophthalmology,
University of Bonn, D-53105 Bonn, F.R.G.

INTRODUCTION

The proteins in human tear fluid form a very complex mixture and can be divided into six main groups: 1) protective proteins: the immunoglobulins (sIgA, IgA, IgG, IgM, IgE; 2) proteins with bacteriostatic or bacteriolytic properties (lactoferrin, tear-specific pre-albumin, lysozyme); 3) proteins derived from the plasma (IgA, IgG, albumin, transferrin); 4) glycoproteins as protease inhibitor (acid α_1-glycoprotein, α_1-antitrypsin, α_1-antichymotrypsin); 5) other functional proteins (ceruloplasmin, α_2-macroglobulin, β_2-microglobulin); 6) enzymes (amylase, peroxydase, plasminogen activator, plasmin, tryptase and LDH derived from conjunctiva). The composition of tear fluid proteins, their concentration and molecular weights, are summarized in Table 1. The main proteins in human tear fluid, synthesized in the lacrimal gland and at high concentrations present in tear fluid are: 1) secretory immunoglobulin A (sIgA), 2) lactoferrin (LF), 3) tear-specific pre-albumin (TSPA) and 4) lysozyme (LYS). Concentrations are given in Table 1.

This study was to analyze tear fluid proteins, and especially sialomucins (glycoproteins glycated with Gal 2-3-NANA) by PHAST gel SDS-electrophoresis. We followed the method of Kuizenga et al.[21] of SDS electrophoresis on minigels, but modified it by application of the gel composition given by Michov[22,23,24] for self cast gels. These low cost gels were specially designed for rapid separation on a microscale. Overall protein staining was done with Coomassie Blue. The glycoproteins amongst the tear proteins (Table 1) can be stained with the periodic acid Schiff reagent[25]. However, this general staining of glycoproteins requires a relatively large amount of proteins and does not discriminate between glycosylation with individual carbohydrates. To overcome this difficulty, tear proteins and glycoproteins in this study were analyzed by staining with Coomassie Blue in combination with western blotting and subsequent staining with lectins.

Table 1. Composition, concentration and molecular weights of proteins from normal human tear fluid.

Protein Constituents	Glycoprotein Function	Intra-Lacrimal Synthesis	Concentration in mg/100 ml	Molecular Weight	References
Secretory IgA	+	+	10.6[1]; 13.27[2,3,4]; 20-110[5]: 32.8 ± 21.9[6]	385.000 Da	1,2,3,4,5,6.
IgA, derived from Serum	-	-	0.03[2,3,4]	160.000 Da	2,3,4,7.
IgG, derived from Serum	-	-	0.3[1]; 0.50[2,3,4]; 0.9 ± 0.6;	150.000 Da	1,2,3,4.
Lysozyme	-	+	169.9[4]; 170[5]; 84[6]; 329,7 ±42,9[10]	14.600 Da	6,8,9,10
Serum Albumin	-	-	2.32[1]; 3.4[2,3,4]; 4,2[10]	69.000 Da	1,2,3,4,10.
Transferrin derived from Serum	-	-	0.10 ± 0,01[10,12,13]	90.000 Da	10,12,13.
Tear-Specific Pre-Albumin	-	+	167.7 ± 18,8[8,10]	17.600 Da[14]	8,10,14.
Tear Lactoferrin	+	+	291 ± 149[6]; 174.1 ± 19.3[15];	82.000 Da[15]	6,15.
IgA Secretory Piece	+	+	79.3 ± 13.9[10]	65.000 Da	10.
Ceruloplasmin	+	+	4.0[13]	135.000 Da	12,13.
Acid α1-Glycoprotein	+	+		44.100 Da	12,13.
IgE	+	+	0.0014[16]	196.000 Da	16.
α1-Antitrypsin	+	+	2.6[1]; 1.50[17]	54.000 Da[17]	1,17.
α1-Antichymotrypsin	+	+	1.40[1]	68.000 Da	1,18.
α2-Macroglobulin	+	+	0.06[1]	725.000 Da	1.
Haptoglobin	+	+	0.10[1]	100.000 Da	1.
Peroxidase	-	+	0.67 ± 0.01[10]		10,19.
β2-Microglobulin	+	+	1.0[1];1.1[6]	11.800 Da	1,6.
Protein G	+	+		31.000 Da[11]	11.
IgM	+	+	0.2[1]; <0.5[6]; 0.29 ± 0.06[10]	900.000 Da	1,6,10.
Total Protein	+	+	1000		20.

MATERIALS AND METHODS

Collection of normal human tear fluid

Unstimulated tears (7 males and 10 females) were collected with capillary tubes from normal healthy volunteers. Their ages ranged from 20 to 35 years (mean 28 yrs).

Electrophoretic analyses

Micro-immunoelectrophoresis of tear fluid was performed according to Bours[26] and minigel electrophoresis according to Michov[22,23,24].

SDS-PAGE was performed on Minigels, using an automated PHAST electrophoresis system of Pharmacia. An SDS stock solution was made containing 7.58% TRIS.HCl, 0.5% SDS and 0,0125% NaN_3. A sample buffer was made containing 1.0ml SDS stock solution, 3mg GPTA, 10mg NaN_3, 10mg bromophenolblue and bidistilled water to a final volume of 100ml. Tear samples ($5\mu l$) were diluted with $5\mu l$ sample buffer and preincubated at room temperature (non-reduced samples, under non-dissociating conditions) before electrophoresis. Reduction of tear samples performed under dissociating (denaturing) conditions, including standard molecular weight markers, was performed in a sample buffer containing 1% dithiothreitol at 100°C for 3min. From the samples $1.0\mu l$ was applied automatically onto the gel with a PHAST-gel sample applicator. Total tear protein concentration applied on each lane ranged from 2 to $5\mu g$. The low range molecular weight markers were from Bio-Rad (161-0304 normal, 161-0305 prestained). Electropho-resis was performed for approximately 35min, following the manufacturer's instructions. We used self-cast gels, made according to the system of Michov[22,23,24] in a TRIS-formate-taurinate buffer system. The stacking gel (S10) of pH 8.07 contained per 100ml: TRIS-Base 4.56g, formic acid 0.91ml, acrylamide 4.80g, bis-acrylamide 0.20g, SDS 0.06g, glycerin 87% 34.48ml. The pH is 8.07. For polymerization of the stacking gel were used: 1.8ml S10, $1.2\mu l$ TEMED and $2.6\mu l$ ammoniumperoxydisulfate of 40g/100ml (APS). The separating gel contained T10-T15 acrylamide monomer, and was poured with the help of a gradient mixer (Pharmacia/LKB Ultrograd 11300, or Pharmacia/LKB 8100-1, respec-tively). The polymerization solution (T10) of pH 8.07, for the running gel contained per 100ml: TRIS-Base 4.56g, formic acid 0.91ml, acrylamide 8.64g, bis-acrylamide 0.36g, SDS 0.06g, glycerin 87% 11.49ml. For polymerization of the separating gel were used: 3ml T10, $2.2\mu l$ TEMED and $2.4\mu l$ APS. The polymerization solution (T15) of pH 7.61, for the running gel contained per 100ml: TRIS-Base 3.47g, formic acid 0.91ml, acryl-amide 14.40g, bis-acrylamide 0.60g, SDS 0.06g and glycerin 87% 11.49ml. For polymeri-zation of the separating gel was used: 3ml T15, $2.2\mu l$ TEMED, $1.6\mu l$ APS. The recipient vessels of the gradient mixer were filled with 3ml of the light solution T10 and 3ml of the heavy solution T15, and the gel was allowed to solidify. The cathode buffer of pH 8.47 contained: TRIS-Base 57.10g, taurine 80.30g, SDS 2.00g and bidistilled water to a final volume of 1 liter. The anode buffer of pH 7.78 contained TRIS-Base 124,80g, formic acid 30.5ml, SDS 2.00g and bidistilled water to a final volume of 1 liter. Agar electrode strips were used in anode buffer (pH 7.78) and cathode buffer (pH 8.47) according to Michov[24]. After electrophoresis the gels were stained with Coomassie Brilliant Blue and destained in 10% acetic acid containing 30% methanol in a Development Unit, accessory to the PHAST System, according to the manufacturer's instructions. Diffusion blotting with lectins was performed in the following buffer: TRIS.HCl 50mmol/l, NaCl 150mmol/l, $MgCl.6H_2O$ 1mmol/l, $MnCl_2.4H_2O$ 1mmol/l, $CaCl_2.2H_2O$ 1mmol/l.

RESULTS

Micro-immunoelectrophoresis of tear fluid, developed with three monovalent and one polyvalent antiserum, revealed one prominent precipitin line for albumin and secretory IgA each (Figs. 1b,e). Secretory IgA and serum IgA appeared to have identical electrophoretic mobilities (Figs. 1d,e). For IgG two precipitin lines were detected in tears as well as in human serum (Figs. 1e,f). Furthermore, in tears at least two additional lines appeared in the spectrum, developed with polyvalent antiserum directed towards the proteins of human whole serum (Fig. 1c).

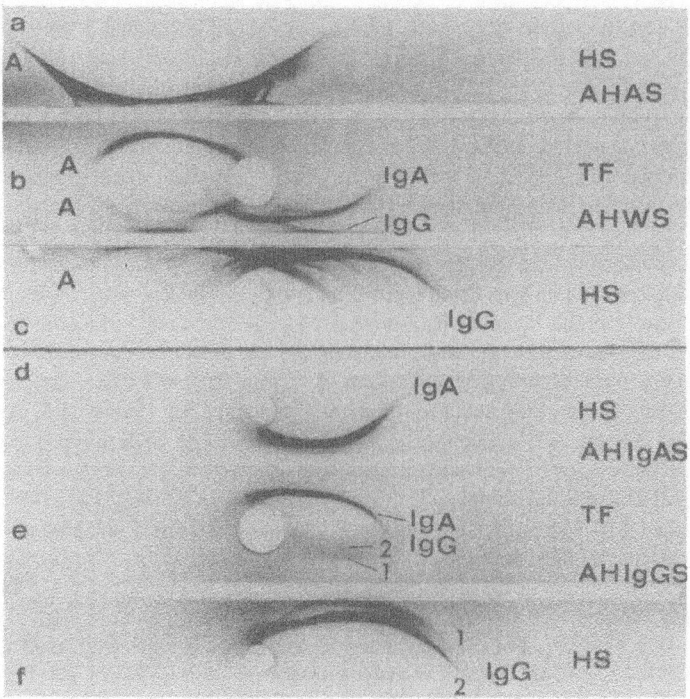

Fig. 1(a-f). Microimmunoelectrophoresis of human tear fluid against various antisera. a,c,d,f) human serum (HS), b,e) tear fluid (TF). AHWS = anti-human whole serum, AHIgAS = anti-human IgA serum, AHIgGS = anti- human IgG serum, A = albumin, IgA = immunoglobulin-A, IgG = immunoglobulin-G.

Figure 2 shows SDS electrophoresis in reduced form of six tear specimen (1-6). The protein composition of human tear fluid shows considerable individual variation as can be seen in the differences between lanes {1,6}, {2,4} and {3,6}. Remains of the sIgA were localized at the interface between the stacking and separating gel. The major tear protein constituents, e.g. sIgA, lactoferrin (LF), tear-specific pre-albumin (TSPA) and lysozyme (LYS) were also clearly separated in this Minigel System. The LF band was separated into at least two bands. Reduction of sIgA produced 3 bands, with MW of 85kDa (IgA secretory piece, SP), 64 kDa (IgA heavy chain α) and 28kDa (IgA light chain $\kappa\lambda$). A number of unidentified bands appeared in the reduced form: a double band at 45kDa, a prominent unknown band (U) at 32kDa (lanes 1,6) and two weak bands at 21 and 19kDa.

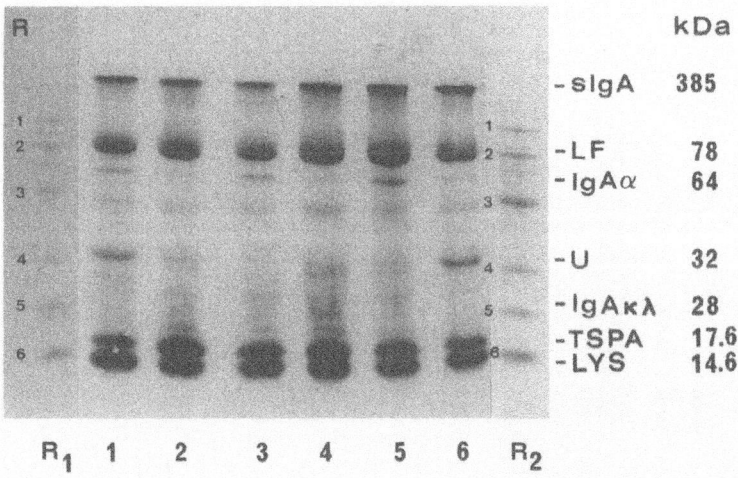

	kDa
-sIgA	385
-LF	78
-IgAα	64
-U	32
-IgAκλ	28
-TSPA	17.6
-LYS	14.6

R_1 1 2 3 4 5 6 R_2

Fig. 2. SDS-PAGE in reduced form (R) of normal human tear fluid ($0.5\mu l$, diluted 1:1 to $1.0\mu l$, lanes 1-6). s-IgA = secretory immunoglobulin-A, LF = lactoferrin, IgAα = immunoglobulin-A, heavy chain, U = unidentified component, IgAκλ = immunoglobulin-A light chain, TSPA = tear-specific pre-albumin, LYS = lysozyme. R_1, R_2 = reference proteins as molecular weight standards, low range. R_2 = pre-stained markers, identical to R_1. R_1 and R_2 are composed of (1) phosphorylase-b (97.4kDa), (2) serum albumin (66.2kDa), (3) ovalbumin (45kDa), (4) carbonic anhydrase (31kDa), (5) trypsin inhibitor (21.3kDa), (6) lysozyme (14.4kDa).

Figure 3a shows SDS electrophoresis under non-reducing conditions. sIgA was found at the interface between stacking and separating gel. LF was localized at 78kDa, albumin (AL) between 66 and 45kDa and protein G at about 32-35kDa. TSPA was identified as the major band just above LYS.

To detect lectin-binding tear proteins, samples under non-reducing conditions were used for blotting with digoxigenin labeled lectin probes. Tear samples from the same gel (Fig. 3a) were treated for blotting with MAA (Fig. 3b). This showed the SP of IgA at 85kDa and sIgA itself at 385kDa.

Fig. 4 shows tear protein samples in the reduced form. In Fig. 4a the SP at 85kDa and the light IgA chain (α) at 28kDa were positive with MAA. The same samples from Fig. 4a were used for blotting with SNA (lanes 1-4). Here only LF was positive.

DISCUSSION

Our study has shown that sIgA and IgA components are proteins glycated with Gal(2-3-NANA). The results have to be considered in the light of multiple investigations of other authors[11,21,27-30] with SDS. These authors have analyzed tear proteins by SDS-electrophoresis and separated the tear proteins in non-reduced form into a number of components (e.g. sIgA, LF, secretory piece SP, protein G, TSPA, LYS). However, several prominent bands remained unidentified. IgG for example, which is an important constituent of tear fluid, is synthesized in the lacrimal gland and present in moderate quantities (Table 1)[1,2,3]. It could easily be detected[19] by immuno-electrophoresis (Fig.1) and other immunologic methods[1,2,3], but was not traced by SDS-electrophoresis[11,21,29,30]. Also IgM in non reduced form[1,6,10] at a concentration of about 0,3 mg/100 ml (Table 1) could not be detected by

321

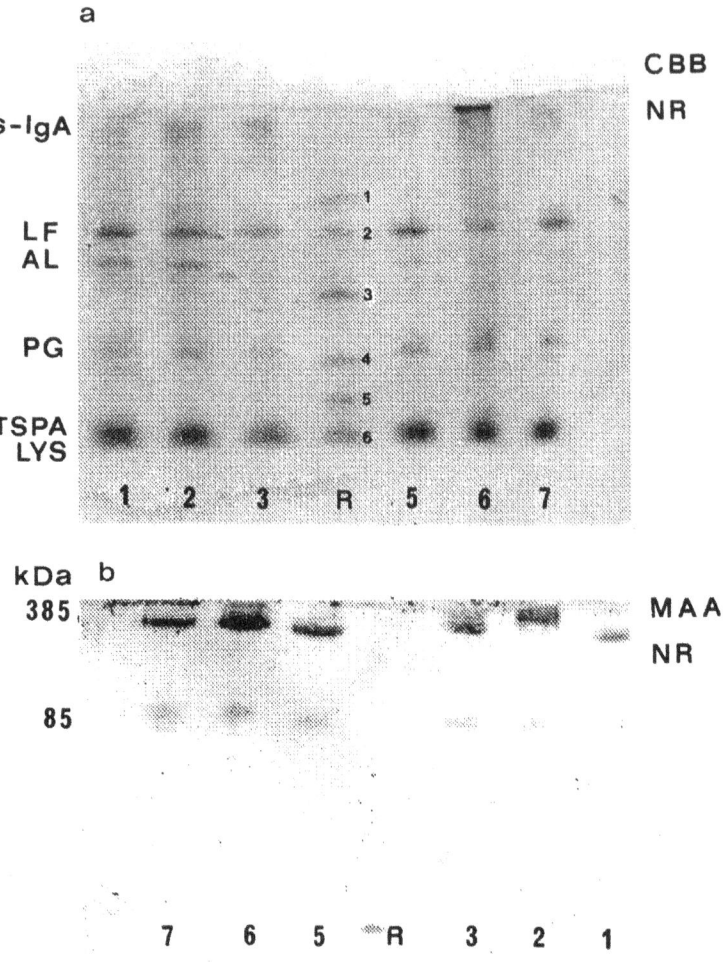

Fig. 3(a,b). SDS-PAGE in non-reduced form (NR) of normal human tear fluid (1.0μl): a) stained with Coomassie Brilliant Blue (CBB), lanes 1-7; b) after blotting with MAA, lanes 7-1. R = reference proteins as molecular weights standards, low range. sIgA = secretory immunoglobulin-A, LF = lactoferrin, AL = albumin, PG = protein G, TSPA = tear-specific pre-albumin, LYS = lysozyme. The component at 85 kDa in b) is the IgA secretory piece.

SDS-electrophoresis. Our investigative strategies try to overcome these problems in combining different electrophoretic techniques.

Among the proteins of human tears, a number of tear-specific proteins are glycated. This was first described by Halken and Bjerrum et al.[27,28]. They showed in the profiles several distinct lectin-bound proteins, with the lectins PHA, PSA, WGA and SBA but did not identify the stained bands satisfactorily. Kuizenga et al.[11] discovered by lectin blotting a number of components positive with 7 different lectins. They found that the reduced composing elements of sIgA were positive in reduced form with the lectins CON-A, PNA,

PHA-E, WGA, Jacalin and PSA. This means that sIgA is glycated with Man/ Glc, Gal/NAcGal and GlcNAc. In addition to these results we have found that sIgA was also glycated with Gal(2-3-NANA) (Figs. 3b,4a). Glycation of tear proteins and especially with

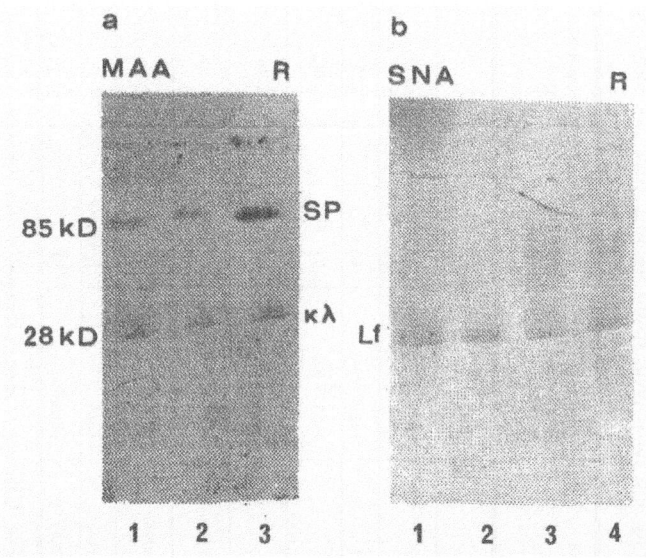

Fig. 4(a,b). SDS electrophoresis in reduced form (R) of normal human tear fluid, lanes 1-3 and 1-4, after blotting with a) MAA and b) SNA. SP = secretory piece, κλ = IgA light chain, LF = lactoferrin.

Gal(2-3-NANA) is of interest for current hypotheses on tear film attachment to the corneal surface[31-34]. In this context other authors[11,28] have reported a variety of data on glycation of sIgA and LF (Table 2).

Since the techniques applied in the referred literature and in this report are somewhat onesided, they should be comple-mented in future by non-denaturing approaches, e.g. by HPLC[35] and by more sensitive methods with a higher resolving power, like isoelectric focusing[36] and isotachophoresis[37], to elucidate and explain all unidentified components of tear fluid in a satisfactory way.

CONCLUSIONS

Secretory IgA itself and the structural elements from sIgA (Secretory Piece, IgA Heavy Chain α and IgA Light Chain κλ) were all stained positive with lectins binding to the following carbohydrates: Man/Glc, Gal/NAcGal and NAcGlc. Furthermore, positive affinity was shown with the lectin MAA which is specific for Gal(2-3-NANA). Thus, glycation of sIgA differs basically from that of lactoferrin, since the latter, after western blotting, reacts with the Gal(2-6-NANA)-specific SNA. These results are considered important for corneal tear attachment and investigations on dry eye syndromes.

Table 2. Carbohydrate specificity of glycated tear proteins, by blotting and subsequent lectin staining after SDS-electrophoresis.

Nr.	Lectin	Source Taxonomic Name	Common Name	Carbohydrate Specificity	Positive Reaction in Non-Reduced Form	Positive Reaction in Reduced Form	Reference/ Figure
1.	CON-A	Canavalia ensiformis	Jack Bean	Man/Glc	sIgA, LF	LF, SP, IgAα, LYS	11.
2.	PNA	Arachis hypogea	Peanut	GalNAc/Gal	sIgA, LF	LF, SP, IgAα, LYS	11.
3.	SBA	Glycine maximus	Soybean	GalNAc/Gal	negative	LYS	11,28.
4.	PHA-E	Phaseolus vulgaris	Kidney bean	GalNAc	sIgA, LF	LF, SP, IgAα, LYS	11,28.
5.	WGA	Triticum vulgaris	Wheat Germ	GlcNAc	sIgA, LF	LF, SP, IgAα, LYS	11,28.
6.	JACALIN	Artocarpus integrifolia	Jacalin	Gal/GalNAc	sIgA, LF	LF, SP, IgAα, LYS	11.
7.	PSA	Pisum sativum	Pea	Man/Glc/GlcNAc	sIgA, LF	LF, SP, IgAα, LYS	11,28.
8.	MAA	Maackia amurensis	a bean*	Gal(2-3-NANA)	sIgA	IgAα, SP	3b.
9.	SNA	Sambucus nigra	Bark from Elder	Gal(2-6-NANA)	negative	LF	4a.

Legend: Man = mannose, Glc = glucose, Gal = Galactose, GlcNAc = N-acetylglucosamine, GalNAc = N-acetylgalactosamine, NANA = N-acetyl-neuraminic acid, sIgA = secretory IgA, IgAα = sIgA heavy chain (α), SP = sIgA secretory piece, LF = lactoferrin, LYS = lysozyme. *of a Papillonaceae from S.E. Asia and Mongolia.

REFERENCES

1. S. Liotet, V.N. Warnet and A. Schroeder, Étude de la barrière hémato-lacrimale humaine normale. *Journal Franç. d'Ophtalmol.* 5:707(1982).
2. R.L. Lundh, S. Liotet and Y. Pouliquen, Study of the human blood-tear barrier and the biochemical changes in the tears of 30 contact lens wearers (50 eyes). *Ophthalmologica, Basel* 188:100(1984).
3. R.L. Lundh, Biochemical and immunological response of tears of 30 aphakic eyes, half of which had received implants and the other half contact lenses. *Ophthalmologica, Basel* 191:164(1985).
4. N. Stambuk, T. Ćurković, M. Trbojević-Čepe and J. Ožegović, Measurement of intraocular IgA and IgM synthesis and filtration through the blood-aqueous barrier in cataract patients. *Current Eye Res.* 9/Suppl:45(1990).
5. R.A. Sack, K.O. Tan and A. Tan, Diurnal tear cycle: evidence for a nocturnal inflammatory constitutive tear fluid. *Invest. Ophthalmol. Vis. Sci.* 33:626(1992).
6. D. Meillet, J. Glomaud, F. Unanue, M.C. Diemert, A. Galli, P. Le Hoang, F. Rousselie and J. Galli, Protéines sériques et lacrymales au cours du syndrome d'immunodéficience acquise. *Journal Franç. d'Ophtalmol.* 12:499(1989).
7. P.T. Janssen and O.P. van Bijsterveld, Origin and biosynthesis of human tear fluid proteins. *Invest. Ophthalmol. Vis. Sci.* 24:623(1983).
8. A.T. Sapse, B. Bonavida, W. Stone and E.E. Sercarz, Human tear lysozyme. III. Preliminary study on lysozyme levels in subjects with smog eye irritation. *Am. J. Ophthalmol.* 66:76(1968).
9. A. Temel, H. Kazokoglu, Y. Taga, Tear lysozyme levels in contact lens wearers. *Ann. Ophthalmol.* 23:191(1991).
10. R.J. Fullard and L. Snyder, Protein levels in nonstimulated and stimulated tears of normal human subjects. *Invest. Ophthalmol. Vis. Sci.* 31:1119(1990).
11. A. Kuizenga, N.J. van Haeringen and A. Kijlstra, Identification of lectin binding proteins in human tears. *Invest. Ophthalmol. Vis. Sci.* 32:3277(1991).
12. A.S. Josephson and D.W. Lockwood, Immunoelectrophoretic studies of the protein components of normal tears. *J. Immunol.* 93:532(1964).
13. A.T. Sapse, B. Bonavida, W. Stone and E.E. Sercarz, Proteins in human tears. I. Immunoelectrophoretic patterns. *Arch. Ophthalmol.* 81:815(1969).
14. K. Felgenhauer, Protein filtration and secretion at human body fluid barriers. *Pflügers Arch.* 384:9(1980).
15. R.M. Broekhuyse, Tear lactoferrin: a bacteriostatic and complexing protein. *Invest. Ophthalmol. Vis. Sci.* 13:550(1974).
16. M.R. Allansmith, G.S. Hahn and M.A. Simon, Tissue, tear and serum IgE concentrations in vernal conjunctivitis. *Amer. J. Ophthalmol.* 81:506(1976).
17. M. Zirm, Proteins in aqueous humor. *Advances in Ophthalmol.* 40:100(1980).
18. M. Zirm and O. Schmut, Immunologische Untersuchungen des Kammerwassers und deren Ergebnisse. *Wiener Klin. Wochenschr.* 88:343(1976).
19. N.J. van Haeringen, Clinical Biochemistry of tears. Survey of Ophthalmol. 26:84(1981).
20. F. Meijer and N.J. van Haeringen, Comparison of three techniques for the determination of protein content in human tears. *Clin. Chim. Acta* 209:209(1992).
21. A. Kuizenga, N.J. van Haeringen and A. Kijlstra, SDS-Minigel electrophoresis of human tears. *Invest. Ophthalmol. Vis. Sci.* 32:381(1991).
22. B.M. Michov, Electrophoresis in one buffer at two pH values. Electrophoresis 10:686(1989).
23. B.M. Michov, Electrophoresis in an expanded stationary boundary. Electrophoresis 11:289(1990).
24. B.M. Michov, A TRIS-formate-taurinate buffer system for the SDS electrophoresis in homogeneous polyacrylamide gel slabs. *GIT Fachzeitschrift für das Laboratorium* 36/7:746(1992).
25. J. Bours, M.H.J. Ahrend and W. Breipohl, The presence of ß-, ßs- and γ-crystallins in the water-insoluble crystallin complex of the ageing bovine lens, *in*: "Eye Lens Membranes and Ageing", G. Vrensen and J. Clauwaert, ed., Topics in Aging Research in Europe 14:341(1991).
26. J. Bours, The presence of lens crystallins as well as albumin and other serum proteins in chick iris tissue extracts. *Exp. Eye Res.* 15:299(1973).
27. P. Halken, T.C. Bøg-Hansen and J.U. Prause, Human tear glycoproteins, *in:* Lectins, T.C. Bøg-Hansen, E. van Driessche, ed., de Gruyter, Berlin, Vol. 5:609(1996).
28. K. Bjerrum, P. Halken and J.U. Prause, The normal human tear glycoprotein profile detected with lectin probes. *Exp. Eye Res.* 53:431(1991).
29. A. Kijlstra, A. Kuizenga, M. van der Velde and N.J. van Haeringen, Gel electrophoresis of human tears reveals various forms of tear lactoferrin. *Current Eye Res.* 8:581(1989).

30. A. Kuizenga, T.R. Stolwijk, E.J. van Agtmaal, N.J. van Haeringen and A. Kijlstra, Detection of secretory IgM in tears of IgA deficient individuals. *Current Eye Res.* 9:997(1990).
31. W. Breipohl, W. Naib-Majani, F. Sinowatz, T. Naguro and A. Wegener, Sialomucin expression in the human accessory lacrimal gland, *in:* "Sjögren's Syndrome - State of the Art", eds. M. Homma, S. Sugai, T. Tojo, N. Miyasaka and M. Akizuki, Proc. of the 4th Internatl. Symposium, Kugler, Amsterdam, New York, 1994, pp. 553.
32. W. Breipohl, W. Naib-Majani, U. Sterzinski, Classification of glycoprotein expression in human conjunctival, main and accessory tear gland cells. Abstract. *Invest. Ophthalmol. Vis. Sci.* 35:1795(1994).
33. W. Breipohl, M. Spitznas, F. Sinowatz, O. Leib, W. Naib-Majani and A. Cusomano, Galactose-binding sites in the acinar cells of the human accessory lacrimal gland. *in:* "Lacrimal Gland, Tear Film, and Dry Eye Syndromes: Basic Science and Clinical Relevance", eds. D.A. Sullivan, D.A. Dart et al., New York, Plenum Press, 1994, pp. 45.
34. W. Breipohl, J. Strobel, W. Naib-Majani, C. Herberhold, M. Hamdi-Ibrahim, C. Reitz, Sialomucin expression in human conjunctival and nasal goblet cells. (Submitted, 1994).
35. R.J. Fullard, Identification of proteins in small tear volumes with and without size exclusion HPLC fractionation. *Current Eye Res.* 7:163(1988).
36. G. Wollensak, E. Murr, A. Mayr, G. Bayer, W. Göttinger and G. Stöffler, Effective methods for the investigation of human tear film proteins and lipids. *Graefe's Arch. Clin. Exp. Ophthalmol.* 228:78(1990).
37. J. Bours and H.J. Födisch, Isotachophoresis of human fetal lens crystallins with increasing gestational age. *Ophthalmic Res.* 18:369(1986).

THE CORNEAL EFFECTS OF 2-(2-NITRO-4-TRIFLUOROMETHYL-BENZOYL)-CYCLOHEXANE 1,3-DIONE (NTBC) IN THE RAT

Mervyn Robinson

Zeneca Central Toxicology Laboratory
Alderley Park
Macclesfield
Cheshire
SK10 4TJ
England

INTRODUCTION

2-(2-Nitro-4-trifluoromethylbenzoyl)-cyclohexane-1,3-dione (NTBC) is a triketone which was originally discovered at the Western Research Centre of Zeneca Ag Products (Prisbylla et al., 1993). The purpose of this paper is to report and describe the ophthalmoscopic and histopathological changes in the cornea of rats when dosed orally with this compound by gavage and to compare them with the changes described by Burns et al. (1976) when rats are dosed with 5% tyrosine in a low protein diet.

MATERIALS AND METHODS

NTBC was synthetised at Zeneca Western Research Centre, Richmond, California, USA and had a purity of 91.5% w/v. The dosing vehicle was Kraft Wesson 100% corn oil supplied by Kraft Foods Ltd.

Male Alpk:APfSD (Wistar-derived) rats were obtained from the Barriered Animal Breeding Colony at Alderley Park, Macclesfield, Cheshire, UK at 35 days old and acclimatised to their environment conditions for 1 week prior to the study start. They were randomly allocated to their experimental group and housed 4 per cage on a multiple housing rat rack and fed CT1 diet (Special Diets Services, Witham, Essex, UK) ad libitum via an automatic nozzle in the cage.

The room temperature was controlled at approximately 21°C with a relative humidity of approximately 50%. Lighting was controlled by a time clock to provide a 12 hour light/dark cycle.

Study 1 consisted of 1 control group and 3 treatment groups, each containing 20 rats as follows: group 1 dosed 0mg/kg/day NTBC (corn oil control), group 2 dosed 2mg/kg/day NTBC, group 3 dosed 10mg/kg/day NTBC, group 4 dosed 40mg/kg/day NTBC.

At week 14, all rats dosed with 2mg/kg/day NTBC which showed the presence of ocular lesions were divided into groups A and B (continued dosing and discontinued dosing respectively) and were placed on a recovery phase of the study until termination at week 21. Allocation to group A or B was by alternate ear number in order to eliminate bias. Two rats dosed at 2mg/kg/day had normal eyes at week 14 and were placed in group A . All rats in the recovery phase (groups A and B) were terminated at week 21. All other rats were terminated at week 14.

Study 2 consisted of 70 rats dosed with 10mg/kg/day NTBC. Rats with corneal lesions as observed by ophthalmoscopy were killed at intervals so that a range of lesion ages could be obtained. The selection and termination procedure was such that a sufficient number of rats with early lesions was achieved.

Rats were dosed daily 7 days per week by gavage for the appropriate duration of the study. Dosing was carried out by using disposable plastic syringes and a plastic nelaton catheter 8FG 10cm long with a 14G stub adaptor. The dosing volume was 0.5ml/100g bodyweight.

The eyes of all rats were examined by a Fison's indirect ophthalmoscope after pupillary dilatation with 0.5% tropicamide (Mydriacyl, Alcon Laboratories, Watford, Herts, UK) at the following times for study 1: all rats predose, weeks 2, 3, 4, 5, 6, 8, 10, 12 and 14; rats on recovery phase weeks 15, 17, 18, 20, 21; and for study 2: daily for the first week of dosing and thereafter at regular intervals and at least once per week.

Any rat requiring removal from the study due to adverse clinical signs and all rats at the appropriate termination day were killed by exsanguination under deep halothane Ph. Eur. (Fluothane, Zeneca Pharmaceuticals, Macclesfield, Cheshire, UK) anaesthesia.

All rats in study 1 dosed with 0, 10, or 40mg/kg/day NTBC were killed at week 14. Rats dosed at 2mg/kg/day NTBC were terminated at week 21. The eyes of rats dosed at 2mg/kg/day NTBC were removed, fixed in Davidson's solution, routinely processed, paraffin wax embedded, cut at 5μm and then stained with haematoxylin and eosin. All sections were examined by light microscopy.

Rats in study 2 were removed from the study sequentially and the eyes treated as above. For rats which showed the presence of small focal lesions of 1 or 2 days duration by ophthalmoscopy the eyes were embedded whole after removal of the lens and step sections at 100μm intervals were taken and stained.

RESULTS

Ophthalmoscopy

The incidence of corneal lesions in study 1 up to 14 weeks is shown in Table 1. The incidence was treatment related but not dose related. With time the incidence increased in all groups with a maximum incidence of 18/20 at 14 weeks in the group dosed at 2mg/kg. In some rats the changes were unilateral, in others they were bilateral.

Table 1   Incidence of Corneal Lesions up to 14 Weeks in Rats in Study 1

	Dose Level of NTBC (mg/kg/day)			
Duration	0	2	10	40
Prestudy	1/20	0/20	0/20	0/20
2 weeks	2/20	5/20	8/20	2/20
3 weeks	1/20	10/20	9/20	5/20
4 weeks	1/20	14/20	15/20	9/20
5 weeks	1/20	15/20	15/20	8/20
6 weeks	1/20	16/20	15/20	8/19
8 weeks	1/20	16/20	16/20	11/19
10 weeks	2/20	17/20	16/20	11/19
12 weeks	1/20	17/20	16/20	12/19
14 weeks	1/20	18/20	16/20	13/19

The nature of the lesions was that of opacity which varied in severity from partial or hazy opacity to complete opacity and varied in extent from very small lesions of 1mm diameter (figure 1) to involvement of the whole corneal surface. In the more extensive lesions vascularisation was evident (figure 2).

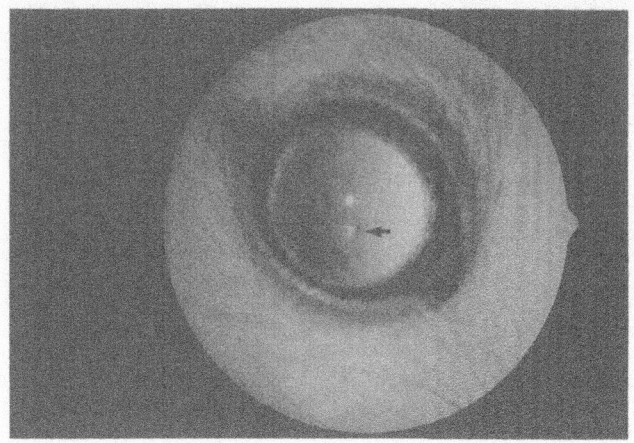

Figure 1. Early Small Focal Corneal Opacity (arrow)

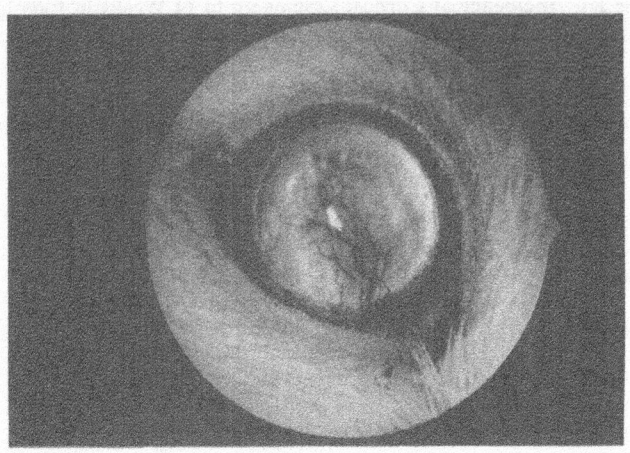

Figure 2.   Large Corneal Opacity with Vascularisation.

With increasing time the lesions initially tended to become more extensive and more severe, although at the later time points some natural reversal of severity was evident. At week 14 the eyes of rats dosed at 2mg/kg/day showed a spectrum of changes including opacity, hazy opacity, vascularisation and in 2 rats ghost vessels. Although the groups A and B were slightly different in terms of incidence of individual lesions, they were largely comparable.

At week 21 just prior to termination, the eyes of rats in group A (continued dosing) were similar to those at week 14 although the opacity in some eyes had become more hazy (Table 2).

In contrast the eyes of rats in group B (discontinued dosing) showed a marked reversal of lesions at week 21 with all rats showing the absence of opacity, hazy opacity or vascularisation, all eyes being either normal or showing ghost vessels only. In group A, of the rats which were normal at week 14, one had developed lesions by week 21 whereas one remained normal throughout.

Table 2   Ophthalmoscopic Findings in Rats Dosed 2mg/kg/day NTBC at Weeks 14 and 21 in Study 1

Ophthalmoscopic Finding	Group A (continued dosing)		Group B (discontinued dosing)	
	14 weeks	21 weeks	14 weeks	21 weeks
Number of animals	11	10*	9	9
Opacity	7	5	3	0
Hazy opacity	2	5	7	0
Vascularisation	9	8	6	0
Ghost vessels	0	0	2	5
No abnormalities	2	1	0	4

* 1 rat removed from study and killed at week 18 due to misdosing

Histopathology

In study 1 the marked differences between the eyes of group A (continued dosing) and B (discontinued dosing) observed by ophthalmoscopy were confirmed by histopathology (Table 3).

Varying degrees of keratitis were present in the majority of rats in group A consisting of one or more of the following features: polymorphonuclear leukocyte infiltration of the corneal epithelium, stroma or Descemet's membrane, the presence of blood vessels in the stroma, hyperplasia of the epithelium, vacuolar degeneration of the epithelium and eosinophil infiltration into the stroma (figure 3).

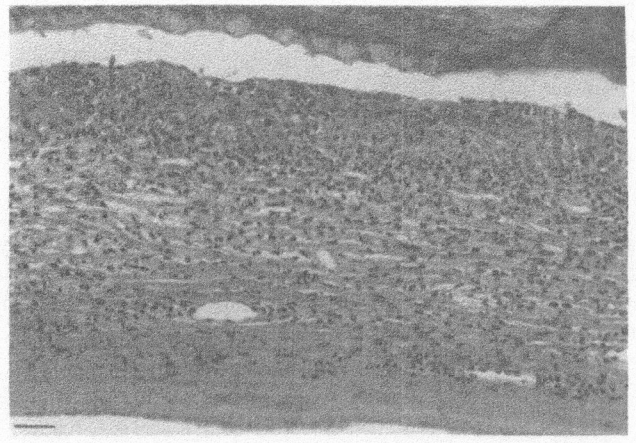

Figure 3.   Histology of Cornea with Marked Keratitis. Bar = 30μ

In contrast the range of changes in the cornea of rats in group B was much reduced and the only changes remaining were residual vascularisation and eosinophil infiltration in the stroma. Features of active keratitis were no longer present and hyperplasia of the corneal epithelium was absent except for minimal change in one rat.

Table 3   **Histopathological Findings in the Cornea of Rats Dosed 2mg/kg/day NTBC in Study 1**

Histopathological Finding	Group A (continued dosing)	Group B (discontinued dosing)
Number of animals	8*	9
Keratitis left eye	6	0
Keratitis right eye	7	0
Vascularisation left eye	5	4
Vascularisation right eye	6	7
Hyperplasia epithelium left eye	5	1
Hyperplasia epithelium right eye	6	0
Polymorphs stroma left eye	6	0
Polymorphs stroma right eye	7	0
Polymorphs epithelium left eye	4	0
Polymorphs epithelium right eye	3	0
Polymorphs Descemet's left eye	1	0
Degeneration epithelium left eye	4	0
Eosinophils left eye	1	2
Eosinophils right eye	6	1

* 1 rat removed from study at week 18

In study 2 the range of corneal changes was similar to those in study 1 with the following additional features. There was a focal disruption or disorganisation of the normal and regular layers of the epithelium. Typically this appeared as a small inverted triangular shaped lesion with the base of the triangle towards the periphery (figure 4).

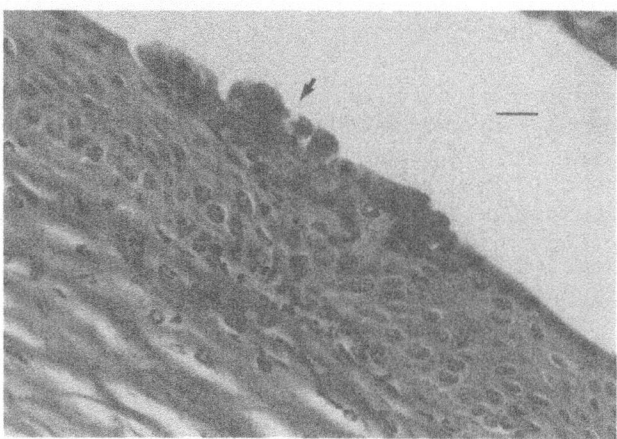

Figure 4.   **Early Corneal Change with "V"-Shaped Area of Disorganisation of Epithelium (arrow).   Bar = 20μ**

Affected cells lost the morphology of their normal counterparts so that the cells at the periphery were more rounded than normal and showed increased eosinophilia. In some cells the nuclei appeared condensed and degenerate. The normal epithelium consisted of four, or at most five, cells whereas the epithelium in the disorganised focal lesion sometimes contained six or seven cells. Frequently in section the epithelium showed separation from the underlying stroma at the point of disorganisation. Although it is considered that this was largely the result of artefactual separation during processing, it nevertheless suggests an altered degree of cellular adhesion during life.

In most eyes with corneal opacities, areas of epithelial disorganisation were accompanied by polymorph infiltration of the outer stroma immediately adjacent to the altered epithelium. In a small number of rats the only change present was the epithelial disorganisation. In these latter rats the lesions were 1 day old whereas in those with associated inflammatory changes the lesions were several days old.

In addition, in the eyes of a large number of rats there were inflammatory cells at the filtration angle often associated with polymorph infiltration of Descemet's membrane. In at least 2 rats the degree of uveitis was such as to result in synechiae and/or proteinaceous effusion into the anterior chamber.

DISCUSSION

The results indicate that NTBC induces corneal opacity with or without accompanying vascularisation at doses of 2-40mg/kg/day by oral gavage within 2 weeks of dosing. Lesions were either unilateral or bilateral. With increasing time the incidence of lesions increased so that after 14 weeks of dosing a maximum of 18/20 rats were affected. A clear dose response was not apparent since the incidence of lesions at 40mg/kg/day was less than at 2 or 10.

Histological examination of lesions of differing ages indicates that the first change to occur was disorganisation of the corneal epithelium. This was rapidly followed by inflammatory changes in the epithelium, stroma and Descemet's membrane. In some cases the anterior uvea was also affected.

When young rats are dosed orally with 5% L-tyrosine in a low protein diet a keratopathy develops within 24-36 hours (Burns et al., 1976). This is characterised ophthalmoscopically by the presence of pinpoint corneal opacities which soon develop into snowflake-like opacities. These changes are then followed by vascularisation. These gross features are therefore similar to those induced by NTBC. Histologically the changes described in the present study also closely resemble those described by Burns and co-workers (1976) although the severity of the dietary induced keratopathy would appear to be greater. No evidence of the crystal formation in the corneal epithelium described by Burns was seen in the present material.

It has been shown that NTBC inhibits 4-hydroxyphenylpyruvate dioxygenase (HPPD) (Lock et al., 1994, Ellis et al., 1993; 1994). This is the second enzyme in the normal catabolic cascade of tyrosine in mammals. Furthermore Lock et al., 1994 have demonstrated an increase in plasma tyrosine when rats are given a single oral dose of NTBC by gavage. The plasma tyrosine levels returned to normal 3 days later.

It is therefore concluded that the mechanism of NTBC toxicity to the cornea is associated with HPPD enzyme inhibition with a subsequent rise in plasma tyrosine levels which in turn induce the corneal opacity and keratitis.

REFERENCES

Burns, R.P., Gipson, I.K., and Murray, M.J., Keratopathy in tyrosinemia, Birth defects. 12:169 (1976).

Ellis, M.K., Whitfield, A.C., Gowans, L.A., Auton, T.R., Provan, W.M., Lock, E.A., and Smith, L.L., 4-Hydroxyphenylpyruvate diogenase: a target for the polyketonic herbicide 2-(2-nitro-4-trifluromethylbenzoyl)-cyclohexane-1,3-dione (NTBC). ISSX Proceedings. 4:135 (1993).

Ellis, M.K., Whifield, A.C., Gowans, L.A., Auton, T.R., Provan, W.M., Lock, E.A., and Smith, L.L., Inhibition of 4-hydroxyphenylpyruvate dioxygenase by 2-(2-nitro-trifluoromethylbenzoyl)-cyclohexane-1,3-dione (NTBC) and 2-(2-chloro-4 - methanesulphonylbenzoyl)-cyclohexane-1,3-dione (CMBC). Toxicol. Appl. Pharmacol. In press (1994).

Lock, E.A., Ellis, M.K., Provan, W.M., and Smith, L.L., The effect of NTBC on the enzymes involved in tyrosine catabolism in the rat, The Toxicologist. 14:221 (1994).

Prisbylla, M.P., Onisko, B.C., Shribbs, J.M., Adams, D.O., Liu, Y., Ellis, M.K., Hawkes, T.R., and Mutter, L.C., The novel mechanism of action of the herbicida triketones, Proceedings of the Brighton Crop Protection Conference: Weeds, 2:731 (1993).

EXACERBATION OF SPONTANEOUS RAT CORNEAL OPACITIES IN A POLYMORPHONUCLEAR ELASTASE INHIBITOR TOXICITY STUDY

J.P. Gillet[1], G. De Burlet[1], S. Molon-Noblot[1], L.D. Wise[2], G. Durand-Cavagna[1], and P. Duprat[1]

[1]: Merck Sharp & Dohme-Chibret Laboratories, Research Centre,
Department of Safety Assessement
Route de Marsat - BP 134 - 63 203 RIOM Cedex (France)

[2]: Merck Research Laboratories,
Department of Safety Assessment
West Point, Pennsylvania, 19486 (USA)

INTRODUCTION

Spontaneous corneal deposits, characterized by the presence of multiple basophilic granules at the basis of the corneal epithelium, are well described in different rat strains (1, 19) but in the literature a variation in terminology is found: i.e. corneal degeneration (1), corneal opacities (12), corneal dystrophy (19) or band keratopathy (33). This pathology is not unique to the rat but has been described in various other laboratory animals such as mouse (34), rabbit (11, 13) and dog (associated to hyperadrenocorticism, 31), as well as in man in which comparison is often done with band keratopathy (1).

Experimentally, corneal deposits have been observed following anomaly of diet composition, with vitamin D3 in excess in rats (32) and in rabbits (9, 25), in certain housing conditions (34), or after drug or toxic administration in man (2, 18) and in animals (12, 13, 16, 30, 33).

Here are described corneal opacities due to an exacerbation of spontaneous corneal deposits in rats receiving L-680,833, a Polymorphonuclear Elastase Inhibitor (PMNEI), a class of compounds for which some preclinical effects were reported (to date especially digestive effects (6)) but no ocular. Relation with spontaneous opacities observed in our rat population and with corneal changes observed in other species of laboratory animals is also presented.

MATERIAL AND METHODS

Animals and housing conditions

Sprague-Dawley rats of the Crl:CD® (SD) BR strain from Charles River France were used. At the beginning of the study, they were approximately 6 weeks old and their body weight ranged from 129 to 282 g. They were housed in wire mesh stainless steel suspended individual cages, and were given rodent chow (UAR O4C) and water *ad libitum.*

Dosing regimen

The compound, L-680,833, a PMNEI which includes a Beta Lactam cycle in its structure, was daily administered (volume 5 ml/kg body weight) by gavage to 15 rats per sex per group as a suspension in 0.5% aqueous methylcellulose at dosages of 0 (control), 50, 150, 300 mg/kg/day during 19 consecutive weeks.

Examinations

As part of the routine evaluations conducted in preclinical safety studies, ophthalmic examinations were performed on study weeks 7, 12, 16 and 18 with an indirect ophthalmoscope after 0.5% tropicamide (Mydriaticum® Chibret) instillation.

Routine serum biochemical analyses were done, as well as total calcium (Weeks 12 and 18) and alkaline phosphatase activity (Weeks 4, 7, 12 and 18), since previous cases of corneal opacities were sometimes related to variations in calcium metabolism and/or alkaline phosphatase activity in the literature (19, 22).

All rats, including those found dead or sacrificed before the scheduled termination of the study (after at least 126 oral doses), were subjected to a full necropsy. Eyes were fixed in a 10% formaldehyde neutral buffered solution except five to be used for electron microscopy which were immersed in 2% paraformaldehyde + 2.5% glutaraldehyde cacodylate buffered fixative.

Paraffin sections were hematoxylin and eosin (HE)-stained and selected sections were stained according to Von Kossa reaction for calcium detection and were evaluated under light microscopy. For electron microscopy, semi-thin sections were toluidine blue-stained and ultra-thin sections were uranyl acetate and lead citrate-contrasted for ultrastructural examination (Jeol 1200 EX electron microscope at 80KV).

RESULTS

Antemortem results

Corneal opacities were found in the mid- and high-dose groups at indirect ophthalmoscopic examination. They occupied the palpebral aperture region of the cornea, and most often were bilateral. In addition to, or in place of the spontaneous dust-like particles commonly observed in our Sprague-Dawley strain, drug-induced corneal lesions were defined as rough linear streaks, as outlined by retroillumination. In some cases these opacities were superimposed on a spontaneous lesion already observed in previous examination(s), while in other typical drug-related lesions they were first observed. Incidence and severity of these drug-induced opacities are reported in Table 1.

Table 1 : Incidence of drug-related corneal opacities

Study Week	4	7	12	16	18
Control	0/30	0/30	0/30	0/30	0/30
L-680,833 :					
50 mg/kg/day		0/30	0/30	0/30	0/30
150 mg/kg/day		0/30	5/30 (1)	8/30 (3)	8/30 (5)
300 mg/kg/day	0/30	14/29 (13)	21/26 (18)	21/23 (18)	21/23 (17)

Number of animals in a group is given according to the early deaths (30 rats per dose group at the beginning of the study).
Number in parentheses represent rats with bilateral corneal opacities.

Opacities were observed first at Study Week 7 examination, their incidence increased up to Study Week 12 and then plateaued. In two rats (one from the high-dose group, another from the mid-dose group), vascularization took place unilaterally around the lesion. In one of these two rats which died before termination, microscopic examination revealed a keratitis. In the other rat, sacrificed at the scheduled necropsy, the opacity and vascularization were gone two weeks later (confirmed by the absence of microscopic changes) indicating the possibility of reversibility of the lesion.

Serum calcium levels did not increase but rather slightly decreased in females in the mid- and high-dose group when compared to those of controls as indicated in Table 2. However, there was a statistically significant (P<0.05) increase of serum alkaline phosphatase in low-, mid-, and high-dose female groups and in mid- and high-dose male groups (Table 2).

Table 2 : Changes in serum biochemical parameters
(% above or below controls)

	Females				Males			
Study Week	4	7	12	18	4	7	12	18
Total Calcium								
50 mg/kg/day			0	-2			0	0
150 mg/kg/day			-2S	-4S			-1	0
300 mg/kg/day			-2S	-4S			-2	-4
Alkaline Phosphatase								
50 mg/kg/day	+26	+25S	+38S	+53S	+11	+7	+10	+14
150 mg/kg/day	+41S	+45S	+72$\underline{S}$	+97$\underline{S}$	+18	+23S	+26S	+24
300 mg/kg/day	+74$\underline{S}$	+116$\underline{S}$	+149$\underline{S}$	+213$\underline{S}$	+41S	+67$\underline{S}$	+69$\underline{S}$	+103$\underline{S}$

S : statistically significant (P < 0.05) through the indicated dose
$\underline{S}$: statistically significant (P < 0.0001) through the indicated dose

Microscopic examinations

Microscopically, drug-induced corneal opacities appeared as thick basophilic deposits mostly at the basis of the corneal epithelium, often at the level of the basal lamina. Since drug-related and spontaneous lesions could be found in the same eye, the drug-induced linear streaks appeared as an exacerbation of the fine granular basophilic spontaneous stippled lesion commonly seen in laboratory rats. In addition there was also necrosis of single scattered epithelial cells, often in the vicinity of large deposits, which are usually not found in the spontaneous lesion, except in old animals. Compared to controls, increase of severity was also reflected by keratitis (corresponding to antemortem vascularization) characterized by newly formed blood vessels surrounded by a few inflammatory cells in the stroma. Below the deposits, in the anterior stroma, stromal reaction, indicated by increased number of keratocytes and/or fibroblasts, was noted in almost all the cases of drug-related lesion. Von Kossa-reaction showed scanty positivity in the most severe cases, indicating that calcification is not an early process, but more probably a consequence of a local metabolic disturbance. Ultrastructurally, electron dense deposits appeared with an "agathe-like" shape in a shifted basement membrane and often in the anterior part of the stroma (see picture). Confirming the light microscopic pattern, occasional necrotic cells were also found in the epithelium as well as polymorphonuclear infiltration and fibroplasia in the outer stroma. Moreover, electron microscopy showed that drug-induced linear deposits resulted from accumulation and coalescence of fine granular deposits similar to the spontaneous one and that the former was thus an exacerbation of the latter.

DISCUSSION

Corneal opacities seen with L-680,833, particularly at the ultrastructural level, showed a strong similarity with spontaneous lesions described in the literature (1, 4, 19) and with those commonly observed in the Sprague Dawley rat strain used in this laboratory whose incidence is indicated in Table 3. Most of the spontaneous corneal changes were very slight, but their severity slightly increased with time.

Table 3 : Percent of control rats with corneal opacity (years 1989, 1990, 1991)

Class of age (weeks)	3-6	7-10	15-20	21-30	31-60	61-97
% Corneal changes :						
M	15	58	65	48	28	27
F	23	45	49	34	14	36

In aged rats (77-97 weeks old), linear corneal opacities, associated or not with vascularization were also observed (24): linear opacities were seen in rats of both sexes with an incidence around 10-12% (Table 4).

Table 4 : Percent of control rats with corneal opacity (aged rats)

Age	77 weeks		97 weeks	
Number of animals per sex	43 F	42 M	56 F	41 M
Punctate opacities %	38	15	48	14
Linear opacities %	4	12	0	10
Opacities with vascularization %	0	12	0	2

The ultrastructural localization in a stromal area correponding to the Bowman's membrane, which does not exist in rat (23), was also consistent with current descriptions. Thus, the aspect and the evolution of the spontaneous corneal changes observed in our rat population suggest that the drug-related changes induced by subacute oral administration of L-680,833 are an exacerbation of the spontaneous phenomenon.

Furthermore, the opacities presently described were similar to those related to dietary excess of vitamin D3 or related to mild hypercalcemia (18, 31). The clearing observed in one rat, after an episode of vascularization, was also noted in rabbits affected by band kerotopathy (11). The increase of serum alkaline phosphatase activity was consistent with results from experimentation on diabetic mice (22). However some differences remain from previous descriptions in animals :

- compared to another drug-induced corneal dystrophy, i.e. morphine-induced (12), the L-680,833-induced lesions were less severe since vascularization was only observed in two rats instead of being a quasi constant feature (up to 82%) in morphine-treated rats despite of shorter duration;

- compared to spontaneous lesion in a close species, the mouse, severity was again lower after L-680,833 administration: in the mouse corneal necrosis onsets as soon as 3 weeks of age (34). There, difference might come from quality of the environment as underlined by Van Winckle and Balk (34), as well as from a species difference since even among rat strain susceptibility to corneal opacities is quite variable (1).

L-680,833-induced corneal opacities in rat morphologically resembled early changes seen in man with band keratopathy (26, 27), with a basophilic granular deposit remaining between cells of normal epithelium. Afterwards, the human lesion increased more than L-680,833-induced change, but this could be an influence of the different lifespans between the two species. In man, iatrogenic induction of corneal dystrophies is known after drug administration (2, 3, 5, 7), after corneal graft (10) or in the course of ocular pathology related or not to a systemic disease (3, 26).

In all described human or animal cases, the mechanism of apparition of corneal changes remained unclear, and the differences from one species to another most probably represented biological variability:

- cornea is in a fragile physiological equilibrium, with a constant liquid flux from the aqueous humor to the epithelium, compensating evaporation, especially at the palpebral aperture. Every modification in the flux gives 2 to 3% variation in corneal thickness (21). In addition, the rat has large eyes with an important corneal area and, thus, is more subjected to dehydratation;

- a disturbance of local metabolism, by local or general cause, can modify the flux: increased evaporation can be due to palpebral hypomobility related to hallucinogenic circumstances with subsequent sedation (12) or to drug-induced hyperexcitability and hyperactivity causing increased palpebral aperture for example. Secondarily, increased evaporation may account for deposition of various substances. According to O'Connor (26) evaporation is accompanied by loss of CO_2 and an increased pH, enhancing calcium

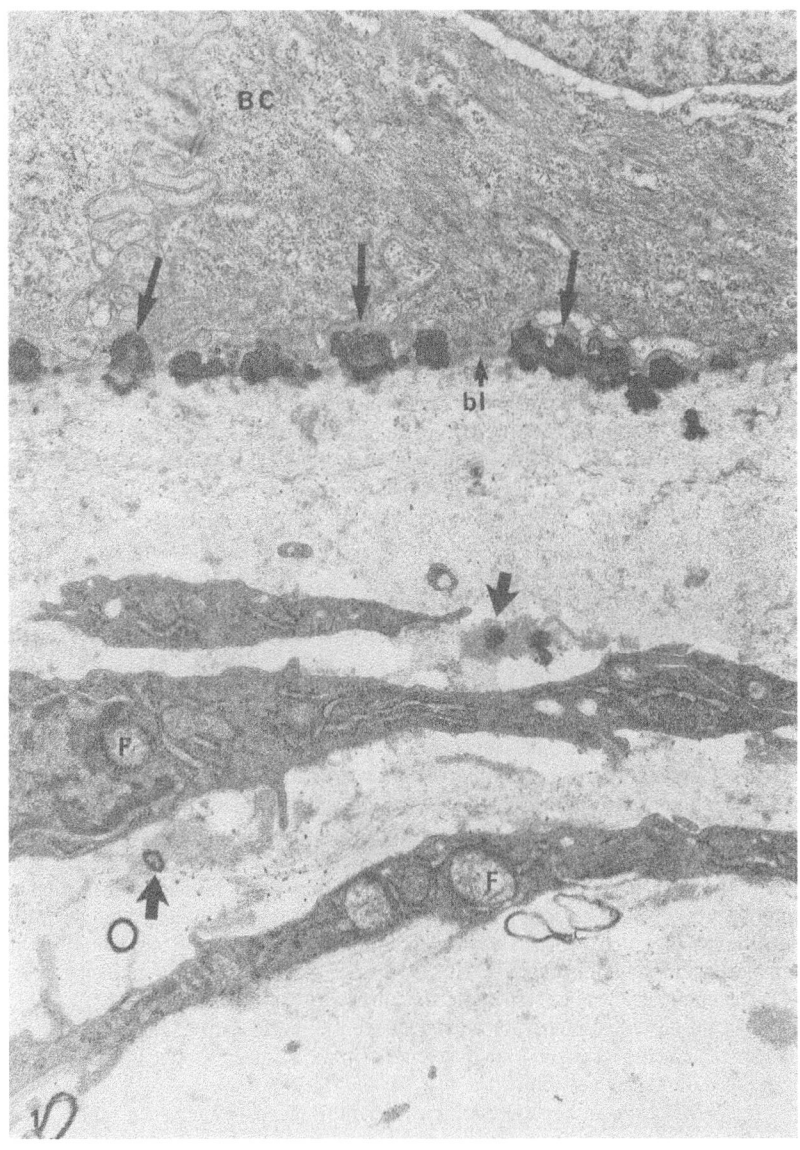

Figure 1. After 19 weeks of treatment with L-680,833 (300 mg/kg/day), accumulation of electron dense deposits (arrows) is observed in the epithelial basal lamina of the cornea. Isolated deposits are also visible in the anterior portion of the stroma close to the fibroblast (F). BC: Basal cell layer X 5000.

deposition in the semi crystalline structure represented by the basement membrane network and hemidesmosomes. In addition, the increased serum level of alkaline phosphatase activity may have played locally a role that has to be taken into account. In the posterior part of the cornea, lactic acid coming from anaerobic metabolism decreases pH and may have prevented calcium deposition (26).

In conclusion, corneal deposits are a common process in numerous species and diseases. In the case of L-680,833, previous studies with PMNEI had demonstrated a marked general toxicity (6) but were not known as oculo-toxic. Two indirect mechanistic possibilities can be discussed for the present drug-induced case in the rat:

- a disturbance of general homeostasis with local consequences on liquid corneal flux and/or the role of increased serum alkaline phosphatase,

- a behavioural modification (that we could not see without a deeper behavioural analysis) inducing a palpebral hypomobility with consecutive increased corneal evaporation.

Further studies will be useful to elucidate the pathogenesis of these L-680,833-induced corneal opacities and evaluate their potentiality as an animal model of human band keratopathy. However, since no eye abnormalities were observed in dogs and cynomolgus monkeys in studies with comparable dosages of this compound, and since these opacities appeared to be the exaggeration of a spontaneous rat specific ocular changes, they are of no toxicological concern for men.

REFERENCES

1. R. Belhorn, G.E. Korte, and D. Abrutyn. Spontaneous corneal degeneration in the rat. *Lab. Anim. Sci.* 38: 46-50 (1988).
2. P.S. Binder, J.K. Deg, and F.S. Kohl. Calcific band keratopathy after intraocular chondroitin sulfate. *Arch. Ophthalmol.* 105: 1243-1247 (1987).
3. D.E. Braverman and W.E. Snyder. A case report of band keratopathy. *Metab. Ped. System. Ophthalmol.* 10: 39-41 (1987).
4. H. Bruner, W.F. Keller, K.A. Stitzel, L.J. Sauers, P.J. Reer, P.H. Long, R.D. Bruce, and C.L. Alden. Spontaneous corneal dystrophy and generalized basement membrane changes in Fischer-344 rats. *Toxicol. Path.* 20: 357 (1992).
5. C.A. Burns. Indomethacin, reduced retinal sensitivity, and corneal deposits. *Am. J. Ophthalmol.* 66: 825-835 (1968).
6. C.P. Chengelis, S. Levin, and C. Cook. Subchronic toxicity study of SC-39026, an elastase inhibitor, in rats. *The Toxicologist*, 29th S.O.T. Meeting, 10: 282 (1990).
7. A.S. Crandall, N.S. Levy, H.D. Hoskins, and J.R. Welch. Characterization of subtle corneal deposits. *J. Toxicol. Cut & Ocul. Toxicol.* 3: 263-269 (1984).
8. J.W. Cursino and B.S. Fine. A histologic study of calcific and noncalcific band keratopathies. *Am. J. Ophthalmol.* 82: 395-404 (1976).
9. D.J. Doughman, G.A. Olson, S. Nolan, and R.G. Hajny. Experimental band keratopathy. *Arch. Ophthalmol.*, 81: 264-271 (1969).
10. R.J. Duffey and J.A. LoCascio. Calcium deposition in a corneal graft. *Cornea*, 6: 212-215 (1987).
11. J.W. Econom, A.M. Silverstein, and L.E. Zimmerman. Band keratopathy in a rabbit colony. *Invest. Ophthalmol.*, 2: 361-368 (1963).
12. R.J. Fabian, J.M. Bond, and H.P. Drobeck. Induced corneal opacities in the rat. *Br. J. Ophthalmol.* 51: 124-129 (1967).
13. B.S. Fine, J.W. Berkow, and S. Fine. Corneal calcification. *Science.* 162: 129-130 (1968).
14. J. Friend, Y. Ishii, and R.A. Thoft. Corneal epithelial changes in diabetic rats. *Ophthal. Res.* 14: 269-278 (1982).
15. A. Garner. Histochemistry of corneal granular dystrophy. *Br. J. Ophthalmol.* 53: 799-807 (1969).
16. R. Guillet, J. Wyatt, R.B. Baggs, and C.K. Kellog. Anesthetic-induced corneal lesions in developmentally sensitive rats. *Invest. Ophthalmol. & Vis. Sci.* 29: 949-954 (1988).
17. K. Hayashi, G. Frangieh, L.A. Hanninen, G. Wolf, and K.R. Kenyon. Stromal degradation in vitamin A-deficient rat cornea. *Cornea.* 9: 254-265 (1990).

18. R. Kennedy and P. Roca. Atypical band keratopathy in glaucomatous patients. *Am. J. Ophthalmol.*, 72: 917-922 (1971).
19. P.E. Losco and C.M. Troup. Corneal dystrophy in Fischer 344 rats. *Lab. Anim. Sci.* 38: 702-710 (1988).
20. S. Mishima and D.M. Maurice. The effect of normal evaporation on the eye. *Exp. Eye Res.* 1: 46-52 (1961).
21. S. Mishima. Some physiological aspects of the precorneal tear film. *Arch. Ophthalmol.* 73: 233-240 (1965).
22. R. Mittl., M.A. Galin, W. Opperman, et al. Corneal calcification in spontaneously diabetic mice. *Invest. Ophthalmol.* 9: 137-145 (1970).
23. S. Molon-Noblot and P. Duprat. Anatomy of the ocular surfaces, cornea and conjunctiva, rat and mouse. *In* : "ILSI Monographs on pathology of laboratory animals. Eye and ear", T.C. Jones, U. Mohr, and R.D. Hunt, eds, 3-16 (1991).
24. S. Molon-Noblot, J.P. Gillet, R.A. Owen, G. Durand-Cavagna, and P. Duprat. Ultrastructure of spontaneous corneal changes in rats. *Electron Microscopy* 3: 689-690 (1992).
25. J. Obenberger, J. Cejkova, and I. Brettschneider. Experimental corneal calcification. *Ophthal. Res.* 1: 175-186 (1970).
26. G.R. O'Connor. Calcific band keratopathy. *Trans. Am. Ophthal. Soc.* LXX: 58-79 (1972).
27. Y. Pouliquen, C. Haye, J. Bisson, and G. Offret. Ultrastructure de la kératopathie en bandelette. *Arch. Ophtal. (Paris)* 27: 149-158 (1967).
28. M. Radnot. Data on the occurrence of calcification in the eye tissues. *Brit. J. Ophthalmol.* 32: 47-54 (1948).
29. L.F. Rich, M.E. Beard, and R.P. Burns. Excess dietary tyrosine and corneal lesions. *Exp. Eye Res.* 17: 87-97 (1973).
30. D.L. Roerig, A.T. Hasegawa, G.J. Harris, K.L. Lynch, and R.I.H. Wang. Occurrence of corneal opacities after acute administration of 1-alpha-acetylmethadol. *Toxicol. & Appl. Pharmacol.* 56: 155-163 (1980).
31. C. Taradach, B. Regnier, and J. Perraud. Eye lesions in Sprague Dawley rats: type and incidence in relation to age. *Lab. Anim.* 15: 285-287 (1981).
32. D.A. Ward, C.L. Martin, and I. Weiser. Band keratopathy associated with hyperadrenocorticism in the dog. *J. Am. Anim. Hosp. Assoc.* 25: 583-586 (1989).
33. I. Weisse, H. Kreuzer, E. Stender, W. Frölke, and D. Meyer. Band keratopathy in rats due to increased dietary content of vitamin D3. *Concepts Toxicol.* 4: 164-178 (1987).
34. T.J. Van Winckle and M.W. Balk. Spontaneous corneal opacities in laboratory mice. *Lab. Anim. Sci.* 36: 248-255 (1986).

THE COMET ASSAY: A RELIABLE AND SENSITIVE METHOD FOR

THE DOCUMENTATION OF UV-B INDUCED DNA DAMAGE

W. Breipohl, C. Penzkofer, W. Naib-Majani, M. Rauwolf,
O. Leip, A. Augustin, and M. Leyendecker

Department of Ophthalmology
University of Bonn
D-53105 Bonn, F.R.G.

INTRODUCTION

Evidence exists that ultraviolet radiation, drugs, chemicals, and inherent mechanisms directly or via the generation of inflammatory mediators and oxygen free radicals can exert effects on DNA damage and repair[1,2,3]. Thus the evaluation of DNA damage and the investigation of factors influencing its quantification are of prime interest for pharmaceutical, clinical and basic scientific reasons [4,5,6]. Previous approaches towards the quantification of DNA damage in lens epithelial cells lacked a systematic analysis of individual factors such as cell origin, cell cycle phase, Go synchronization, and the interaction between these factors.

To overcome these gaps in our knowledge and as a first in a series of investigations this study describes the application of the DNA comet assay technique[5,7-9] for the quantification of UV-B induced DNA damage in cultured bovine lens epithelial cells.

MATERIALS AND METHODS

Passage I cells of bovine lens epithelium (central anterior pole region and preequatorial (peripheral) region) have been cultured on uncoated Falcon dishes (3.5 cm diameter; seeding density was 35×10^3 cells per dish) for three days (exponential growth phase). Then UV-B (maximal emission 290 - 310 nm) was applied (70 J/m^2) to cells washed in PBS. After radiation cultures were briefly washed with Earle's solution. This was followed by gentle trypsinization (500 μl of 0.05% trypsin (Biochrom-Seromed/1:250)) for about three to five minutes and resuspension in 1 ml Earle's. The suspension was centrifuged in Eppendorf caps for 5 minutes at less than 100 g after which the sediment with the cells was resuspended in 75μl of 0.5% agarose (BDM; Electran - agarose, low gelling temperature (37°C)).

Further the DNA comet assay technique was applied at 4°C and (as far as possible) processed in the dark. Technical details were in general as defined by others[7-9]. In brief: Frosted histological glas slides were coated with $125\mu l$ 0.5% agarose (Merck; analytical nucleic acid electrophoresis grade, gelling at 56-60°C) and briefly stored at 4°C. After gelling of the coating agarose the slides were covered with those trypsinized and in $75\mu l$ agarose resuspended cells and stored for 10 minutes at 4°C. Then another layer from $125\mu l$ of 0.5% agarose was transferred on top of the previous two layers resulting in an agarose sandwich with the suspended cells in the middle layer. After gelling of the third layer the slides were exposed at 4°C to strongly alkaline lysis buffer (pH 10)[5] for 60 minutes, washed 45 minutes in electrophoresis buffer, and electrophoretically treated (225 mA and 25 V) for 10 minutes. Following electrophoretic separation the sandwiches were treated with neutralizing buffer before cell DNA was stained with ethidium bromide, photographed with an Olympus fluorescence microscope, and evaluated with the help of an image analytical system (Leitz Quantimet 500). The definition of the comet, its use and the distance of DNA fragment migration was as explained in Figure 1.

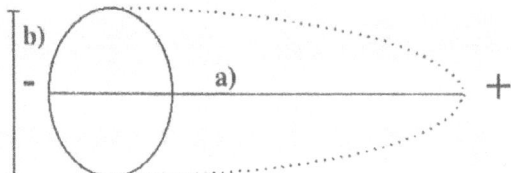

Figure 1. Diagram to explain how the comet length (a), nuclear diameter(b), DNA migration distance outside the nuclear area (a-b), and comet length ratio (a:b) was calculated. DNA fragments migrate towards the anode (+) and away from the cathode (-), ratio of comet length and nuclear diameter = a:b

RESULTS

Due to methodological conditions, DNA damage is given in pixels. Different absolute pixel values do not necessarily reflect different amounts of DNA damage as calibration of the morphometric device differed. What has to be compared is the increase in pixels between controls and UV-B irradiated cells, or the shifts in the ratios of comet length and nuclear diameter.

In preceeding methodological test series (details not shown) it could be seen that DNA fragmentation in cultured bovine lens epithelial cells can be evaluated with the help of the comet assay technique. DNA fragmentation was best documented with electrophoresis times of 10 minutes and an UV irradiation dose of 70 J/m^2. Thus these conditions were applied in the present study as well.

The interference of DNA fragmentation with cell origin (preequatorial versus central anterior pole cells), proliferating potential and cell cycle phase respectively was documented in two sets of experiments.

Experimental set 1: Control and UV-B irradiated lens epithelial cells not separated according to preequatorial (i.e. mitotic active epithelial region) and central (i.e. mitotic silent epithelial region) origin, differed greatly in their DNA damage (Figure 2). The irradiated group had a mean comet length by far (+263%) exceeding the mean of the control group.

Analysis of individual cell comets in the controls revealed that about 10% of the comets greatly deviated from the group's mean in excessively exceeding it (Figure 3). The respective analysis of the irradiated cells revealed a higher percentage of excessively deviating comets from the mean in both directions (i.e. above and below) (Figure 4).

	Ratio comparison	Comet length (in Pixel)
control	1,30 ± 0,68	33,97 ± 18,36
UV-B	3,77 ± 0,95	89,51 ± 22,57

Figure 2. Mean comet length and ratio (comet length divided by nuclear diameter) in non UV-B versus UV-B irradiated bovine lens passage I epithelial cells in culture. The mean comet length increases to 263% after UV-B irradiation. The ratio increases to 290%. Central and preequatorial cells have not been separated.

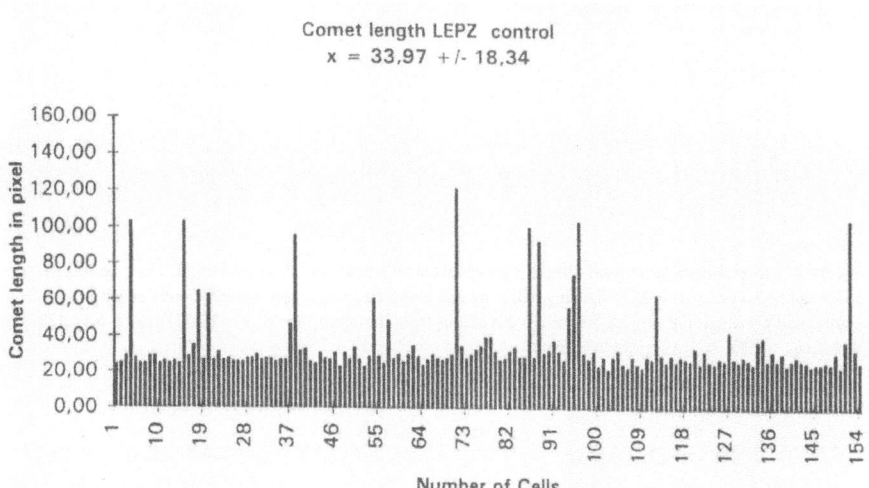

Figure 3. Morphometric documentation of individual comet lengths in UV-B untreated bovine passage I lens epithelial cells (n = 154). During culturing and harvesting cells were not differentiated into those from central and preequatorial region. About 10% of the cells show comets greatly deviating from the mean of 33,97 +/- 18,34 in <u>one</u> direction only. LEPZ = lens epithelial cells.

Experimental set 2: To check whether the above reported individual comet length deviations from the groups and the 263% increase in comet length after UV-B irradiation reflect differences in cell origin and cell kinetics (i.e. proliferative potential), the comet assay technique was applied concomitantly to passage-I cells from central versus peripheral epithelial origin. It could be shown that non irradiated bovine passage I lens epithelial cells of preequatorial origin had less intense ("spontaneous") DNA damage in comparison to central cells. However, UV-B radiation induced an increase in DNA damage, the extent of which was clearly cell origin related. In peripheral cells the increase amounted to 552%, while in central cells it increased by 147% "only" (Figure 5).

To further check the influence of the proliferative potential and cell cycle phase on DNA susceptibility to UV-B additional experiments used Go synchronized cells. Synchronization was achieved by serum depletion for 36 h and checked by BrdU / anti-BrdU immunfluorescence microscopy. UV-B irradiation induced DNA damage of central synchronized cells exceeded that of non synchronized cells (+569% versus +147%). UV-B irradiation of syn-

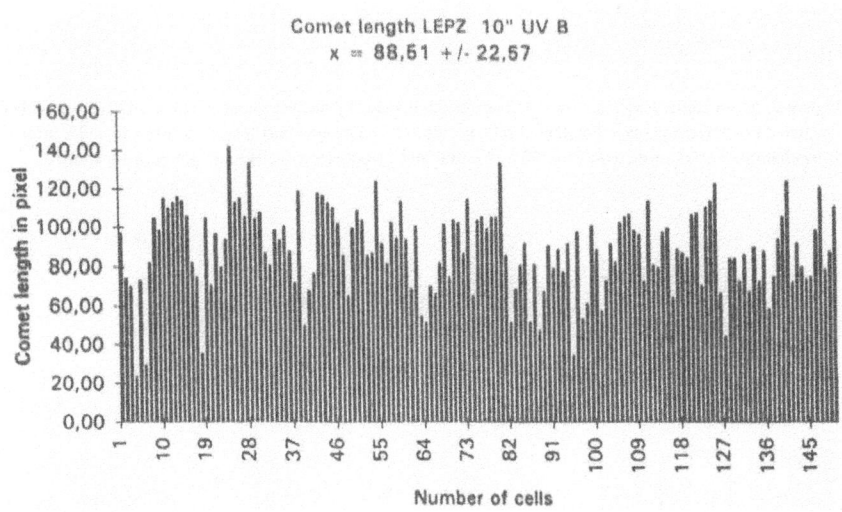

Figure 4. Morphometric documentation of individual comet lengths in UV-B treated (70 J/m²) bovine passage I lens epithelial cells (n = 151). During culturing and harvesting cells were not differentiated into those from central and preequatorial region. Excessive deviations from the mean (88,51 +/- 22,57) can be found in both directions. LEPZ = lens epithelial cells.

	Ratio comparison	Comet length (in Pixel)
control center	5,44 ± 2,52	89,76± 37,42
control periphery	2,98 ± 1,91	45,11 ± 30,78
UV-B center	8,11 ± 1,80	131,56 ± 17,24
UV-B periphery	20,55 ± 5,87	249,14 ± 47,05

Figure 5. Table to document mean comet length (with standard deviation) in untreated versus UV-B irradiated bovine passage I lens epithelial cells of central and preequatorial origin. Untreated peripheral cells have a lower comet length mean than their central counterparts. UV-B irradiation (70 J/m²) reverses this ratio leading to a higher mean comet length in the peripheral cells. The mean comet length increases after UV-B to 147% and 552% in the central and peripheral cells respectively. The ratios increase to 149% and 690%.

chronized preequatorial cells caused the same increase in DNA damage as in non synchronized preequatorial cells (+555% versus +552%). These values also document that the extent in DNA fragmentation increase was no longer different between preequatorial

(+555%) and central (+569%) cells after synchronization (Figure 6). Interestingly the incidence of ("spontaneous") DNA fragmentation in untreated peripheral control cells was always less in comparison to non irradiated central cells (Figures 5,6).

The respective alterations of the ratios (comet length divided by nuclear diameter) followed the same trends as described for the comet lengths. However, absolute values differed slightly.

	Ratio comparison	Comet length (in Pixel)
control center	1,67 ± 0,88	188,07± 97,83
control periphery	1,01 ± 1,65	169,44 ± 96,10
UV-B center	10,25 ± 2,97	1069,77 ± 221,05
UV-B periphery	9,14 ± 3,11	940,25 ± 197,98

Figure 6. Table to document mean comet length (with standard deviation) in synchronized (36 h serum depletion) untreated and irradiated bovine lens epithelial cells of central and preequatorial origin. No differences in the amount of DNA damage can be observed between central and peripheral Go cells. UV-B irradiation (70 J/m²) leads to a 569% and 555% increase of comet length in the central and peripheral cells respectively.

DISCUSSION

Previous investigations showed more vigorous proliferation of passage-I bovine lens epithelial cells with preequatorial origin in comparison to cells with central origin[10]. In addition UV-B induced an increase in nuclear number per cell[11]. This study extends those investigations documenting that UV-B leads to DNA fragmentation in lens epithelial cells, in a cell origin and cell cycle phase dependent manner. The extent of DNA damage was measured and quantified by the DNA comet assay technique[5,7-9].

A wide variety of environmental, chemical and physiological conditions affect the structure of DNA and its repair mechanisms. A potent environmental agent to affect the DNA, its replication and repair in the eye is UV radiation[5-7]. It has also been described that UV radiation provokes peroxidation of membrane lipids which themselves can provoke DNA damage as well[1,6,12]. To differentiate between DNA damage directly induced by UV-B and damage caused by UV-B induced oxgen free radicals it appeared necessary to quantify first the overall effects of UV-B on DNA. However, so far nobody had documented the extent of overall UV-B induced DNA damage in relation to the effects on lens epithelial cell proliferation.

As reported for ionising radiation, proliferating and especially S-phase cells are more vulnerable than Go cells[13]. Therefore we assumed also a cell cycle dependent shift in UV-B vulnerability of DNA. The differentiation between "spontaneous" DNA, cell cycle phase and UV-B evoked DNA damage appears crucial. It could be speculated that occasionally (ca. 10%) observed long comets in the non UV irradiated control cells (Figure 2) could be due to both, UV influences from the natural environment (day light, room light) and tissue culture (e.g. hypoxy) or preparatory tissue sampling conditions. Environmental UV effects to influence the outcome of the experiments can be neglected, because, as far as possible, experiments were performed in the dark. DNA fragmentation linked to cell cycle i.e., observation of comets in controls, has been assumed as negligible, as no effect of cell cycle position was observed following alkaline lysis[8].

For two main reasons, our data not corroborate with the latter assumption. First, peripheral passage I cells, have a higher proliferation index when compared to central cells[10]. In addition, experimental set 2 revealed a higher increase of DNA damage in peripheral than in central cells. Thus one could speculate that the amount of (perhaps S-phase) cells, characterized by higher susceptibility to UV induced DNA damage, could be higher in peripheral than central cells. Concomitantly, shorter comets of cells in an irradiated entity could well reflect the percentual amount of cells in a given cell cycle phase characterized by less UV-B sensitivity (Figure 4). Second, if our assumption on a cell cycle influence on UV-B inducible DNA damage is justified, then synchronization of cells in any given phase of the cell cycle should lead to the same increase of DNA damage by UV in central and peripheral cells. Indeed, the higher peripheral UV-B susceptibility of preequatorial in comparison to central lens epithelial cells (Figure 5) was no longer observed after synchronization of the cells in Go prior to UV irradiation (Figure 6).

As can be calculated from the values given in Figures 2, 5, and 6, the ratios (comet length divided by nuclear diameter) increase with the same tendency as the comet lengths. However, the ratio increases are always above those of the comet lengths. One could speculate that this tendency could be related to results observed earlier: that nuclear diameters do also change after UV-B irradiation of lens epithelial cells in culture[11]. Unfortunately the influence of regionality in cell origin on changes in nuclear diameter after UV-B irradiation has not yet been investigated, to conclusively answer this speculation.

However, regionality in lens epithelial cell behavior, and especially so in proliferation in vivo was related to the local expression for external (fibrocytic) growth factor receptors[14]. In contrast, no regionality could be found regarding the expression of internal growth regulators, e.g., the growth suppressor gene p53 which is of prime importance for the regulation of the generation cycle (Breipohl and Naib-Majani, unpublished).

Growing evidence accumulates that the interactions between UV, growth factors, growth factor receptors and growth suppressors intimately depend on DNA-damage inducible genes like gadd, MyD and others, which - in a hitherto poorly understood way - are influenced also by UV[12,15-18]. Thus our data on UV-B inducible DNA damage, here evaluated with the help of the comet assay technique, appear a promising first step towards a better understanding of such interactions. With this type of investigations we anticipate especially deep insights into the interactions between DNA damage induced by UV and other environmental factors[6] on one side, and cell proliferation, DNA repair, and regional growth control on the other side.

SUMMARY

This investigation has documented UV-B induced DNA damage in cultured passage I bovine lens epithelial cells. DNA fragmentation in these cells, was measured and quantified by the DNA comet assay technique. As shown, the extent of DNA fragmentation is influenced by both, cell cycle phase and regional origin. Non irradiated lens epithelial cells descended from the preequatorial epithelial region were less vulnerable than cells whose predecessors were taken from the central epithelial region. UV-B irradiation (70 J/m^2) reversed this ratio into its opposite. Synchronization by serum depletion abolished the regional differences in UV-B inducible DNA damage. The results are considered important for our understanding on the principles of DNA vulnerability, repair, growth regulation and regionality in lens epithelial cells and assumingly others.

Acknowledgments

Support by the EU programme "The role of membranes in lens ageing and cataract" is gratefully acknowledged.

REFERENCES

1. Andley, U.P., Lewis, R.M., Reddan, J.R. Kochevar, I.R. Action spectrum for cytotoxicicty in the UV-A- and UV-B wavelength region in cultured lens epithelial cells, *Invest. Ophthalmol. Vis. Sci.* 35:367-373 (1994).
2. M.V. Riley S. Susan, M.J. Peters, C.A. Schwartz, The effects of UV-B irradiation on the corneal endothelium, *Current Eye Research* 6:1021-1033 (1987).
3. M.V. Riley, S.A. Elgebaly, The release of a neutrophil chemotactic factor from UV-B irradiated rabbit corneas, *Current Eye Research* 9:677-682 (1990).
4. L.A. Applegate, R.D. Ley, DNA damage is involved in the induction of opacification and neovascularization of the cornea by ultraviolet radiation, *Exp. Eye Res.* 52:493-497 (1991).
5. N.J. Kleiman, A. Spector, DNA single strand breaks in human lens epithelial cells from patients with cataract, *Current Eye Res.* 12:423-431 (1990).
6. A. Spector, G.-M. Wang, R.-R. Wang, The prevention of cataract caused by oxidative stress in cultured rat lenses. II. Early effects of photochemical stress and recovery, *Exp. Eye Res.* 57:659-667 (1993).
7. N.P. Singh, M.T. McCoy, R.R. Tice, E.L. Schneider, A simple technique for quantification of low levels of DNA damage in individual cells, *Exp. Cell Res.* 175:184-191 (1988).
8. P.L. Olive, D. Wlodek, R.E. Durand, J.P. Banáth, Factors influencing DNA migration from individual cells subjected to gel electrophoresis, *Exp. Cell Res.* 198:259-287 (1992).
9. V.J. McKelvey-Martin, M.H.L. Green, P. Schmezer, B.L. Pool-Zobel, M.P. De Meo, A. Collins, The single cell gel electrophoresis assay (comet assay): a European review, *Mutation Res.* 288:47-63 (1993).
10. W. Breipohl, M. Leyendecker, O. Leip, H. Akiyoshi, Investigations on cell proliferation of bovine lens epithelial cells, submitted (1995).
11. O. Leip, W. Breipohl, H. Akiyoshi, T. Naguro, M. Leyendecker, C. Penzkofer, C., Effects of UV-B radiation on cultured bovine lens epithelial cells, Abstract, *XXVII Intern. Congr. Ophthalmol.* Toronto (1994).
12. A.J. Fornace, Mammalian genes induced by radiation; activation of genes associated with growth control, *Annu. Rev. Genet.* 26:507-526 (1992).
13. M. Molls, C. Streffer, The influence of G_2 progression on X-ray sensitivity of two cell mouse embryos, *Int. J. Radiat. Biol. Relat. Stud. Phys. Chem Med.* 46:355-365 (1984).
14. R. deJong, J.W. McAvoy, Distribution of acidic and basic fibroblast growth factors (FGF) in the foetal rat eye: implications for lens development, *Growth Factors* 6:159-177 (1992).
15. T. Kartasova, P.v.d. Putte, Isolation, characterization, and UV-stimulated expression of two families of genes encoding polypeptides of related structure in human epidermal keratinocytes, *Mol. Cell. Biol.* 8:2195-2203 (1988).
16. Q. Zhan, K.A. Lord, I. Alamo jr., M. C. Hollander, F. Carrier, D. Ron, K. W. Kohn, B. Hoffman, D.A. Liebermann, A.J. Fornace jr., The gadd and Myd genes define a novel set of mammalian genes encoding acidic proteins that synergistically suppress cell growth, *Mol Cell. Biol.* 14:2361-2371 (1994).
17. Q. Zhan, F. Carrier, A.J. Fornace jr., Induction of cellular p53 activity by DNA-damaging agents and growth arrest, *Mol. Cell. Biol.* 13:4242-4250 (1993).
18. A.J. Fornace jr., D.W. Nebert, M.C. Hollander, J.D. Luethy, M. Papathanasiou, J. Fargnoli, N.J. Holbrook, Mammalian genes coordinately regulated by growth arrest signals and DNA-damaging agents, *Mol. Cell Biol.* 9:4196-4203 (1989).

SPONTANEOUS OCULAR FINDINGS
AND ESTHESIOMETRY / TONOMETRY MEASUREMENT
IN THE GÖTTINGEN MINIPIG
(CONVENTIONAL AND MICROBIOLOGICALLY DEFINED)

Olivier Loget

Pharmakon Europe
Domaine des Oncins - BP 0118
69593 L'Arbresle Cédex
France

SUMMARY

Gross examinations, ocular reflexes, esthesiometry, indirect ophthalmoscopical and biomicroscopical examinations and tonometry were performed in eighteen 6 to 8 week old microbiologically defined and in fourty-nine 2 to 10 month old conventional Göttingen minipigs. Ophthalmological findings often consisted of embryonic remnants (hyaloid artery, pupillary membrane) which seemed to decrease in incidence with time, although this decrease was not confirmed by statistical analysis. The most important findings were either considered to be congenital in origin or of undetermined etiology. The most noteworthy findings were, in decreasing order of incidence, as follows : hyaloid artery remnants (microbiologically defined : 83.3 %, conventional : 76.5 %), tigroid fundus (microbiologically defined : 72.2 %, conventional : 75.5 %), slight lens opacities (microbiologically defined : 38.9 %, conventional : 41.8 %) and pupillary membrane remnants (microbiologically defined : 33.3 %, conventional : 21.4 %). These findings did not affect the visual capabilities of the pigs.

INTRODUCTION

Since the use of miniature swine to replace or to complement the dog or monkey as experimental models in toxicity studies is likely to increase, a better knowledge of their anatomical, physiological and histopathological characteristics is needed. In this study, the normal ocular pattern of the Göttingen minipig is described, in order to be able to differentiate between spontaneous and induced ophthalmological abnormalities which may occur in subsequent toxicity studies. Consequently, the same examinations were performed as those required for toxicity studies in non-rodent species.

MATERIALS AND METHODS

Eighteen (nine males and nine females) young microbiologically defined Göttingen minipigs and fourty-nine (nineteen males and thirty females) older conventional minipigs (Ellegaard Göttingen Minipigs ApS, Sorø Landevej 302, DK-4261 Denmark) were examined. The examination of the young microbiologically defined minipigs was carried out on delivery at customer's facility (Leo Pharmaceutical Products, 55 Industriparken, DK-2750 Ballerup, Denmark). That of the older minipigs was performed at the clinic of the supplier's veterinarian (Dr. P. Skydsgaard, DVM, PhD).

The ocular reflexes (corneal palpebral, pupillary direct and consensual) were evaluated. (In the case of the microbiologically defined minipigs, the pupillary reflex was checked, a few days after the main examinations, by Dr. Jens Lichtenberg, DVM, Toxicologist, Leo Pharmaceutical Products). After esthesiometry (Cochet-Bonnet esthesiometer) and macroscopic examination of the eye and its adnexae, the pupils were dilated with 0.5 % tropicamide (Mydriaticum, MSD Chibret, Paris). Two drops were instilled into each eye about 15 minutes before examination. Then indirect ophthalmoscopical and slit lamp biomicroscopical examinations were performed using a binocular indirect ophthalmoscope (Heine Omega 100 with a double aspheric 20 D lens) and a Kowa SL 5 slit lamp biomicroscope. Prior to the ophthalmoscopical and biomicroscopical examinations, the head light source of the indirect ophthalmoscope was used to observe the external ocular adnexae, the anterior segment and the vitreous body. Retinography was performed using a fundus camera (Kowa RC2 with 25 Asa films : Koda Chrome 25). Thereafter, following corneal anesthesia (Novesine, MSD Chibret, Paris) tonometry was performed with a Tonopen tonometer. All the examinations were performed on non-anesthetized animals restrained in appropriate slings.

Analysis of variance and Student's t-test were performed on the esthesiometry and tonometry results and the three different groups (6 to 8 week old microbiologically defined, 2 to 5 month old and 6 to 10 month old conventional minipigs) were compared for the incidence of the main findings, using a chi-square test.

RESULTS

Gross Findings

Pupillary reflexes occurred slowly and their amplitude was small in conventional minipigs. In microbiologically defined animals, most of the pupillary reflexes were normal, but in two of them the reflex occurred faster and in two others it occurred slowly or very slowly.

Eyelids were thick and did not open very easily. The straight cilia were sometimes so numerous that it was difficult to perform some examinations (esthesiometry, tonometry, biomicroscopy...). Although blepharitis and conjunctivitis were noted in several microbiologically defined minipigs on the day of their arrival at the client's facility, this inflammation disappeared spontaneously, except in four animals.

The caruncle was well developed. The nictitating membrane was usually slightly brown in colour on its free margin. Due to the depth of the orbit, the ocular globe was in a deeper position than in other laboratory species. The sclerae were most often slight and rarely slightly brown pigmented (one conventional and one microbiologically defined minipig in this survey). The irises were brown, brown/blue or blue colored. In some animals, the iris was blue for one eye and brown for the other.

Ophthalmoscopical and Slit Lamp Biomicroscopical Findings

The main findings are described below in decreasing order of incidence and are summarized in Tables 1 to 4 and in Figure 1.

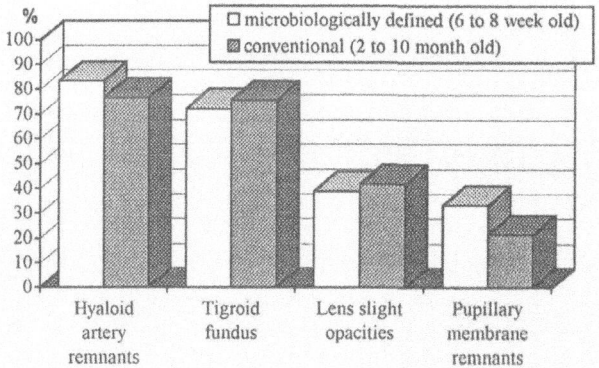

Figure 1. Incidence of main ocular findings.

Hyaloid artery remnants are rests of the artery which, in the foetus, supply blood to the internal eye[1], and most specifically to the posterior lens capsule. After ciliary vessel formation, this artery is supposed to regress progressively until complete disappearance. Sometimes the regression process is not complete. In these cases, parts of the arteries or the glial layer persist. The remnants may form a cord-like structure running from the optic disc to the posterior lens pole, or just consist of parts of this line, most often localized close to the lens. Such findings are described in other species. They are known to occasionally induce posterior capsular cataract, and to sometimes regress with age, in beagle dogs[2, 3] and in Yucatan micropigs[4]. In this survey, no cataract was described but the comparison between 6 to 8 week old microbiologically defined minipigs (83.3 %), 2 to 5 (81.6 %) and 6 to 10 (73.3 %) month old minipigs' eyes showed a quite early trend to decrease (Tables 1, 3, 4).

Tigroid fundus is the name which is given by some authors[4, 6, 7] to a lack of fundus pigmentation making the choroidal vessels visible. This pattern was found in most of the pig eyes examined in this survey (72.2 % in microbiologically defined minipigs and 75.5 % in conventional minipigs, Tables 1, 2). It is known to occur with an incidence of 75 % in Göttingen miniature swine, 25 % in Vietnamese miniature swine[6] and 50 % in Yucatan micropigs[4]. All animals with blue colored irises had this type of fundus.

Pupillary membrane remnants are remnants of a thin mesodermal membrane which seals the foetal pupil. This membrane is supposed to regress before birth. This regression sometimes does not occur completely. The persistent parts of the pupillary membrane can form focal deposits or strands on the anterior part of the lens. In some species, these deposits produce an anterior capsular cataract. This was not the case in the minipigs examined in this survey, although these remnants were often present on the anterior capsule of the lens. As with the incidence of the hyaloid artery remnant, the persistent pupillary membrane is known to decrease with age in beagle dogs[5] and in Yucatan micropigs[4]. This incidence seems to decrease with time in conventional Göttingen minipigs. Moreover, the magnitude of the decrease was higher for the pupillary membrane than for the hyaloid artery. This finding was observed in 33.3 % of the eyes of the 6 to 8 week old microbiologically defined, in 26.3 % of the eyes of the 2 to 5 month old and in 18.3 % of the eyes of the 6 to 10 month old conventional minipigs (Tables 1, 3, 4).

TABLE 1. Ophthalmological findings in 6 to 8 week old microbiologically defined Göttingen minipigs.

OBSERVATIONS	Males (N = 18)		Females (N = 18)		Both sexes (N = 36)	
	n	%	n	%	n	%
GROSS FINDINGS						
Blepharitis	15	83.3	15	83.3	30	83.3
Conjunctivitis	8	44.4	8	44.4	16	44.4
Palpebral papilloma	-	-	1	5.6	1	2.8
Slight brown coloration of the sclera	-	-	1	5.6	1	2.8
CORNEA						
Pinpoint opacities	1	5.6	-	-	1	2.8
Opalescence of the stroma	-	-	-	-	-	-
IRIS						
Blue color	2	11.1	4	22.2	6	16.7
Brown/blue color	2	11.1	2	11.1	4	11.1
Brown color	14	77.8	12	66.7	26	72.2
Pupillary membrane remnants	6	33.3	6	33.3	12	33.3
LENS						
Suture line abnormality	1	5.6	-	-	1	2.8
Focal nuclear opacity	2	11.1	1	5.6	3	8.3
Posterior cortical pinpoint opacities	4	22.2	3	16.7	7	19.4
Posterior capsular opacities	-	-	3	16.7	3	8.3
VITREOUS						
Refringent points	2	11.1	-	-	2	5.6
Hyaloid artery remnants	14	77.8	16	88.9	30	83.3
FUNDUS						
Tigroid fundus	12	66.7	14	77.8	26	72.2
Retinal haemorrhage	-	-	-	-	-	-
Retinal degeneration	-	-	-	-	-	-
Optic disc abnormality	-	-	-	-	-	-

N = number of eyes examined, n = number with finding, % = percentage with finding.

TABLE 2 . Ophthalmological findings in 2 to 10 month old conventional Göttingen minipigs.

OBSERVATIONS	Males (N = 38)		Females (N = 60)		Both sexes (N = 98)	
	n	%	n	%	n	%
GROSS FINDINGS						
Blepharitis	-	-	2	3.3	2	2.0
Conjunctivitis	10	26.3	2	3.3	12	12.2
Palpebral papilloma	-	-	-	-	-	-
Slight brown coloration of the sclera	-	-	1	1.7	1	1.0
CORNEA						
Pinpoint opacities	-	-	1	1.7	1	1.0
Opalescence of the stroma	1	2.6	-	-	1	1.0
IRIS						
Blue color	5	13.2	9	15.0	14	14.3
Brown/blue color	8	21.1	21	35.0	29	29.6
Brown color	25	65.8	30	50.0	55	56.1
Pupillary membrane remnants	9	23.7	12	20.0	21	21.4
LENS						
Suture line abnormality	1	2.6	1	1.7	2	2.0
Focal nuclear opacity	2	5.3	6	10.0	8	8.2
Posterior cortical pinpoint opacities	8	21.1	11	18.3	19	19.4
Posterior capsular opacities	8	21.1	4	6.7	12	12.2
VITREOUS						
Refringent points	2	5.3	1	1.7	3	3.1
Hyaloid artery remnants	30	78.9	45	75.0	75	76.5
FUNDUS						
Tigroid fundus	27	71.1	47	78.3	74	75.5
Retinal haemorrhage	1	2.6	-	-	1	1.0
Retinal degeneration	-	-	1	1.7	1	1.0
Optic disc abnormality	1	2.6	1	1.7	2	2.0

N = number of eyes examined, n = number with finding, % = percentage with finding.

TABLE 3. Ophthalmological findings in 2 to 5 month old conventional Göttingen minipigs.

OBSERVATIONS	Males (N = 26)		Females (N = 12)		Both sexes (N = 38)	
	n	%	n	%	n	%
GROSS FINDINGS						
Blepharitis	-	-	-	-	-	-
Conjunctivitis	8	30.8	-	-	8	21.1
Palpebral papilloma	-	-	-	-	-	-
Slight brown coloration of the sclera	-	-	1	8.3	1	2.6
CORNEA						
Pinpoint opacities	-	-	1	8.3	1	2.6
Opalescence of the stroma	-	-	-	-	-	-
IRIS						
Blue color	4	15.4	1	8.3	5	13.2
Brown/blue color	4	15.4	1	8.3	5	13.2
Brown color	18	69.2	10	83.3	28	73.7
Pupillary membrane remnants	7	26.9	3	25.0	10	26.3
LENS						
Suture line abnormality	-	-	1	8.3	1	2.6
Focal nuclear opacity	-	-	2	16.7	2	5.3
Posterior cortical pinpoint opacities	3	11.5	5	41.7	8	21.1
Posterior capsular opacities	5	19.2	1	8.3	6	15.8
VITREOUS						
Refringent points	1	3.8	1	8.3	2	5.3
Hyaloid artery remnants	21	80.8	10	83.3	31	81.6
FUNDUS						
Tigroid fundus	16	61.5	7	58.3	23	60.5
Retinal haemorrhage	1	3.8	-	-	1	2.6
Retinal degeneration	-	-	1	8.3	1	2.6
Optic disc abnormality	1	3.8	-	-	1	2.6

N = number of eyes examined, n = number with finding, % = percentage with finding.

TABLE 4. Ophthalmological findings in 6 to 10 month old conventional Göttingen minipigs.

OBSERVATIONS	Males (N = 12)		Females (N = 48)		Both sexes (N = 60)	
	n	%	n	%	n	%
GROSS FINDINGS						
Blepharitis	-	-	2	4.2	2	3.3
Conjunctivitis	2	16.7	2	4.2	4	6.7
Palpebral papilloma	-	-	-	-	-	-
Slight brown coloration of the sclera	-	-	-	-	-	-
CORNEA						
Pinpoint opacities	-	-	-	-	-	-
Opalescence of the stroma	1	8.3	-	-	1	1.7
IRIS						
Blue color	1	8.3	8	16.7	9	15.0
Brown/blue color	4	33.3	20	41.7	24	40.0
Brown color	7	58.3	20	41.7	27	45.0
Pupillary membrane remnants	2	16.7	9	18.8	11	18.3
LENS						
Suture line abnormality	1	8.3	-	-	1	1.7
Focal nuclear opacity	2	16.7	4	8.3	6	10.0
Posterior cortical pinpoint opacities	5	41.7	6	12.5	11	18.3
Posterior capsular opacities	3	25.0	3	6.3	6	10.0
VITREOUS						
Refringent points	1	8.3	-	-	1	1.7
Hyaloid artery remnants	9	75.0	35	72.9	44	73.3
FUNDUS						
Tigroid fundus	11	91.7	40	83.3	51	85.0
Retinal haemorrhage	-	-	-	-	-	-
Retinal degeneration	-	-	-	-	-	-
Optic disc abnormality	-	-	1	2.1	1	1.7

N = number of eyes examined, n = number with finding, % = percentage with finding.

Posterior cortical pinpoint lens opacities were observed using the slit lamp biomicroscope. However, it was not possible to see them using the indirect ophthalmoscope; consequently, these findings cannot be considered as cataracts which are opacities visible using standard ophthalmoscopic methods[8]. The incidence of this kind of opacity does not seem to be age-related : it was found in 19.4 % of the eyes of the 6 to 8 week old microbiologically defined minipigs, 21.1 % of the eyes of the 2 to 5 month old and 18.3 % of the eyes of the 6 to 10 month old conventional minipigs (Tables 1, 3, 4).

Other lens opacities were observed with a lower incidence. Posterior capsular opacities consisted most often of pinpoints (only visible by biomicroscopy) but sometimes in plaques. Taradach and Greaves[9] in the dog and Saint-Macary[4] in the Yucatan micropig have already described similar opacities which were not thought to be definitely bound with hyaloid remnants, although all the minipig eyes having hyaloid artery remnants showed this kind of opacity. Some animals presented focal nuclear opacities which have also already been described in the dog[9], in the Sprague-Dawley rat[10] and in the Yucatan micropig[4].

Refringent points in the vitreous were noted in approximately 5 % of the eyes (Tables 1, 3, 4). Other noteworthy findings, including corneal, lens and fundus abnormalities, were observed in less than 5 % of the eyes examined.

Esthesiometric and Tonometric Findings

The esthesiometry and tonometry measurements showed that the minipig seems to have a slightly less sensitive cornea than the rabbit and a slightly higher intraocular pressure than the rabbit, beagle dog, cynomolgus and rhesus macaque which are usually studied in our laboratory. Moreover, the tonometry values were much higher than those reported by Charlin[11] in Yucatan micropigs. However, this marked difference was most probably due to the type of tonometer used.

STATISTICAL EVALUATION

A statistical comparison between 6 to 8 week old microbiologically defined, 2 to 5 and 6 to 10 month old conventional Göttingen minipigs was made. The minimal, maximal and mean values and the standard deviations for the esthesiometry and tonometry results are indicated in Tables 5 and 6.

The esthesiometry values were not very homogeneous statistically. A comparison between sexes was performed within groups, using Student's t-test. The only group which did not show a statistically significant difference ($p >= 0.05$) between sexes was the microbiologically defined group. Consequently, an analysis of variance was performed, each sex considered separately. As this analysis showed that the three groups (8 to 10 week old microbiologically defined, 2 to 5 and 6 to 10 month old conventional) were not homogeneous ($p < 0.001$), each of them was compared to the others, using Student's t-test (each sex considered separately). This comparison showed statistically significant differences between the microbiologically defined minipigs and the two other groups in males ($p < 0.001$ when compared with 2 to 5 month old and $p < 0.01$ when compared with 6 to 10 month old conventional minipigs) and between the 6 to 10 month old conventional minipigs and the two other groups in females ($p < 0.001$). The results are more homogeneous in the microbiologically defined minipigs, although the differences between sexes could be partially attributed to the different numbers of males and females in the other two groups.

The tonometry values were statistically more homogeneous. A comparison between sexes was performed within groups and did not show any statistically significant difference ($p >= 0.05$). Consequently, the statistical analysis of the tonometry results was performed without differentiating between sexes. As the analysis of variance showed a difference between the three groups (p < 0.01), each of them was compared to the others using Student's t-test. This test showed a statistically significant difference between 2 to 5 and 6 to 10 month old conventional minipigs (p < 0.01).

The incidence of pupillary membrane remnants, hyaloid artery remnants and tigroid fundus, was statistically compared between sexes, within each group. This comparison did not show any statistically significant difference. Consequently, further comparison (between groups) was performed without differentiating between sexes. Although the incidence of pupillary membrane and hyaloid artery remnants seemed to decrease with age, this decrease was not statistically significant. The chi-square showed a statistically higher incidence of tigroid fundus in 6 to 10 month than in 2 to 5 month old conventional Göttingen minipigs.

CONCLUSIONS

The evaluation and statistical analysis of the results of this survey permitted definition of the main variants of the minipig's eye and to conclude that most of the abnormalities seen were congenital in origin and similar to those seen in other laboratory species. The incidence and severity of most of these abnormalities generally decreases with age in other species[2,3] as well as in the Yucatan micropig[4]. The statistical analysis did not permit confirmation of this hypothesis within the eye groups examined. A further survey, including older animals (up to several years of age) should be performed to investigate the age-related decrease of hyaloid artery and pupillary membrane remnants.

ACKNOWLEDGMENTS

I would like to thank Mr L. Ellegaard and Dr P. Skydsgaard (Ellegaard Göttingen Minipigs ApS) and Drs J.T. Mortensen, J. Lichtenberg and B.H. Nielsen (Leo Pharmaceutical Products) for access to their minipigs.

TABLE 5. Esthesiometry in Göttingen minipigs (cm).

	Males					Females					Both sexes				
	m	sd	m ± 2 sd	min	max	m	sd	m ± 2 sd	min	max	m	sd	m ± 2 sd	min	max
6 to 8 week old microbio defined															
males : n = 18	2.8	0.5	1.8 3.8	2.0	3.5	2.9	0.6	1.7 4.1	2.0	4.0	2.9	0.6	1.7 4.1	2.0	4.0
females : n = 18															
2 to 10 month old conventional															
males : n = 38	2.2	0.5	1.2 3.2	1.0	3.0	2.6	0.4	1.8 3.4	1.5	3.5	2.4	0.5	1.4 3.4	1.0	3.5
females : n = 60															
2 to 5 month old conventional															
males : n = 26	2.3	0.5	1.3 3.3	1.0	3.0	3.1	0.3	2.5 3.7	2.5	3.5	2.5	0.6	1.3 3.7	1.0	3.5
females : n = 12															
6 to 10 month old conventional															
males : n = 12	2.1	0.6	0.9 3.3	1.0	3.0	2.4	0.4	1.6 3.2	1.5	3.0	2.4	0.4	1.6 3.2	1.0	3.0
females : n = 48															

n = number of eyes examined, m = mean, sd = standard deviation, min, max = minimum, maximum value, microbio defined = microbiologically defined.

TABLE 6. Tonometry in Göttingen minipigs (mmHg).

	Males					Females					Both sexes				
	m	sd	m ± 2 sd	min	max	m	sd	m ± 2 sd	min	max	m	sd	m ± 2 sd	min	max
6 to 8 week old micobio defined males : n = 18 females : n = 18	27.0	4.4	18.2 35.8	20	38	25.3	3.6	18.1 32.5	19	34	26.2	4.1	18.0 34.4	19	38
2 to 10 month old conventional males : n = 38 females : n = 60	26.3	4.9	16.5 36.1	11	39	27.3	3.5	20.3 34.3	21	40	26.9	4.1	18.7 35.1	11	40
2 to 5 month old conventional males : n = 26 females : n = 12	25.3	4.2	16.9 33.7	11	32	25.7	1.9	21.9 29.5	20	28	25.4	3.6	18.2 32.6	11	32
6 to 10 month old conventional males : n = 12 females : n = 48	28.3	5.7	16.9 39.7	19	39	27.7	3.6	20.5 34.9	21	40	27.9	4.1	19.7 36.1	19	40

n = number of eyes examined, m = mean, sd = standard deviation, min, max = minimum, maximum value, microbio defined = microbiologically defined.

REFERENCES

1. L.W. Williams and K.N. Gelatt, Food animal ophthalmology, *in* : "Textbook of Veterinary Ophthalmology", K.N. Gelatt, ed., Lea & Febiger, Philadelphia (1981).

2. D.M. Schiavo and W.E. Field, The incidence of ocular defects in a close colony of Beagle dogs, *Lab. Anim. Sci.* 24:51 (1976).

3. R.W. Bellhorn, A survey of ocular findings in 8 to 10 month old Beagles, *J. Am. Vet. Med. Assoc.* 164:1114 (1974).

4. G. Saint-Macary and C. Berthoux, Ophthalmologic observations in the young Yucatan micropig, *Lab. Anim. Sci.* 44:334 (1994).

5. R.W. Bellhorn, A survey of ocular findings in 16 to 24 month old Beagles, *J. Am. Vet. Med. Assoc.* 162:139 (1973).

6. L. De Schaepdrijver, P. Simoens, L. Pollet, H. Lauwers, J.J. De Laey, Morphologic and clinical study of the retinal circulation in the miniature pig. B : Fluorescein angiography of the retina, *Exp. Eye Res.* 54(6):975 (1992).

7. L.F. Rubin, "Atlas of Veterinary Ophthamoscopy", Lea & Febiger, Philadelphia (1974).

8. R. Heywood, Juvenile cataracts in the Beagle dog, *J. Small. Anim. Pract.* 12:171 (1971).

9. C. Taradach and P. Greaves, Spontaneous lesions in laboratory animals : incidence in relation to age, *Crit. Rev. Toxicol.* 12:121(1984).

10. C. Taradach, B. Régnier, J. Perraud, Eye lesions in the Sprague-Dawley rats : type and incidence in rela-tion to age, *Lab. Anim.* 15:285 (1981).

11. J.F. Charlin, Etude expérimentale chez le microporc d'un substitut du vitré : le collagène IV humain placentaire, *Thèse de Doctorat de Sciences Médicales présentée à la Faculté de Médecine de l'Université de Rouen* (1991).

12. R.W. Bellhorn, Laboratory animal ophthalmology, *in* : "Textbook of Veterinary Ophthalmology", K.N. Gelatt, ed., Lea & Febiger, Philadelphia (1981).

MEASUREMENT OF INTRAOCULAR PRESSURE IN CYNOMOLGUS MONKEYS USING A TONOPEN®

Malcolm Eddie and Peter Lee

Pharmaco LSR
Occold, Eye
Suffolk, IP23 7PX. Great Britain

INTRODUCTION

The Tonopen has been proposed as being a suitable instrument for the measurement of intraocular pressure in a number of laboratory animal species[1-7]. We at Pharmaco LSR have recently used a Tonopen to measure the intraocular pressures of untreated and Pilocarpine treated cynomolgus monkeys at different times of day over several days. This paper presents our methods of data collection and summarises the results obtained.

MATERIALS AND METHODS

A group of four non-juvenile male cynomolgus monkeys received two sham doses of physiological saline by instillation onto the right eye followed, several days later, by instillation of 4.0% pilocarpine (Oftan, Leiras, Finland) on five occasions at 12 hour intervals. Immediately before and at intervals of 1, 2, 4, 6, 8, 10 and 12 hours after each sham dose and after the first and fifth pilocarpine instillations, the intraocular pressure of each eye of each monkey was measured by means of a hand-held Tonopen XL intraocular pressure recorder (Biorad, Ophthalmic Division, Santa Ana, California, USA). An ophthalmic anaesthetic, (Ophthaine, Ciba Geigy) was applied to the eyes of each monkey prior to each occasion of recording. The left eye acted as a contralateral control for the sham and pilocarpine treated eyes.

Throughout the recording procedures the animals were restrained, without sedation, in a custom built 'chair' (Figure 1), allowing the procedure to be quickly and conveniently performed by two or three people. Ten individual pressure recordings were taken from the centre of the cornea of each eye at each timepoint (Figures 2, 3). From these readings the mean individual and group intraocular

Ocular Toxicology, Edited by I. Weisse *et al.*
Plenum Press, New York, 1995

pressures were calculated. Although it was impossible to prevent all movement of the monkey's eyes and head while recordings were being made, clearly abnormal pressure readings due to movement were omitted and further readings obtained to provide ten satisfactory readings from which to calculate the mean intraocular pressure. Dosing, and the intraocular pressure recordings, were performed at approximately the same times on each day, between 8.00 and 20.00 hours.

All the values for the pilocarpine treated animals were obtained 'blind' in the course of investigations into the effects upon intraocular pressure of an NCE.

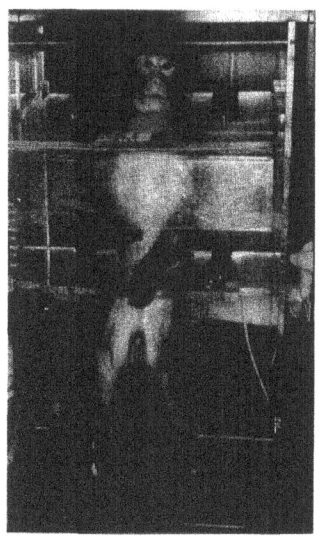

Figure 1
Custom built chair showing
non-juvenile cynomolgus monkey.

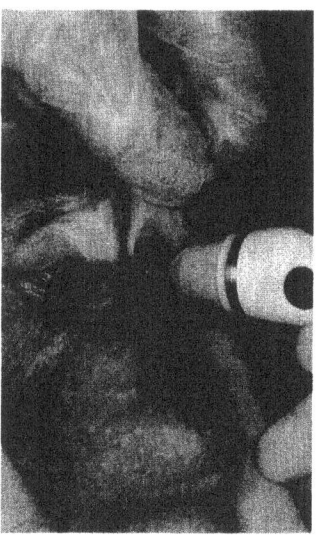

Figure 2
Detail of Tonopen in use.

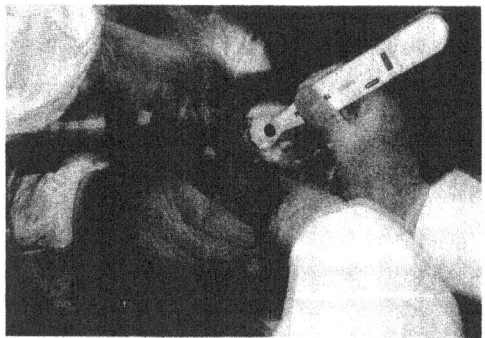

Figure 3
Detail of correct recording procedure.

RESULTS

The group mean intraocular pressures of the left and right eyes are presented in Table 1. The range of mean intraocular pressures in the sham-dosed monkeys (both eyes) was found to be between 15.9 and 19.1 mmHg on the first occasion and between 14.6 and 19.5 mmHg on the second occasion. Following the sham doses we were unable to demonstrate any consistent diurnal variation in intraocular pressures over the time course examined (Figures 4 and 5). The values obtained for the contralateral eyes were similar (not more than 1.5 mmHg on any occasion). The first administration of pilocarpine caused a clear decrease in mean intraocular pressure in the treated eyes relative to the untreated eyes with a differential of between 2.1 and 3.0 mmHg being evident from one to six hours following dosing (Figure 6). Immediately prior to the fifth 12-hourly dose of pilocarpine the mean intraocular pressure of the dosed eyes was 3.0 mmHg below that of the undosed eye, indicating a residual effect from the previous doses. Following the fifth dose the mean intraocular pressure dropped further and at eight hours after dosing was below 10 mmHg, with a differential from the contralateral control eyes of 5.7 mmHg (Figure 7).

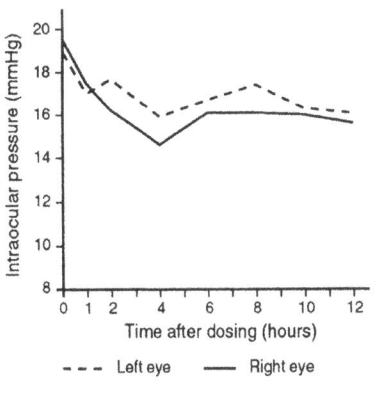

Figure 4. First sham

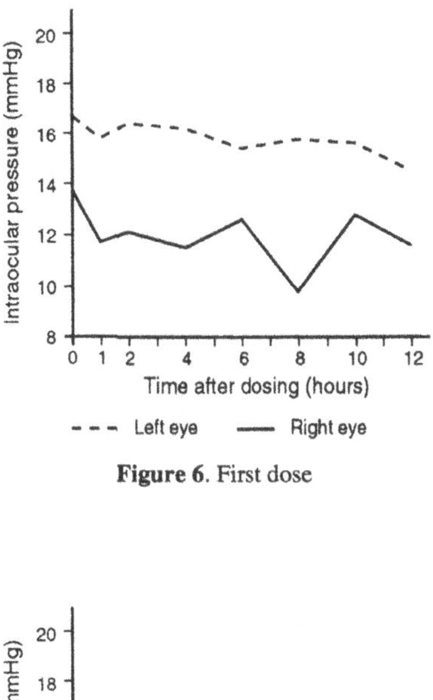

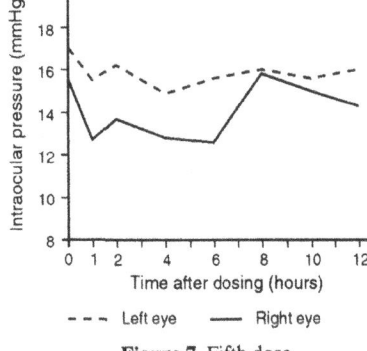

Figure 6. First dose

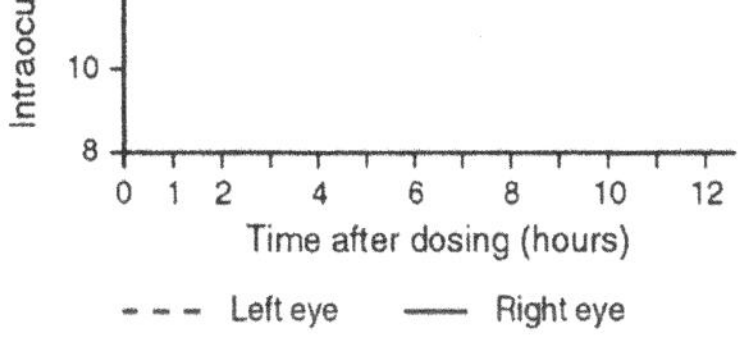

Figure 5. Second sham

Figure 7. Fifth dose

Table 1. Intraocular pressure – group mean values with and without instillation of 4% pilocarpine

Time after dosing (hours)	First sham		Second sham		First dose		Fifth dose	
	R	L	R	L	R	L	R	L
0	16.3 (3.3)	17.8 (1.4)	19.5 (1.7)	18.9 (2.2)	15.5 (2.6)	17.0 (2.7)	13.7 (2.5)	16.7 (1.8)
1	18.4 (1.4)	19.1 (1.2)	17.5 (2.0)	17.0 (3.2)	12.7 (1.1)	15.5 (1.2)	11.7 (2.7)	15.8 (1.7)
2	17.1 (3.1)	16.8 (1.3)	16.2 (3.4)	17.7 (3.2)	13.7 (3.4)	16.2 (3.0)	12.1 (3.3)	16.4 (1.9)
4	16.2 (1.3)	16.8 (1.9)	14.6 (4.7)	15.9 (2.9)	12.8 (3.3)	14.9 (1.3)	11.5 (3.9)	16.2 (2.3)
6	16.8 (2.5)	18.3 (2.4)	16.1 (4.2)	16.7 (3.2)	12.6 (3.5)	15.6 (3.2)	12.6 (2.4)	15.4 (1.9)
8	16.2 (2.9)	15.9 (2.8)	16.1 (2.5)	17.4 (2.8)	15.8 (1.6)	16.0 (1.7)	9.8 (1.9)	15.5 (1.5)
10	16.8 (2.4)	17.7 (1.2)	16.0 (2.4)	16.3 (2.4)	15.0 (1.9)	15.6 (1.9)	12.8 (3.0)	15.6 (2.7)
12	18.0 (1.8)	16.9 (2.5)	15.6 (1.8)	16.1 (1.1)	14.3 (2.3)	16.0 (1.8)	11.6 (3.2)	14.5 (2.0)

CONCLUSIONS

The results show that, using this procedure, the Tonopen is a convenient means of measuring intraocular pressures in unanaesthetised laboratory animals, including the relatively intractable cynomolgus monkey. This technique proved to be sensitive enough to clearly distinguish between pilocarpine-treated and untreated or sham-dosed eyes and, following the sham doses, showed a high degree of similarity between contralateral eyes.

REFERENCES

1. P. Evans, personal communication

2. D.R. Priehs, G.G. Gum, R.D Whitley, and L.E. Moore 'Evaluation of three tonometers in dogs' Am. J. Vet. Res 1990 Oct, 51(10) pp. 1547-50

3. P.E. Miller, J.P. Pickett, and L.J. Majors 'Evaluation of two applanation tonometers in horses', Am. J. Vet. Res. 1990 Jun, 51(6) pp. 935-7

4. P.E. Miller, J.P. Pickett, L.J. Majors, I.D. Kurzman 'Evaluation of two applanation tonometers in cats', Am. J. Vet. Res 1991 Nov 52(11) pp. 1917-21

5. J. Dziezyc, N.J. Millichamp, and W.B. Smith 'Comparison of applanation tonometers in dog and horses' J. Am. Vet Med Assoc. 1992 Aug 1, 201(3) pp 430-3

6. A. Mermoud, G. Baerveldt, D.S. Minckler, M.B. Lee, and N.A. Rao 'Intraocular pressure in Lewis rats' Invest. Ophthalmol Vis Sci 1994 Apr 35(5) pp 2455-60

7. C.G. Moore, S.T. Mline, J.C. Morrison 'Noninvasive measurement of rat intraocular pressure with the Tonopen' Invest. Ophthalmol Vis Sci 1993 Feb 34(2) pp363-9

LEAD-INTOXICATION OF DOPAMINERGIC CELLS IN THE RETINA

Konrad Kohler[1], Helmuth Lilienthal[2], and Eberhart Zrenner[1]

[1]Department of Pathophysiology of Vision and Neuroophthalmology,
Division of Experimental Ophthalmology, University Eye Hospital
D - 72076 Tübingen, Germany
[2]Medical Institute of Environmental Hygiene
D - 40225 Düsseldorf, Germany

INTRODUCTION

Inorganic lead is a major environmental pollutant which causes alterations in behaviour and cognitive performance, especially on learning, in both animals and humans (Bushnell and Bowman, 1979; Lilienthal et al., 1986; Davis et al., 1990). If lead is taken up in early developmental stages of life, its effects on brain functions are long-lasting and persist even after cessation of exposure (Hammond and Dietrich, 1990).

Lead intoxication of the visual system is well known and has been extensively described. Visual processing deficits are generated by a direct action of lead on the visual cortex but lead also induces severe alterations in the physiology, morphology and biochemistry of the photoreceptors in the retina (for a review see Fox, 1992). ERG as well as morphological studies have shown that lead selectively affects rods with little or no effects on cones. Lead also competitively and reversibly inhibited isolated retinal Na,K-ATPase.

In the CNS a neurotoxic effect of lead on the catecholaminergic system has been reported. With respect to the catecholamines, the data point to a selective action of lead, with the midbrain and the diencephalon being prime targets. In these brain areas lead exposure results in alterations in the concentration of dopamine and in addition in a reduction in the activity of the dopamine synthesising enzyme tyrosine hydroxylase (McIntosh et al., 1989).

Here we report a lead induced decrease in tyrosine hydroxylase-content in neurones of the rhesus monkey retina, with persistence beyond the end of lead exposure.

MATERIAL AND METHODS

In three experimental groups (0, 350, 600 ppm lead exposure) the retinas of three animals were examined and in each retina the peak fluorescence intensities of ten tyrosine hydroxylase (TH)-immunoreactive cells were measured.

Lead Treatment

Rhesus monkeys were pre- and postnatally exposed to 0, 350, or 600 ppm (parts per million) of lead acetate in the diet over 9 years. These doses resulted in an averaged daily oral intake of 0, 42, or 70 mg lead calculated for an adult animal. The doses were sub-toxic, and neither the body weight nor the haematological parameters were influenced by lead exposure. Blood lead levels during this period are shown in Figure 1A.

Lead exposure was followed by a 32 month period of lead free diet. During this period blood lead levels decline to nearly those of the untreated controls (Figure 1B).

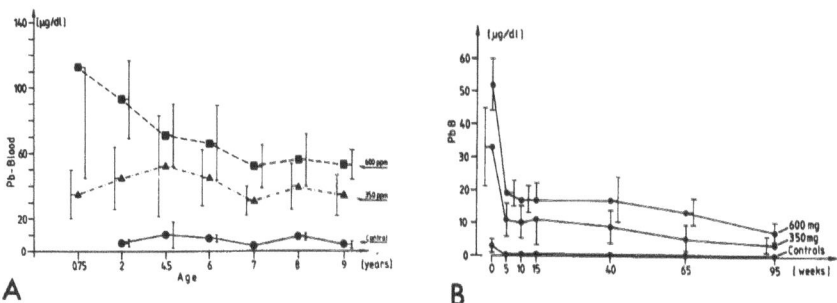

Figure 1. The graphs show blood lead levels in control animals and in those exposed to 350 ppm or 600 ppm lead acetate during the first nine years of postnatal development (A) and blood lead levels during the following 32 month of lead free diet (B). Means are given and the standard deviations are included.

Tyrosine hydroxylase immunocytochemistry

The animals were sacrificed after the lead free period. The eyes were immediately enucleated and hemisected along the ora serrata. The vitreous was removed and the eye cup was fixed in 2% paraformaldehyde, 2% glutaraldehyde in 0.1M phosphate buffer (PB, pH 7.4) for 24 hours. The fixed retina was dissected, washed in PB and prepared for cryo sectioning.

For tyrosine hydroxylase detection a monoclonal antibody (Incstar) developed in mouse against TH was used. Preincubation of cryostat sections was carried out in 10 % normal goat serum. Sections were then incubated with TH-antibody in a 1:500 dilution over night. The TH-antibody reaction was visualised with a FITC-conjugated anti-mouse IgG.

Measurement of Fluorescence Intensity

A computer-assisted confocal laser scanning microscope (Zeiss LSM 10) was used to measure FITC-fluorescence in TH-immunoreactive cells. Maximal fluorescence intensity of a stained cell was adjusted in the conventional mode at the microscope and the cell was then immediately scanned with the adjusted focus to prevent bleaching of the peak intensity by repeated scans. Thereafter focus-series (0.5 μm steps) were recorded using a programmed scanning operation. Fluorescence intensity was detected with a photomultiplier and converted into grey levels ranging from 0 (black) to 256 (white). The background was always set as zero. Means and standard deviations were calculated. To determine statistically significant differences between the means analysis of variance followed by t-test was used.

RESULTS

The morphology of TH-immunoreactive neurones in the rhesus monkey retina was described in detail by Mariani and Hokoc (1988). They showed that a bright and a weak fluorescent cell type is present in these animals. In our experiments both cell types were present in the control group which was not treated with lead. The bright fluorescent type is shown in Figure 2A. Cell bodies of this type with a diameter of 15 ± 1.8 µm were located in the innermost row of the inner nuclear layer (INL). Their cytoplasm was strongly immunoreactive for TH, so that in most of the cells the dark non-fluorescent nucleus was outshone by cytoplasmic fluorescence. Several large, bright, fluorescent processes originated from a cell body and arborized in the outermost part of the inner plexiform layer (IPL). The processes form a dens network up to 6 µm thick directly below the row of somata. Fine fibres extended from the network towards the INL, occasionally reaching the outer plexiform layer (OPL). To quantify the immunoreaction, fluorescence intensity was measured in the cell bodies of the bright fluorescent type. In the TH-immunoreactive cells of control animals the peak fluorescence intensity, given in grey levels of the photomultiplier, reached 226 ± 21.

The second immunoreactive cell type could be easily distinguished from the first by its less-bright fluorescence, location in the retina, and smaller cell bodies (12 ± 1.3 µm; not shown). As this cell type disappeared in the lead treated animals its fluorescence was not quantified.

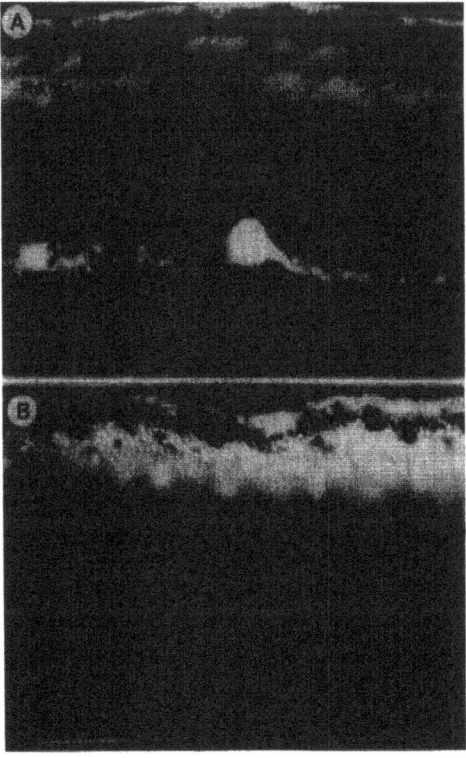

Figure 2. Micrographs of TH-immunoreactive cells in a retina of an untreated control animal (A) and in a retina of a monkey exposed to 600 ppm lead over nine years with a subsequent 32-month period of lead-free diet (B). Note the decrease in fluorescence intensity in the cell bodies (arrows) and in the fibre layer (arrowheads). An unlabeled amacrine cell (asterisk) is surrounded by stained fibre. The outer segments of the photoreceptors (PhR) show an unspecific fluorescence. INL: inner nuclear layer, IPL: inner plexiform layer, calibration bar: 30 µm

371

In animals exposed to 350 ppm lead fluorescence intensity decreased, so that in all of the cell bodies the darker nucleus could be observed within the cytoplasm; moreover the fibre layer was less immunoreactive. However, fibres in the INL were still visible. The weak fluorescent cell type disappeared to a large extend. Peak fluorescence intensity reached 121 ± 44 grey levels.

Figure 2B shows a TH-immunoreactive cell from an animal exposed to 600 ppm lead. The dark nucleus is surrounded by a small ring of fluorescence within the cytoplasm. The dense network of the fibre layer has turned into single immunoreactive spots, and no ascending fibres could be observed in the INL. The weakly fluorescent cell type was no longer detectable in these retinas. The peak fluorescence intensity was reduced to 50 ± 22 grey levels.

Figure 3 gives an overview of the peak fluorescence intensities of TH-immunoreactive cells in the different experimental groups. Compared to the control animals both lead treated groups show a highly significant reduction in fluorescence intensity (t-test p< 0.001) and the effects of different lead exposure are clearly dose dependent.

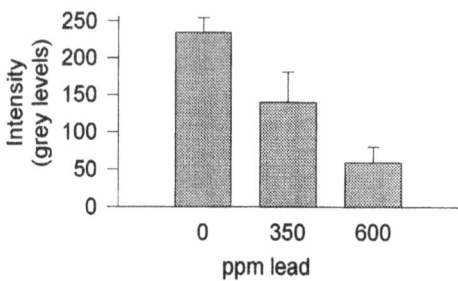

Figure 3. Histogram summarising the effects of the different lead exposures on TH immunoreaction in monkeys with 0 ppm, 350 ppm, and 600 ppm lead exposure. The lead effects are dose dependent and highly significant (p < 0.001) compared with the 0 ppm control. The peak fluorescence intensity is given in grey levels ranging from 0 (black) to 256 (white).

DISCUSSION

In the retinas of lead-exposed rhesus monkeys TH-immunocytochemistry revealed a photometrically confirmed decrease in the relative levels of the enzyme tyrosine hydroxylase as quantified photometrically. Moreover, there appeared to be a disintegration in the wiring diagram of these catecholamine-containing neurones, as shown by the total loss of TH-immunoreaction in the weakly immunoreactive cell type and by fading immunoreactive processes in the catecholaminergic fibre network. Lead is well known to inhibit a large number of enzymes, probably by binding to sulfhydryl groups (Valle and Ulmer, 1972). It is therefore not surprising that TH may by one of these enzymes.

In the hypothalamus a lead-related reduction of tyrosine hydroxylase activity has been reported in association with alterations in steady-state catecholamine levels (Meredith et al., 1988). Since the retina is a genuine part of the diencephalon, it may be affected by lead in the same way as diencephalic brain regions. Furthermore, in the mesolimbic brain lead has been reported to reduce dopamine synthesis (Lasley and Lane, 1988).

We have recently shown that b-wave amplitudes increased under scotopic conditions in the same lead-treated groups of monkeys examined histologically in this study, whereas b-wave latencies remained unchanged (Lilienthal et al. 1994). The increase in b-wave amplitudes measured 26 months after termination of lead exposure corresponds well to an increase measured during the treatment phase (Lilienthal et al., 1988). Keeping in mind that lead may affect catecholaminergic neurochemistry and that dopamine is the main catecholamine in the retina, these lead-induced ERG-alterations deserve closer examination with respect to dopaminergic ERG effects. In rabbits and humans, dopamine and the dopamine precursor L-DOPA reduce the b-wave (Cavalacci et al., 1980), whereas dopamine antagonists such as haloperidol increased the b-wave amplitude in cats without affecting latencies (Schneider and Zrenner, 1991). This indicates that lead induces similar effects as dopamine antagonists.

In the rhesus monkey retina, TH-immunoreactive cells are amacrine cells (Mariani and Hokoc, 1988), which exert a massive synaptic input on the so-called AII amacrines (see Witkovsky and Deary, 1991, for a review). The rod pathway, which has no direct access to ganglion cells, is linked via the AII amacrines to the 'on' and 'off' ganglion cells of the cone system. Dopamine is therefore an essential modulator of scotopic signals. AII amacrines are surrounded by a ring of dopaminergic fibres emerging from the TH-immunoreactive fibre plexus. This was also observed in the retinas of our untreated control group (Figure 2A). In the lead-treated animals, these rings are vigorously reduced (350 ppm lead) or totally absent (600 ppm lead).

We do not know whether the retinal cells are able to reestablish a full and healthy TH-content after lead exposure is terminated and whether the synaptic wiring is affected irreversibly by lead-induced intoxication. Although TH-immunoreactive cells have some capacity to restore their TH-synthesis after intoxication the receptive fields of these "reanimated" cells are smaller, and arborisation of processes less pronounced.

The lead induced alterations in ERG signals, the changes in the morphological situation of the TH-immunoreactive cells, and the general decrease of TH-content in these cells strongly support the idea that lead induces a decrease in dopaminergic neurotransmission within the retina . It is especially remarkable that this effect is so long-lasting and even persisted when blood lead levels declined nearly to those of the untreated control group.

REFERENCES

Bushnell, P.J., and Bowmann R.E., 1979, Persistence of impaired reversal learning in young monkeys exposed to low levels of dietary lead, *J. Toxicol. Environ. Health* 5:1015.

Cavalacci, G., Perossini, M, and Wirth, A., 1980, The interest of electroretinography in Parkinsonism, *Doc. Ophthalmol. Proc. Ser.* 23:121.

Davis, J.M., Otto, D.A., and Weil, D.E., 1990, The comparative developmental neurotoxicity of lead in humans and animals, *Neurotoxicol. Teratol.* 12:215.

Fox, D.A., 1992, Visual and auditory system alterations following development or adult lead exposure: a critical review, *in*: "Human lead Exposure", H.L. Needleman, ed., CRC Press, London.

Hammond, P.B., and Dietrich, K.N., 1990, Lead exposure in early life: health consequences, *Rev. Environ. Contamin. Toxicol.* 115:91.

Lasley, S.M., and Lane, J.D., 1988, Diminished regulation of mesolimbic dopaminergic activity in rat after chronic inorganic lead exposure, *Toxicol. Appl. Pharmacol.* 95:474.

Lilienthal, H.G., Winneke G., Brockhaus A., and Molik B., 1986, Pre- and postnatal lead-exposure in monkeys: effects on activity and learning set formation, *Neurobehav. Toxicol. Teratol.* 8:265.

Lilienthal, G.H., Lenaerts, C., Winneke, G, and Hennekes, R., 1988, Alteration of the visual evoked potential and the electroretinogram in lead-treated monkeys, *Neurotoxicol. Teratol.* 10:417.

Lilienthal, H.G., Kohler, K., Turfeld M., and Winneke G., 1994, Persistent increases in scotopic b-wave amplitudes after lead exposure in monkeys, *Exp. Eye Res.* 59:203.

McIntosh, M.J., Meredith, P.A., Moore M.R., and Goldberg, A., 1989, Action of lead on neurotransmission in rats, *Xenobiotica* 19:101.

Mariani A.P. and Hokoc J.N., 1988, Two types of tyrosine hydroxylase immunoreactive amacrine cells in the rhesus monkey retina, *J. Comp. Neurol.* 276:171.

Meredith, P.A., McIntosh, M.J., Petty, M.A., and Reid, J.L., 1988, Effects of lead exposure on rat brain catecholaminergic neurochemistry, *Comp. Biochem. Physiol.* 89:215.

Schneider, T., and Zrenner, E., 1991, Effects of D-1 and D-2 dopamine antagonists on ERG and optic nerve response of the cat, *Exp. Eye Res.* 52:425.

Vallee, B.L., and Ulmer, D.D., 1972, Biochemical effects of mercury, cadmium and lead, *Ann. Rev. Biochem.* 41:91.

Witkovsky, P., and Dearry, A., 1991, Functional roles of dopamine in the vertebrate retina, *in:* "Progress in Retinal Research" Vol. 11, N. Osborne and G. Chader, ed., Pergamon Press, Oxford.

INDEX

The manufacturer's authorised representative in the EU is Springer
Nature Customer Service Centre GmbH, Europaplatz 3, 69115 Heidelberg,
Germany. If you have any concerns regarding our products, please
contact ProductSafety@springernature.com

Printed and bound by CPI Group (UK) Ltd, Croydon, CR0 4YY

23/04/2026

02095622-0003